AGING ISSUES, HEALTH AND FINANCIAL ALTERNATIVES

OLDER DRIVERS IMPAIRED BY MULTIPLE MEDICATIONS

AGING ISSUES, HEALTH AND FINANCIAL ALTERNATIVES

Additional books in this series can be found on Nova's website under the Series tab.

Additional E-books in this series can be found on Nova's website under the E-books tab.

TRANSPORATION ISSUES, POLICIES AND R & D

Additional books in this series can be found on Nova's website under the Series tab.

Additional E-books in this series can be found on Nova's website under the E-books tab.

AGING ISSUES, HEALTH AND FINANCIAL ALTERNATIVES

OLDER DRIVERS IMPAIRED BY MULTIPLE MEDICATIONS

LISA M. PERKINS
AND
DANIELLE J. WHITE
EDITORS

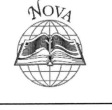

Nova Science Publishers, Inc.
New York

Copyright © 2011 by Nova Science Publishers, Inc.

All rights reserved. No part of this book may be reproduced, stored in a retrieval system or transmitted in any form or by any means: electronic, electrostatic, magnetic, tape, mechanical photocopying, recording or otherwise without the written permission of the Publisher.

For permission to use material from this book please contact us:
Telephone 631-231-7269; Fax 631-231-8175
Web Site: http://www.novapublishers.com

NOTICE TO THE READER

The Publisher has taken reasonable care in the preparation of this book, but makes no expressed or implied warranty of any kind and assumes no responsibility for any errors or omissions. No liability is assumed for incidental or consequential damages in connection with or arising out of information contained in this book. The Publisher shall not be liable for any special, consequential, or exemplary damages resulting, in whole or in part, from the readers' use of, or reliance upon, this material. Any parts of this book based on government reports are so indicated and copyright is claimed for those parts to the extent applicable to compilations of such works.

Independent verification should be sought for any data, advice or recommendations contained in this book. In addition, no responsibility is assumed by the publisher for any injury and/or damage to persons or property arising from any methods, products, instructions, ideas or otherwise contained in this publication.

This publication is designed to provide accurate and authoritative information with regard to the subject matter covered herein. It is sold with the clear understanding that the Publisher is not engaged in rendering legal or any other professional services. If legal or any other expert assistance is required, the services of a competent person should be sought. FROM A DECLARATION OF PARTICIPANTS JOINTLY ADOPTED BY A COMMITTEE OF THE AMERICAN BAR ASSOCIATION AND A COMMITTEE OF PUBLISHERS.

Additional color graphics may be available in the e-book version of this book.

LIBRARY OF CONGRESS CATALOGING-IN-PUBLICATION DATA

ISBN 978-1-61209-374-1

Published by Nova Science Publishers, Inc. † New York

CONTENTS

Preface		**vii**
Chapter 1	Multiple Medications and Vehicle Crashes: Analysis of Databases *National Highway Traffic Safety Administration*	**1**
Chapter 2	A Pilot Study to Test Multiple Medication Usage and Driving Functioning *National Highway Traffic Safety Administration*	**263**
Index		**379**

PREFACE

Research results indicate that older adults have a higher rate of fatality and injury in motor vehicle crashes than any other age group except for teenagers. With the aging of the American population, concern arises regarding potential increases in rates of crash involvement and injury. This new book examines the association of the impairing effects of multiple medication use, drug/drug interactions and drug/disease interactions on motor vehicle crashes in individuals age fifty years and greater.

Chapter 1- The number of older adults is expected to increase dramatically in the next 25 years. By 2030, over 70 million Americans will be over age 65. This older population will be more mobile than ever. There has been substantial growth in numbers of licensed drivers, and this trend is expected to continue. It is anticipated that there will be an increase in both the number of older drivers and the amount of driving within this age group.

Research results indicate that older adults have a higher rate of fatality and injury in motor vehicle crashes per mile driven than any other age group except for teenagers. With the aging of the American population, concern arises regarding potential increases in rates of crash involvement and injury. In order to devise strategies to address these concerns, it is useful to consider which factors relate to crash involvement among older adults.

Chapter 2- The number of older licensed drivers in the United States is growing at a rate faster than the overall population. As people age, they are more likely to take one or more potentially driver-impairing (PDI) medications. TransAnalytics, LLC, completed a pilot study to gain a better understanding of the safety impact on older drivers of taking multiple PDI medications, providing an update on the prevalence of prescription medications in the older population, and the effects on driving of specific drugs/drug classes. Research activities included a literature review; a data mining exercise; the prioritization of other databases for future data mining; and a field study including on-road evaluations of older drivers who take multiple PDI medications by an occupational therapist, and associated instrumented vehicle observations. The results of this work point to what appear to be relatively stronger, and weaker, strategies for carrying out future studies in this vital area of research.

In: Older Drivers Impaired by Multiple Medications
Editor: Lisa M. Perkins and Danielle J. White

ISBN: 978-1-61209-374-1
© 2011 Nova Science Publishers, Inc.

Chapter 1

MULTIPLE MEDICATIONS AND VEHICLE CRASHES: ANALYSIS OF DATABASES[*]

National Highway Traffic Safety Administration

EXECUTIVE SUMMARY

Introduction

The number of older adults is expected to increase dramatically in the next 25 years. By 2030, over 70 million Americans will be over age 65. This older population will be more mobile than ever. There has been substantial growth in numbers of licensed drivers, and this trend is expected to continue. It is anticipated that there will be an increase in both the number of older drivers and the amount of driving within this age group.

Research results indicate that older adults have a higher rate of fatality and injury in motor vehicle crashes per mile driven than any other age group except for teenagers. With the aging of the American population, concern arises regarding potential increases in rates of crash involvement and injury. In order to devise strategies to address these concerns, it is useful to consider which factors relate to crash involvement among older adults.

Driving is a complex behavior requiring sequences of activities that occur in an intricate and variable environment. Impairments in visual, cognitive, and motor function may affect the driver's ability to drive safely. Many age-related factors may impair driving ability, such as age-related decrements in cognitive and physical functioning, increased prevalence of medical conditions or age-related medical conditions, and increased use of multiple medications.

Because impaired driving is a major cause of motor vehicle crashes (MVC) and injuries, the National Highway Traffic Safety Administration (NHTSA) has long studied the impact of alcohol and illicit drug use on driving ability. NHTSA has also conducted studies to examine the impact of certain legal drugs such as antihistamines, benzodiazepines, and narcotic

---

[*] This is an edited, reformatted and augmented edition of a National Highway Traffic Safety Administration publication.

analgesics. Prior studies (Foley, 1995, Leveille, 1994, Ray, 1992, Hemmelgam, 1997, Hu, 1998, Koepsell, 1994, Sims, 2001, Carr, 2000, Lyman, 2001, Masa, 2000, Edwards, 1995, and McGwin, 2000) addressing drug-crash problems have been limited to selected drugs (typically drugs of abuse or antihistamines, antidepressants, benzodiazepines, or narcotic analgesics) or selected diseases (Alzheimer's, diabetes, epilepsy).

This is the first study to consider the association of the impairing effects of multiple medication use, drug/drug interactions, and drug/disease interactions on motor vehicle crashes in individuals age 50 years and greater. An age cut-off of 50 years was selected to maximize sample size and because age-related changes and corresponding increased medication use begin to occur at this age. Individuals start to receive treatment for high blood pressure, osteoarthritis, hypercholesterolemia, and adult-onset diabetes. Multiple medications (prescription and non-prescription) begin to be used to treat or prevent emergence of age-related conditions.

The major barrier to conducting studies of this nature in the past was costly data collection methods, requiring analysis of blood, saliva, sweat, hair, or urine, police crash reports, arrests, medical examiner reports, hospital reports, self-reported driver surveys, and simulator observations. This study overcomes these constraints by using population databases (the publicly available National Ambulatory Medical Care Survey [NAMCS] and a proprietary patient-level medical insurance claims database).

Methodology

We studied two databases: The NAMCS database and a proprietary insurance claims database (PharMetrics). NAMCS provides statistics on demographic characteristics of patients and services provided, including information on diagnostic procedures, patient management, and planned future treatment. The limitation of this database is that one is not able to link, longitudinally, the medical and pharmaceutical data on a patient-specific basis. We used NAMCS survey data from 1998, 1999, and 2000. There was a total of 71,468 physician/patient visits contained in those three year surveys.

The PharMetrics database is an anonymized, proprietary patient-level medical insurance claims database containing longitudinal medical and pharmaceutical data for thousands of individuals with motor vehicle crash diagnoses and the medications and diseases in a proximal time period to the crash. The PharMetrics Patient-Level Database includes patients enrolled during the time period from January 1998 to March 2002. There were 81,408 cases (patients with a diagnosis code for motor vehicle crashes) and 244,224 age-, sex-, and date-matched controls. Hundreds of drugs and diseases and combinations of drugs and diseases can be studied using a case-control matched pair design or logistic regression analysis of possible associations of medication use among older adults and motor vehicle crashes with this database.

The main objectives of this study were to determine the relative frequency of various combinations of medications used by those who have experienced MVCs and those who have not by analyzing proprietary and non-proprietary databases; and to conduct a case-control study and regression analysis of possible associations between the use of medications (and combinations thereof) and MVCs amongst older drivers.

Results

The results of the study revealed an association between the kinds and number of medications older adults take and the risk of having MVCs. The study suggested that the drugs considered to have an impairing effect on the driving ability of older drivers were the most commonly used by older adults involved in MVCs. Thirty-six percent of the NAMCS survey group over age 50 mentioned use of two or more drugs. More than 58 percent of the over age 50 group mentioned use of one or more potentially driver impairing (PDI) medications. Fourteen percent of the drug mentions involved drug-drug interactions.

The descriptive analysis of the proprietary database identified higher rates of drug use in general than the NAMCS results. Fifty-eight percent of the older adult study subjects received two or more medications. Approximately 64 percent of the older adult study subjects received PDI medications. Nearly 51 percent of the older adult study subjects suffered from potentially driver impairing conditions. We identified 24 percent of the older adult study subjects as concomitantly using medications that are known to interact. Eight percent of the older adult study subjects appeared to be using medicines that presented therapeutic conflicts with diseases/conditions for which they were being treated.

The Case Control Analysis suggested an association between motor vehicle crashes and many potentially driver impairing medications, potentially driver impairing diseases, and various combinations of drugs and diseases. Thirty-five of the 90 potentially driver impairing drug classes had odds ratios over 1.2 ($p < .05$). Seven of the 15 medication classes with the highest odds ratios are classes that have been reported to be especially problematic in older patients.

Seventy-nine of 200 driver impairing disease classes had statistically significant odds ratios over 1.4. Our results supported previous studies that linked NSAIDS, ACE Inhibitors, anticoagulants, antidepressants, and benzodiazepine use with motor vehicle crashes. We also corroborated previous studies that linked depression, alcoholism, arthritis, history of falls, back pain, diabetes, heart disease, stroke, arrhythmias, coronary artery disease, and sleep apnea with motor vehicle crashes. Most of the drug interaction pairings had higher odds ratios for MVCs than when the drugs were used alone. Though we observed some drug-disease conflicts with statistically significant elevated odds ratios, they involved such small numbers of cases and controls that it is difficult to make any conclusions about these increases in risk.

The number of total medications, PDI medications, PDI diseases, drug-drug interactions, and drug-disease conflicts were used as categorical variables in a regression analysis examining their role in MVCs. Study subjects taking one or more medications were found to be 1.43 times more likely to be involved in MVCs than older adults taking no medications. Compared to patients taking no PDI medications, those taking one or two PDI medications were 1.29 times more likely to be involved in MVCs and that risk increases to 1.87 among patients taking three or more PDI medications.

The risk for patients with one or two PDI diseases was 1.49 times greater than that for older adults without any PDI diseases. Three or more PDI conditions further increased the risk for MVCs to 2.20 times that of older adults with no PDI diseases. Drug interactions were also associated with a statistically significant increased risk of MVCs (odds ratio of 1.47 for 1-2 drug interactions and 1.92 with patients with 3 or more drug interactions). The risk for MVCs among study subjects with at least one drug-disease conflict was 1.2 times that for older adults without any drug-disease conflicts.

Discussion/Conclusions

The results of this analysis suggest that both the kinds and number of medication exposures, and the characteristics of diseases/disorders present among study subjects may predict an increase in risk for MVCs among older adults.

As the population continues to age, an increasingly complex interplay of factors will impact driving safety. Older adults will develop chronic diseases that may have driver impairing characteristics such as heart disease with the potential for arrhythmias and syncope; diabetes with the potential for ketoacidosis, hypoglycemia, and retinal deterioration; depression with the potential for cognitive disturbances; back pain and arthritis leading to physical mobility impairment and distracting pain. Layered onto the underlying chronic diseases are the medications used to treat those conditions along with their potential to exacerbate other coexisting conditions, induce side effects, and promote dangerous drug interactions. By demonstrating the potential link between multiple drug therapies and MVCs, this study serves to highlight the need for a thorough examination of the relationships among drugs, diseases, and the older driver.

There are limitations to the data used in the case control study, which make it difficult to gauge the strength of these associations. The main limitations are sample size and the inherent weaknesses of administrative claims data. Particularly, in this study, with the diagnostic outcome being an ICD9-CM "E" code to identify patients who were drivers in a motor vehicle crash, the strength of the association of a PDI drug or condition is only meaningful if the "E" code assignment is accurate. (ICD9-CM codes are used by health care providers to bill for services. "E" codes are used in conjunction with diagnostic and procedure codes to classify external causes of injury and other adverse effects).

Additionally, some effects of medications on driver impairment may abate with continued use. This study did not address the contribution to MVCs associated with de novo exposure (initiation of drug therapy when individuals are most likely to experience side effects) and prolonged exposure to prescribed medications (when individuals may become tolerant to side effects).

From a policy perspective there is a troubling relationship between MVCs, multiple medication use, interactions, medication/disease conflicts, and the aging driver. While older drivers are at increased risk of a crash when they take multiple PDI medications, this study cannot isolate the cause of these crashes and determine the relative contributions of the medication, medical condition and age. Furthermore, this analysis cannot predict whether an individual older driver with an underlying medical condition who takes multiple PDI medications can drive safely.

This study suggests the need for further research to elucidate the complex interplay of factors affecting the aging adult and driving ability. The results of this research supports the intentions of NHTSA to promote the development of educational programs to increase consumer and healthcare provider awareness about the potential driver impairing effects of increasingly complex medical and pharmaceutical therapies in older adult drivers.

I. PROJECT OVERVIEW AND OBJECTIVES

This is the Final Report of a study performed for a contract entitled "Examination of Databases for Multiple Medications/Polypharmacy". This study was conducted by Aida A. LeRoy and M. Lee Morse of Iatrogen, LLC under subcontract to Orchid Biosciences.

Impaired driving is a major cause of motor vehicle crashes and injuries. The National Highway Traffic Safety Administration (NHTSA) has long studied the impairing effects of alcohol and illegal drugs on driving performance. NHTSA has also conducted research on the impairing effects of certain legal drugs such as antihistamines, benzodiazepines, and narcotic analgesics. It is recognized that certain medications may impair driving performance. Many prescription and non-prescription medication labels carry warnings against operating heavy machinery or motor vehicles. Compounding this risk are the effects of multiple medication use. Medications may interact, impairing metabolism, potentiating medication effects, or worsening underlying medical conditions. Older adults are often treated with multiple medications for diseases associated with aging, such as diabetes, cardiovascular disease, and arthritis. Drug interaction effects in older individuals are magnified by age-related changes in liver and kidney function. NHTSA sought to study multiple medication usage in older adults in the context of motor vehicle crashes and public safety. For the purpose of this analysis, older adults were defined as individuals over age 50.

The objectives of this project were to:

a. Determine the relative frequency of multiple medications and medical conditions within the older adult population (over age 50) in both those who have experienced a motor vehicle crash (MVC) and those who have not, by analyzing proprietary and non-proprietary databases; and

b. Conduct a case control study of the associations between the use of medications/medical conditions, and motor vehicle crashes among older drivers.

A. Overview

The number of older Americans is expected to grow dramatically over the next several decades. By 2030, almost 20 percent of the United States population will be 65 years of age or older. In 2000, 35 million persons were age 65 or older. By 2030, with the aging of the baby boomer generation, it is predicted that over 70 million Americans will be 65 years of age or older (Federal Interagency Forum on Aging-Related Statistics, 2000). This aging segment of the United States population is very heterogeneous and varies significantly with respect to health status, economic level, ethnicity, and other demographic variables.

The vast majority of older adults continue to rely on the passenger vehicle for mobility -- either as drivers or as passengers. There has been a dramatic growth in numbers of licensed older drivers and this trend is expected to continue. Also, older drivers in 2001 drove more miles and took longer trips as compared to older drivers in 1995 (Oak Ridge National Laboratory, 2005). As the American population ages, it is expected that there will be an increase in both the number of older drivers and the amount of driving within this age group.

Research results indicate that individuals age 65 and older have higher rates of fatality and injury in motor vehicle crashes **per mile** driven than any other age group except for teenagers (Oak Ridge National Laboratory, 2005). There are a number of reasons for these differences. First, older adults are more fragile and more vulnerable in crashes. Thus, they have higher risks for fatalities and serious injuries (Li et al., 2001). However, the rate of **per person** crash involvement decreases with age until the rate increases in individuals age 85 years and older. Even at this age, the rate per person is lower than for younger drivers (Oak Ridge National Laboratory, 2005). Older drivers are also involved in different types of crashes. Older drivers have different patterns of driving than other drivers, and many tend to self-regulate their driving, for example, by decreasing night-time driving (Kelly, R. et al., 1999). Thus, driving patterns among older adults may reduce the exposure rate of crash involvement in comparison to other drivers.

With the aging of the American population, concern arises regarding projected increases in rates of crash involvement. In order to address these concerns, it is useful to consider which factors relate to crash involvement among older adults. Many age-specific factors may impact driving ability, such as age-related decrements in cognitive and physical functioning, increased prevalence of medical conditions or age-related medical conditions, and increased use of multiple medications (Millar, 1999). It is important to note that age alone does not necessarily predict fatality rates or crash rates. In a University of Michigan study, "able older drivers" had lower rates of fatalities when rates were proportionally corrected for licensed drivers (DOT, 2003). By identifying the risk factors, such as driving conditions, health conditions, treatment, medications, functioning, and exposure, strategies can be developed to minimize the impact on motor vehicle crash-related injuries among older adults.

1. Driving

Driving is a complex behavior and can be considered a higher order instrumental activity of daily living (IADLS) (Morgan, 1995). Driving requires complex sequences of activities that occur in an intricate and rapidly variable environment. This environment includes the environment external to the vehicle as well as the environment within the vehicle, both of which may impact safety. For example, concurrent physical, social, and other demanding tasks may distract the driver and influence driving. Safety is dependent upon environmental conditions, the demands of the situation, and the abilities of the driver. Impairments in visual, cognitive, and/or motor function may impact the driver's ability to drive safely. Within each of these modalities of function, driving may require complex processing and action. For example, cognitive function includes the recall of basic information such as, "where I left my keys," but also decision making skills such as, "How can I react most quickly to a moving object in the roadway?" In this example, motor abilities (such as ease of movement of the foot), visual acuity, and attention processing also influence driving skill. Because of the complex nature of driving, impairment due to age, medical condition, or medication can seriously affect the ability of an older adult to drive safely.

2. Age, Medical Conditions, and Medications

Age

On average, aging brings changes and decrements to visual, cognitive, and motor functioning. For example, changes in the structure of the eye can affect visual perception (Owsley, 1994). However, on an individual basis, age – per se – is not a good predictor of driving abilities. For example, a healthy 75-year-old who wears corrective lenses may be able to drive safely, despite some age-related changes. Behavioral changes, health status, environment, and medical interventions may influence the effects of age-related changes. Generally, around age 50, individuals begin to seek treatment for conditions typically associated with aging, such as hypertension, Type II diabetes mellitus, hyperlipidemia, sleep disturbances, etc.

Medical, Cognitive, and Emotional Conditions

Research has been conducted to examine the association of medical, cognitive, and/or emotional conditions and disabilities with functioning and driving abilities. In general, diagnosis alone is not a good predictor of functioning. The type of condition, the severity of the condition, the management of the condition (medical and pharmaceutical), adaptations to the environment, changes in behavior of the individual, and the age of the individual are all factors that influence whether a particular medical, cognitive, or emotional condition will affect driving functioning. For example, while severe cataracts can affect vision, cataract surgery has been shown to improve vision and is correlated with decreases in crashes (Owsley, 2002). In general, the more severe the medical condition and the greater the presence of medical, cognitive, or emotional comorbidities, the more likely that functioning will be impaired. Naturally, this varies on an individual basis.

Medical, cognitive, or emotional conditions typically affect functioning if they are severe, improperly managed, unmanageable, or affected by other conditions. In this chapter, "potentially driver impairing" (PDI) conditions are defined as conditions that are associated with loss of body control (hypoglycemic coma, seizures, fainting, low blood pressure, blurred vision), central nervous system effects (inattentiveness, sleepiness, dizziness, confusion), or conditions that cause stiffness and pain (arthritis, pain conditions). Examples of such conditions are diabetes mellitus, arthritis, seizures, depression, insomnia, arrhythmias, cardiovascular disease, Alzheimer's, and Parkinsonism, among others. Treatment, however, may ameliorate these conditions and the consequent driver-impairing aspects of the condition.

Medications

While medication treatment offers disease amelioration, it also has the potential for undesirable drug side effects and interactions. In this regard, the older adult faces many challenges. The most evident are the age-related changes in health and physical status. Many among the rapidly growing population over age 65receive medical therapy for several chronic conditions simultaneously, often involving treatment with up to eight different drugs per day in addition to use of over-the-counter drugs (Ellenhorn's Medical Toxicology, 2nd ed). As a result, older adults use a disproportionately high amount of medications: older adults represent 13 percent of the U.S. population but consume about 30 percent of all prescription drugs (Noble: Textbook of Primary Care Medicine).

A number of factors portend an increase in the number of potential drug interactions experienced by older adults including:

- an increase in the number of drugs taken daily,
- alterations in pharmacokinetics,
- long-term drug use,
- alteration in gut surface area,
- decrease in gastric motility,
- decreased gastric acid secretion,
- multiple drugs competing for binding sites on serum albumin,
- multiple drugs competing for metabolic enzymes,
- increase in the proportion of fat to body mass,
- decreased body water,
- reduced liver size with diminished ability to metabolize drugs,
- less efficient renal clearance of drugs, and
- an increase in g-receptor sensitivity, especially to cardiovascular and psychotropic drugs.

Symptoms of drug-induced poisonings, overdoses, drug interactions or side effects are often interpreted as normal signs of aging and thus fail to be linked to a pharmaceutical etiology[1]. Some of these symptoms include:

- disorientation,
- tremors,
- lethargy,
- depression,
- forgetfulness,
- loss of appetite, and
- constipation.

Other effects are extensions of anticipated pharmacologic effects or side effects of normal doses of drugs that are particularly relevant to older adult drivers, such as:

- dizziness,
- drowsiness,
- tremors,
- rigidity,
- confusion,
- hypoglycemia,
- hypotension, and
- blurred vision.

Sedation and confusion are common drug complications in elderly patients, especially from medications with anticholinergic effects and sedative-hypnotics that affect the central nervous system. Willcox et al. (1994) found that "Physicians prescribe potentially inappropriate medications for nearly a quarter of all older people living in the community, placing them at risk of adverse drug effects such as cognitive impairment and sedation." Other disturbances that are common side effects of drugs in older adults include orthostasis (postural hypotension), falls, depression, urinary retention or incontinence, constipation, anorexia, and metabolic abnormalities, such as hypoglycemia, hypokalemia or hyperkalemia, hyponatremia or hypernatremia, and azotemia. McGwin et al. (2000) conducted a population-based case-control study of drivers age 65 and older and found that an increased risk of at-fault involvement in crashes was found for older drivers using common drugs such as non-steroidal anti-inflammatory drugs (NSAIDs), antihypertensive drugs (specifically ACE inhibitors), anticoagulants, or benzodiazepines.

Certain medications, based on their pharmacology, how they are taken, side-effects, etc., may potentially have a negative effect on driving. To qualify as a potentially driver-impairing medication for the purposes of our study, the medication had to be associated with central nervous system side effects, alter blood sugar levels, affect blood pressure, affect vision, or otherwise have the potential to interfere with driving skills.

Examples of "potentially driver impairing (PDI)" medications include:

Drug Class	Possible Effects
Anti-Diabetic Drugs	Hypoglycemia
Anticholinergics	Blurred vision
Narcotic analgesics	Sedation
Anti-hypertensive drugs	Hypotension
Sedative/Hypnotics	Sedation
Antidepressants	Sedation, dizziness
Allergy drugs	Sedation, dizziness
Anti-arrhythmics	Fainting (syncope)
Anticonvulsants	Ataxia, dizziness, sedation
Skeletal Muscle Relaxants	Dizziness, sedation

Recently, Curtis et al. (2004) reported the results of a study to identify inappropriate prescribing for elderly Americans in a large outpatient population. Inappropriate prescribing was defined using the Beers revised list of drugs to be avoided in elderly populations (Beers, 1997). Curtis conducted a retrospective cohort study using outpatient prescription claims. He found that 21 percent of the patients studied filled a prescription for one or more drugs of concern. More than 15 percent of subjects filled prescriptions for two drugs of concern, and 4 percent filled prescriptions for three or more of the drugs within the same year. There is increasing evidence that older adults are being prescribed medications that are known to be problematic based on their age.

Drug-related adverse events are an important cause of emergency department visits and hospitalizations in older adults, and adverse drug events (ADEs) may be responsible for 11-30 percent of hospital admissions (Chan, 2001 and Hanlon, 1997). Nearly 90 percent of all patients admitted were taking one or more over-the-counter or prescribed medications daily, while the average ADE-related hospitalized older adult patient was taking 4.2 drugs, and 13 percent of these admitted patients were taking eight or more medications daily.

ADEs are reportedly responsible for over 10 percent of emergency department visits (Hohl, 2001). In one study, no adverse events were seen in patients taking one or fewer medications. However, in patients taking two to five medications per day, the frequency of ADEs requiring emergency room intervention was 11.5 percent, and for those taking six or more medications daily, the incidence of emergency room visits for ADEs climbed to 16.9 percent. Examination of drug regimens showed that 31 percent of patients also had the potential for at least one adverse drug interaction.

The combination of driver-impairing medical conditions and the use of multiple medications (both impairing and non-impairing) suggests that the aging driver population may be at increased risk for motor vehicle crashes. Our analysis was designed to shed light on the issue of an aging driving population and the impact of diseases and the consequent use of medications. In addition to the inherent side-effects associated with medications, this study also looked at the contribution to motor vehicle crash risk associated with 'problematic medication use' among the older drivers. Problematic use is defined as use that is in therapeutic conflict with other disorders for which the patient is being treated, or other medications the patient is concomitantly receiving.

B. Project Objectives

The objectives of this project are to:

1. Determine the relative frequency of various combinations of medications used by both those who have experienced a motor vehicle crash (MVC) and those who have not by analyzing proprietary and non-proprietary databases; and
2. Conduct a case-control study of possible associations between the use of select medications (and combinations thereof) and MVCs among older drivers (age 50 and older).

II. METHODOLOGY

A. Purpose and Contract Tasks

While many studies have been reported in the literature addressing drug-crash problems and various subsets of drivers, they have been limited to selected drugs (typically drugs of abuse or antihistamines, antidepressants, benzodiazepines, or narcotic analgesics) or selected diseases (Alzheimer's, diabetes, epilepsy). Additionally, these studies have involved costly data collection methods, such as analysis of blood, saliva, sweat, hair, or urine. Some have relied on data taken from police crash reports, arrests, medical examiner reports, research based on data from trauma units and hospitals, and self-reported data from driver surveys. Further, these studies have not looked at the interactions between drugs and diseases.

We conducted an exploratory study to examine the use of a wider array of medication classes and medical conditions and their potential interactions in older adult drivers and association with motor vehicle crashes. We also examined the feasibility of using a national survey database and a longitudinal, patient-specific medical and pharmaceutical claims-linked database for this study. The use of anonymized patient-specific longitudinal databases, absent recall bias (such as insurance claims databases) has served to generate hypotheses in epidemiologic studies involving drugs, medical conditions and outcomes. In addition, data from well-designed national surveys (such as NAMCS) have been successfully used to characterize the use of medicationsin the general U.S. population.

B. Database Discussion

The selection of databases for this project was performed in consultation with NHTSA. We selected two types of databases: A publicly available database (NAMCS) derived from an annual survey sponsored by the Centers for Disease Control/National Center for Health Statistics (CDC/NCHS), and a proprietary patient-level insurance claims database licensed from PharMetrics.

The National Ambulatory Medical Care Survey (NAMCS) is an annual national survey designed to obtain objective, reliable information about the provision and use of ambulatory medical care services in the United States. Findings are based on a sample of visits to non-federally employed office-based physicians that are primarily engaged in direct patient care. Physicians in the specialties of anesthesiology, pathology, and radiology are excluded from the survey.

Specially trained interviewers visit physicians prior to their participation in the survey in order to provide them with survey materials and instruct them on how to complete the forms. Data collection from the physician, rather than from the patient, expands information on ambulatory care collected through other NCHS surveys. Each physician is randomly assigned to a 1-week reporting period. During this period, data for a systematic random sample of visits are recorded by the physician or office staff on an encounter form provided for that purpose. Data are obtained on patients' symptoms, physicians' diagnoses, and medications ordered or provided. The survey also provides statistics on the demographic characteristics of patients and services provided, including information on diagnostic procedures, patient management, and planned future treatment.

The basic sampling unit for the NAMCS is the physician-patient encounter or visit. The NAMCS is not based on a sample of the population. NAMCS is based on a sample of *visits* rather than a sample of people. The data can be used to find out how many ambulatory care visits were made involving a certain diagnosis, but cannot be used to find out how many people have a certain diagnosis.

The absence of patient-specific denominator data significantly reduces the usefulness of survey databases for performing risk/outcomes analysis.

Risk and outcomes analysis requires longitudinally linked medical and pharmaceutical data on a patient-specific basis. To perform the kinds of case-control matched pair logistic regression analyses required to examine the question of medication related motor vehicle crashes in very large populations, patient-specific longitudinal databases are required. There are a number of health care programs that have databases that allow for linkage of medical and pharmaceutical claims data; very few that are available from non-proprietary sources. Those that are nonproprietary (such as State Medicaid programs and other federally funded health care programs) are only available through interagency agreements that are time-consuming to obtain and require extensive data cleaning and manipulation. Thus, we identified proprietary databases that would allow the longitudinal patient-specific medical and pharmaceutical claims linkages for our study.

We solicited proposals from two private companies (PharMetrics and Ingenix) that provide anonymized patient-specific medical and pharmaceutical claims-linked databases. These datasets are derived from hospital, medical and pharmaceutical claims paid through health insurance programs. Services not paid for by the insurance program (such as over-the counter medicines or weight reduction medicines) were not included. Because the sources of the database (geographic location, demographic representation, etc.) are unknown, it can not be determined whether either database can be generalized to the U.S. population of drivers over age 50. Both databases identified a similar number of individuals with ICD9-CM "E"-codes for Motor Vehicle Crashes (PharMetrics had 103,000 patients and Ingenix 70,000 patients). Costs to obtain the databases were the same. The PharMetrics database appeared to have better quality control procedures and they had better customer service. Therefore, we selected PharMetrics as the vendor for the following reasons: 1) larger dataset size, 2) greater ease of identifying individuals enrolled in the insurance plan during our study period, 3) better quality control, 4) equal cost, and 5) more responsive customer service.

The use of administrative claims data for conducting research involving adverse drug reactions and post-marketing drug surveillance has been well described in the literature (Strom and Morse, 1988 and Morse, 1991). Medical record linkage systems merge insurance claims data arising from the dispensing and refilling of prescription medications (which serves as a proxy for consumption) and the provision of medical and hospital services (hospital claims are discharge diagnoses). Gross errors in diagnostic codes and patient demographic data (e.g., age and sex) did not appear to be widespread and generally agreed with patient chart data (Hennessy, 2003 and Quan, 2002), and thus these data systems appear to provide a useful source of healthcare events data (Federspiel, 1976 and Worth, 1996). Administrative claims data has been reported to be particularly useful in studies of inappropriate prescribing for the elderly (Curtis et al., 2004) and have also been demonstrated to be useful in the study of medication use and vehicle crashes (Ray, 1992 and Jacobs, 2004).

Use of administrative health claims data provides advantages when performing certain types of epidemiologic research. For example, pharmaco-epidemiologic research (the association of drug usage with defined outcomes) using administrative health claims databases, has been documented in the literature (Strom, 1984 and Morse, 1991). An important advantage of using this type of database is the ability to link, cost-effectively, patient demographic, medication use, and medical services usage information longitudinally. These databases support the temporal association of one or many drugs to outcomes of medical services. Researchers are not dependent on recall accuracy by the patient or provider. In case control designs, medication use is examined in a defined time period prior to the defined outcome, compared to matched controls using the same age, sex, and time period studied.

The use of administrative claims data is not without challenges. Several studies suggest that structured data validation processes should be instituted when using claims data to identify data limitations and weaknesses (Hennessey, 2003 and Roos, 1996). Administrative data were found to have diagnoses and conditions that were highly specific (e.g., diabetes mellitus) but that vary greatly by condition in terms of sensitivity (e.g., severe, moderate, or mild). To yield the most informative diagnostic profile from claims data, some researchers have suggested that all physician billings for patients be examined (Wilchesky, 2004). Useful clinical information in claims databases generally resides in *data patterns* rather than in data elements and requires a quality control system that elevates the correctness of data relations above the validity of single facts. The use of massive data sets requires that quality control corresponds to the nature of the high-level information that is derived from large databases (Walker, 2001).

Claims databases are also constrained by missing data (not reported or collected). For example, with respect to consumption, it is only possible to know what medications were dispensed when patients fill prescriptions, but not whether patients actually ingest medicines. (Methodologically this would generally bias against an association between the drug and the outcome). Moreover, the use of medications not reimbursable by the drug program (e.g., OTC herbals, non-formulary medicines) will not be recorded in the database and thus the contribution of these medicines to the outcome being assessed cannot be evaluated. Similar constraints exist for diagnostic data as well. Medical services for non-covered conditions or events will not appear in the database. This may be particularly problematic for motor vehicle crashes where a third-party liability is established and medical claims are paid by the 'at fault' driver's insurance company (claims processed outside the database participating insurer). Motor vehicle crash data included in our study must have resulted from the payment of an emergency room or hospital service bill within the insurance system we are accessing in order to be observed as a medical event.

The following sources of error and study design influences must be considered when evaluating the results of an analysis using an administrative claims database:

- Reporting error
  - This type of error can bias in either favor of (when diagnoses are reported that increase payment fees) or against (under-reporting) the hypothesis.
- Ascertainment error (correctly billed but incorrectly diagnosed):
  - If this error is effectively symmetrical it should have limited effect on the hypothesis.
- Detection bias (prolonged periods of eligibility or frequent visits yield increased opportunity to detect):
  - This bias can skew towards reinforcing the hypothesis; but age, sex, and time period matching (requiring case and controls to have identical observation periods) can minimize this bias.

Given the limitations of administrative medical claims databases, we consider the primary utility of this study to be the generation of hypotheses regarding associations between medication use and motor vehicle crashes.

We used both the NAMCS and the PharMetrics databases to determine the frequency of medication use and patterns of use and diagnosis among individuals over age 50. An age cutoff of 50 years was selected to maximize sample size and because age-related changes and corresponding increased medication use begin to occur at this age. Individuals start to receive treatment for high blood pressure, osteoarthritis, hypercholesterolemia, and adult-onset diabetes. Multiple medications (prescription and non-prescription) begin to be used to treat or prevent emergence of age-related conditions.

1. Non-Proprietary Database

a. Database Description

NAMCS provides detailed prescription drug and disease mentions collected and reported by a panel of physicians. It is a national probability sample survey of visits to office-based physicians. The survey is designed to meet the need for objective, reliable information on the provision and use of ambulatory medical care services in the United States. We chose NAMCS from 1998-2000 to obtain information on drug use characteristics and disease prevalence for the U.S. population. These years were complete and readily available at the start of the project. The NAMCS data is provided either unweighted or weighted (data projected to the entire U.S. population).

b. Quality Control

The National Center for Health Statistics, Centers for Disease Control and Prevention (CDC) conducts a thorough system of data completeness checks, data edits, and quality control for NAMCS data collection and process. Field staff conducts checks of the survey information for completeness. Clerical edits are performed upon receipt of the data. Patient records are manually reviewed and ambiguous entries are reclassified. In addition, computer edits for code ranges and inconsistencies are performed. Further, all medical and drug coding is subjected to a two-way 10-percent independent verification procedure. Non-response rates for age and sex are five percent or less. Missing data items are inputted by randomly assigning a value from a patient record form with similar characteristics (National Center for Health Statistics, 1998, 1999, 2000).

After obtaining the NAMCS data, we also performed a series of quality control procedures:

- Reviewed at random 200 records from the raw data file for completeness, and reasonableness before loading data into our SAS file system;
- Verified the number of records for each year's data in our files against NAMCS documentation;
- Reviewed frequency report by 10-year age group and for both weighted and non-weighted datasets for out-of-range values (outliers);
- Verified all drug class codes and ICD-9 CM codes matched their respective reference files;
- Verified the Number of Medications field against drug class fields 1 to 6 to ensure consistency;
- Excluded 10,765 visits from the original 71,468 physician/patient visits representing individuals too young to drive (under age 16);
- Excluded 2,491 patients from the 60,703 physician/patient visits from the previous step because they had diagnoses inconsistent with their sex.
- We identified the motor vehicle crash E-code Group, which resulted in a final number of 548 physician/patient visits (unweighted) and 16,500,227 (weighted) physician/patient visits.

Included ICD9-CM Codes	Excluded ICD9-CM Codes
E810-E816 (Motor Vehicle Traffic Accidents) E819-E823 (Motor Vehicle Non-Traffic Accidents) only with the subdivisions: Driver .0, Motorcyclist .2, and Unspecified .9.	Passenger .1 and .3 Occupant of Streetcar .4 Rider of Animal .5 Pedal Cyclist .6 Pedestrian .7, and Other Occupant .8.

Figure 1. ICD9-CM "E" Codes for Motor Vehicle Crashes

c. Eligibility

All office-based physician visits in the NAMCS sample between 1998 and 2000 were included in the analysis. In total, there were 23,339 sample visits for 1998; 20,760 sample visits for 1999; and 27,369 sample visits for 2000 (total of 71,468 physician/patient visits). We limited Motor Vehicle Crash E-codes to those that involve *motor vehicles* and including ICD9-CM codes (Figure 1):

d. Preparation of NAMCS Analysis File

We used the National Drug Code Directory Classes used by NAMCS to identify all medications reported in the survey. A table of medication classes containing potentially driver impairing medications (Appendix I) was defined. To qualify as a driver-impairing medication the medication had to be associated with central nervous system side effects, alterations in blood sugar levels, changes in blood pressure, impaired vision, or otherwise have the potential to interfere with driving skills. We also defined potentially driver impairing diseases (Appendix II). These conditions are associated with loss of body control (hypoglycemic coma, seizures, fainting, low blood pressure, blurred vision), central nervous system effects (inattentiveness, sleepiness, dizziness, confusion), or conditions that cause stiffness or pain (arthritis, pain conditions). We also prepared tables of drug interaction conflicts (Appendix III), and drug-disease conflicts (Appendix IV). Drug interaction conflicts were determined from drug interaction compendia and drug literature. Drug-disease conflicts are based on side effects of drugs that contribute to or are contraindicated by underlying medical conditions. These conflicts are obtained from drug compendia, manufacturer literature, and primary medical journal references.

The 1998, 1999, and 2000 data were loaded into the SAS file system separately and merged into a single file for analysis. In total, there were 71,468 sample visits (23,339 sample visits for 1998; 20,760 for 1999; and 27,369 for 2000).

We subdivided this database into individuals 16-49 years of age and individuals over age 50. We also divided the population into those with a mention of motor vehicle crashes and those without.

NAMCS presents the results in their database as unweighted, reflecting just the data collected, and weighted, which extrapolates to the U.S. population as a whole. The unit of analysis in the NAMCS survey is the physician visit, not the patient. The total number of physician visits is 58,212 (unweighted) and 1,880,862,898 (weighted). The number of physician visits among the Motor Vehicle Crash E-code patients is 548 (unweighted) and 16,500,227 (weighted). The breakdown of physician visits (weighted) among the Over Age

50 Motor Vehicle Crash E-code patients was 4,457,588 and among the Age 16-49 patients was 12,042,639 visits.

e. Database Queries: Descriptive Analysis

We designed a number of queries to conduct a thorough descriptive analysis of the NAMCS database. Queries were performed to identify the frequencies of age, sex, medications dispensed, concomitant drugs used, and co-morbidities, both for the entire cohort, for patients with Motor Vehicle Crash mentions, both weighted, and unweighted. We analyzed numbers and types of medications in general, driver impairing medications, driver impairing diseases, drug-drug conflicts, and drug-disease conflicts. The Motor Vehicle Crash-Involved category was narrowly defined to include the E-codes for *motor vehicle* crashes only where the patient was the *driver, motorcyclist, or unspecified.* We excluded *passenger, occupant of streetcar, rider of animal, pedal cyclist, pedestrian,* and *other occupant.* (See Figure 1). We performed the following queries with results by number of physician visits by age and sex:

Query 1: Number of Physician Visits
Query 2: Number of Medications
Query 3: Number of Specific Combinations of Drug Classes
Query 4: Number of Potential Driver Impairing Medications
Query 5: Number of Conflict Medications
Query 6: Number of Specific Potential Driver Impairing Disease Groups
Query 7: Number of Potential Driver Impairing Disease Groups
Query 8: Number of Disease-Drug Conflicts

2. Proprietary Database

a. Database Description

The PharMetrics Patient-Level Database includes patients enrolled during the time period from January 1998 to March 2002. Individuals with E-codes for motor vehicle crashes and three controls for each case provide information about patient demographics, number of medications dispensed, patterns of medication combinations, and disease prevalence for patients with and without motor vehicle crashes in the enrollment population. Occurrences of drug-drug conflicts and drug-disease conflicts were also examined. The first phase of the analysis of the proprietary data utilized the same descriptive queries that were used for the non-proprietary dataset. The second phase of the analysis of the proprietary dataset was a matched-pair case control study.

b. Quality Control

PharMetrics followed an extensive data quality review procedure that used over 100 quality measures. Key demographic, service date, diagnosis and medication variables were included in the review process. Key variables from each data submission were compared to expected ranges based on PharMetrics' production database norms. Data that deviated from norms were either excluded from the production database or sent back for correction and re-submission. Each variable on every record was evaluated.

We also performed the following QC measures:

- Checked and reconciled the number of records loaded against PharMetrics' documentation.
- Performed basic field audits for anticipated types, value ranges, and formats.
- Generated a frequency for every character variable (e.g., sex) and checked out-of-range values.
- Calculated a mean, minimum, and maximum for all numeric variables (e.g., age, days drug supplied, quantity dispensed, etc.) and checked outliers.
- Validated data against specified inclusion/exclusion criteria.
- Developed diagnostic and drug ranking reports and examined them for reasonableness given the demographic nature of underlying population (e.g., geriatric diseases and commonly used medications)

The database we obtained from PharMetrics is a patient-level insurance claim database. The PharMetrics patient-level database is an integrated set of fully adjudicated medical and pharmaceutical claims for all covered medical and pharmaceutical services. It includes both inpatient and outpatient diagnoses and procedures, and both standard and mail order prescription records. This database is a longitudinal, anonymized, patient-specific medical and pharmaceutical claims-linked database. We selected an insurance claims database because it provided the ability to analyze medication usage and disease treatments and their temporal relationship to the motor vehicle crash. In total, there were 81,408 cases and 244,224 controls.

c. Eligibility

Data contained in the proprietary database included patients enrolled during the time period from January 1998 to March 2002. Cases were defined as all patients with one or more claims with an ICD9-CM code indicative of a motor vehicle crash (See Figure 1) and with at least six months of continuous enrollment prior to their first claim(s) with a crash code. Three control patients were randomly matched to each case patient. For each control, a match number was provided that linked the control to the case. Matching was based on the following matchingcriteria:

- No claims with any of the motor vehicle crash codes listed in Appendix V.
- Age (as of January 1998), within 5 years of the age of the case
- Sex (case matched to control)
- At least 6 months of continuous enrollment prior to the Case study subject's first claim with a crash code
- There were a total of 81,408 cases and 244,224 controls.

d. Refinement Steps

We performed extensive quality control, data cleaning and refining steps with results as follows:

- Excluded 25 case patients from the original 81,408 case patients due to either missing sex or more than two possible sexes, leaving 81,383 patients.
- Removed 9,891 case patients from the 81,383 case patients from the previous step due to missing year of birth, leaving 71,492 patients.
- Excluded 20,461 case patients under age 16 from the 71,492 case patients from the previous step, resulting in 51,031 patients.
- Removed 146 case patients from the 51,031 case patients from the previous step because their motor vehicle crash code(s) were apparently used to justify physical therapies they received leaving 50,885 case patients with all E-Codes. Note: If a patient had a procedure code of '97001', '97002', '97039', '98940', '98941', '98942', '98943', 'Q0086', and 'S9131' (codes for physical therapy or chiropractic services) on the same date as the event, AND there was no ER visit on the event date, a day immediately before or after the event date, the MVA E-code was apparently used to justify the physical therapies or chiropractic services.
- Fifty-three (53) case patients were excluded because of wrong sex diagnoses, which left 50,832 case patients.
- Inclusion of only patients with Motor Vehicle Crash E-codes listed above resulted in a total of 33,519 cases. Among them we have 5,378 cases of age 50 or above. The ratio of cases to controls is 1 to 3. Therefore, we have 16,134 controls of age 50 or above.

e. Database Queries: Descriptive Analysis

The following queries, which describe the frequencies of age, sex, medications dispensed, concomitant drugs used, and co-morbidities, were conducted according to the design used for the non-proprietary dataset. For each query, one set of tables was generated by number of patients by age and sex.

Query 1: Number of Patients.
Query 2: Number of Medications
Query 3: Number of Specific Drug Combinations
Query 4: Number of Driver Impairing Medications
Query 5: Number of Drug Interaction Conflicts
Query 6: Number of Specific Potential Driver Impairing Disease Groups
Query 7: Number of Potential Driver Impairing Disease Groups
Query 8: Number of Disease-Drug Conflicts

f. Methodology for Case-control Analysis

A McNemar-matched pair case-control design was employed to obtain odds ratio measures of potential MVC risk and to conduct a conditional logistic regression analysis using the proprietary database. The McNemar is a statistical test designed to describe the strength of an association between an outcome and an intervention among sets of a matched pair of subjects. Pairing with the intervention subject can occur with one (e.g. 1:1) or multiple controls (e.g. 1:2. 1:3, 1:4, etc.). In general, the greater the number of control pairings, the narrower the confidence interval around the 'best guess estimate' of the association measured. Data contained in the proprietary database included patients enrolled during the time period

January 1998 to March 2002. Individuals with E-codes for motor vehicle crashes with the restricted definition and three controls for each case were selected. Each case was matched with three controls by age and sex. Three controls represented the maximum number of controls available from the database, and thus provided the maximum sensitivity available for this population sample. In order to control seasonal factors, controls had the same event date as their corresponding cases.

More specifically, cases were defined as all patients with one or more claims with an ICD9-CM code indicative of a motor vehicle crash (see Figure 1) and with at least six months of continuous enrollment prior to their first claim(s) with a crash code. Three control patients were randomly matched to each case patient. For each control, a match number was provided that linked the control to the case. Matching was based on the following matching criteria:

- No claims with any of the motor vehicle crash codes listed in Appendix V.
- Age (as of January 1998), within five years of the age of the case.
- Sex (case matched to control).
- At least six months of continuous enrollment prior to the Case study subject's first claim with an crash code.

Medical history claims during the 60-day window prior to the MVC event date were analyzed using the odds ratio and conditional logistic regression analysis methodologies. We analyzed the numbers and types of medications in general, driver impairing medications, driver impairing diseases, drug-drug conflicts, and drug-disease conflicts.

Odds ratios for driver impairing drugs, driver impairing disease groups, drug-drug conflicts, and drug-disease conflicts were calculated without controlling other factors. We computed their corresponding 95 percent confidence intervals and p-values against the null hypothesis that the odds ratio was equal to one.

Table 1. Regression Analysis Variables

Variables	Values
Number of Medications	No Medications
	1 or more
Number of Driver Impairing Medications	No Impairing Drugs
	1 – 2
	3 or more
Number of Driver Impairing Diseases	No Impairing Diseases
	1 – 2
	3 or more
Number of Drug-Drug Conflicts	No Drug-Drug Conflicts
	1 – 2
	3 or more
Number of Drug-Disease Conflicts	No Drug-Disease Conflicts
	1 or more

In addition to the McNemar analysis, we built a model to predict motor vehicle crash (MVC) risk, SAS PROC PHREG with a forward selection option was used to conduct an unconditional logistic regression. We defined the dependant variable as 1 for cases and 0 for controls. Independent variables included number of medications used, number of driver impairing medications used, number of driver impairing disease groups, number of drug-drug conflicts, number of drug-disease conflicts, and baseline driver impairing medical conditions. Number of medications used and number of driver impairing medications used were determined to have multi-colinearity and only number of driver impairing medications was left in the logistic regression model. Number of driver-impairing medications used, number of driver-impairing disease groups, and number of drug-drug conflicts have three computational values while number of medications used and number of drug-disease conflicts have two categories.

Reference groups for number of medications, number of driver impairing medications, number of driver impairing diseases, number of drug-drug conflicts, and number of drug-disease conflicts were 'No Medications', 'No Impairing Drugs', 'No Impairing Diseases', 'No Drug-Drug Conflicts', and 'No Drug-Disease Conflicts' respectively. Odds ratios and 95 percent confidence intervals were computed for those variables with and without control of other variables.

3. Eligibility and Case-Control Matching Procedures

- Case group: All patients with one or more claims with an ICD9-9-CM code indicative of a motor vehicle crash (see Figure 1) AND at least six months of continuous enrollment prior to the first claim with a crash code.
- Control group: Three patients were randomly matched to each case patient. For each control, a match number was provided that linked the control to the case. Matching was based on the following matching criteria:
  - No claims with any of the motor vehicle crash codes listed in Appendix V.
  - Age (as of January 1998), within 5 years of the age of the case.
  - Sex same as the case patient.
  - At least 6 months of continuous enrollment prior to the first claim date with a crash code of the corresponding case patient.

In addition, only patients with drug benefits were included for study, as evidenced by the presence of at least one paid pharmacy claim during the period of observation. Patients aged 65 years and older were included only if they were part of a Medicare Risk plan, as full medical and pharmacy utilization data was required for this analysis.

4. Preparation of Analysis File

A case file, a control file, and a crosswalk file, which links each control patient to each case patient, were prepared for analysis. The case file and control files contained the Patient ID and information about enrollment, demographics, medical claims, and pharmacy claims. The crosswalk file contained the case Patient ID, control Patient ID and match number. We also prepared files for medication classes, potential driver impairing medications (Appendix

I), potential driver impairing diseases (Appendix II), drug interactions conflicts (Appendix III), and drug-disease conflicts (Appendix IV).

III. RESULTS

A. Non-proprietary Database: Descriptive Analysis

1. General Findings: Descriptive Analysis

a. Demographics

The NAMCS dataset contained both unweighted and weighted numbers and percentages. The weighted numbers are projected to the whole U.S. population while the unweighted is the actual numbers obtained from the survey. This chapter will summarize the weighted findings for physician visits for patients with the Restricted Definition of E-codes for Motor Vehicles.

Over Age 50 individuals represented 27 percent of physician visits. Females represented 50.4 percent of the over 50 age group, but only 49.6 percent of the 16-49 age group (see Figure 2 and Appendix VI, Table 1b).

b. Number of Medications

For the over 50 age group, within the NAMCS database, 61 percent of visits had medication mentions. Of those, 25 percent had mentions of only one drug and 36 percent had mentions of between 2 and 6 drugs (see Figure 3). In contrast, in the Ages 16-49 group, 51 percent of visits had medication mentions (19 percent had mentions of only one drug, while 32 percent of the visits had mentions of between 2-6 drugs). The survey did not list mentions of more than six drugs. (See Appendix VI, Table 2b). As expected, a greater percentage of visits for the over 50 age group had mentions of drug use than did visits for the Ages 16-49 group (61% versus 51% respectively).

c. Frequently Used Medication Classes

The most frequently mentioned medication classes in the over 50 age group visits (see Appendix VI, Table 2b), in descending order by frequency of use, are listed below (See Table 2). An * identifies the Potentially Driver-Impairing Drug Classes. Both groups received frequent mentions of potentially impairing drug classes. The older adult group adds cardiovascular medication mentions to their top ten list, while the younger group has more anti-asthmatic and anticonvulsant medication group mentions. Both had mentions of use of pain relievers, muscle relaxants and antidepressants. Skeletal Muscle Relaxants, Antidepressants, and Anti-anxiety Agents are considered to be inappropriate for use in individuals over 65 (Beers, 1997).

The most frequently mentioned medication classes in the Under Age 50 Group visits (See Appendix VI, Table 2b), in descending order by frequency of use, is listed above. (See Table 2). An * identifies the PDI medication classes.

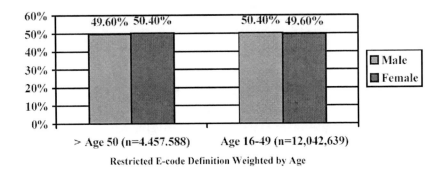

Figure 2. Non-Proprietary Database Demographics

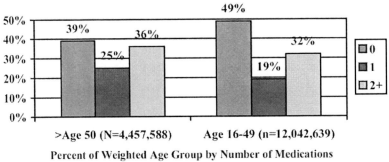

Figure 3. Non-Proprietary Database Number of Medications by Age Strata

Table 2. Most Frequently Used Medication Classes

Medication Classes	Weighted > Age 50 Group (n=4,457,588)	Weighted Age 16-49 Group (n=12,042,639)
*ANTIARTHRITICS	19%	16%
*SKELETAL, MUSCLE RELAXANTS	15%	15%
*ANALGESICS, NARCOTIC	14%	12.4%
*NSAID	10%	11%
ANALGESICS, NON-NARCOTIC	8%	10%
*ANTIDEPRESSANTS	7.5%	7%
*DISORDERS, ACID/PEPTIC	7%	4%
*ANTI-ANXIETY AGENTS	6%	2.4%
*BETA BLOCKERS	5%	--
*ACE INHIBITORS	4.7%	--
*ANTICONVULSANTS	--	2%
ANTIASTHMATICS/BRONCHODILATORS	--	1.7%

d. Most Frequent Drug Combinations

The most frequently appearing mentions of drug combinations in the Over Age 50 Group visits are provided in descending order of frequency in Table 3. (See also Appendix VI, Table 3b). The Over 50 age group received mentions of use of multiple medication classes, many which interact to potentiate driver impairing effects. For example, narcotic analgesics used with muscle relaxants, antidepressants, or antianxiety agents will result in potential sedated and confused reactions.

e. Use of Potentially Driver Impairing (PDI) Medications

The survey data was further analyzed to identify the rate of mentions of use of medications that we defined as being potentially driver impairing. (Appendix VI, Table 4b).

More than 58 percent of the Over Age 50 Group visits mentioned one or more PDI medications. Twenty-seven percent had mentions of one PDI medication and close to one-third (31%) had mentions of two or more PDI drugs. Over 48 percent of the Under Age 50 Group visits received one or more PDI medication mentions. Twenty percent had mentions of one PDI medication, and 28 percent had mentions of two to six PDI medications. (See Figure 4).

Table 3. Most Frequently Appearing Drug Combinations in the Over Age 50 Group

Most Frequently Appearing Drug Combinations by Percent in the > Age 50 Group (n=4,457,588)	
Drug Combinations	
• Narcotics, Antianxiety Agents, Antiarthritics, Skeletal Muscle Relaxants	2.7%
• Nacotics, Antiarthritics, GI Disorder, Anti-Hyperlipidemic Agents, Skeletal Muscle Relaxants	2.3%
• Ace Inhibitor Hypotensive, Narcotics, Antidepressants	2.0%
• Alpha Agonists, Antidiarrheal agents, GI Disorder, Diuretics, Homeopathic drugs, Potassium Supplements	1.8%
• Narcotics, Antianxiety Agents, Antidepressants, Antihypertensives, Calcium Metabolism, Thyroid Hormones	1.4%
• Ace Inhibitor Hypotensive, Steroids, Non-narcotic Analgesics, Antiarrhythmics, Topical	1.4%
• Ace Inhibitor Hypotensive, Antiarthritics, Beta Blockers	1.3%

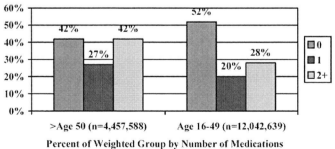

Figure 4. Use of Driver-Impairing Medications

Table 4. Appearance of Driver Impairing Medical Conditions

Medical Condition	Weighted > Age 50 Group (n=4,457,588)	Weighted Age 16-49 Group (n=12,042,639)
Hypertension	7.7%	--
CNS Excitation	6.8%	6.8%
Peripheral Neuropathy	2.6%	--
Ankylosing Spondylitis	2.1%	--
Psychoses	2.1%	1.4%
Diabetes Mellitus I and II	1.8%	--
Depression	1.6%	0.97%
Head Trauma	-	1.2%
Alcoholism	1.4%	--
Congestive Heart Failure	1.4%	--
Thyroid Disease	--	0.5%
Anxiety Disorder	--	0.45%
Bipolar Disorder	--	0.3%

f. Appearance of Potentially Driver Impairing (PDI) Medical Conditions

We performed additional analysis to identify the percentage of individuals in the motor vehicle crash (MVC) group visits (weighted) with mention of potentially driver impairing medical conditions. (Appendix VI, Table 6b).

Although both older and younger individuals with the definition of motor vehicle crashes received mentions of potential driver impairing diseases, the older adults had greater percentages of physician mentions of Driver Impairing Medical Conditions. (See Table 4).

g. Drug Interactions and Drug Disease Conflicts

We performed further analyses to determine whether the use of multiple medications, which increase the risk of drug interactions and drug/disease conflicts, were mentioned more frequently in the crash involved individuals' visits (Appendix VI, Tables 5b and 8b). We looked for drug interaction mentions that result in increased driver impairing effects (e.g., a drug interferes with the metabolism of the other drug and results in increased blood levels and side effects) and disease/drug interactions that can result in aggravation of a driver impairing disease (e.g., a drug can cause hypoglycemic effects in a diabetic) or a disease that can influence the side effects of a PDI drug (e.g., hepatic dysfunction can impair metabolism of a drug and thus increase side effects).

In terms of the number of drug-drug conflicts, visits with older patients seem to be more likely to have more drug mentions with drug-drug conflicts (14%). Only five percent of the drug mentions in the Age 16-49 group visits were drug/drug conflicts. We were not able to detect drug/disease conflicts in this dataset.

B. Proprietary Database: Descriptive Analysis

1. General Findings: Descriptive Analysis

a. Demographics

The total number of cases is 33,605. The number of **Over Age 50 Cases** in the motor vehicle crash E-code group is 5,398 or 16 percent of the total. The number and percent of Over Age 50 females in the case group is 2,842 or 52.6 percent and the Over Age 50 males group has 2,556 patients or 47.4 percent (See Figure 5). The remainder of the case group (28,205 patients) is between age 16 and 49. Females represent 54.9 percent and males 45.1 percent. There are three age- and sex-matched controls for each case. (Appendix VII, Tables 1a and 1b).

b. Number of Medications

In the **Over Age 50 Case Group**, the number of prescriptions per crash victim ranged between zero and 36 prescriptions in the 60-day period immediately precedent to their motor vehicle crash (the Event Window). Twenty-eight percent of the **Over Age 50 Case Group** received no prescriptions, and 14 percent received one prescription. Fifty-eight percent of the **Over Age 50 Case Group** received two or more prescriptions (See Figure 6). Sex differences were apparent since 65 percent of **Over Age 50 Case Group** females used two or more prescriptions in the 60-day analysis period in contrast to 51 percent of males. (Appendix VII, Table 2a and 2b).

In the **Over Age 50 Control Group** the number of prescriptions per person ranged between zero and 30 prescriptions in a 60-day period. Thirty-six percent of the Over Age 50 Controls received no prescriptions, 15 percent received one prescription and 49 percent received two or more prescriptions. Fifty-four percent of females received two or more prescriptions compared to 43 percent of males. (See Figure 6).

Over Age 50 Case Group patients tended to have a higher rate of drug utilization as evidenced by the fact that 36 percent of **Control** patients Over Age 50 used no prescriptions compared to 28 percent of **Case** patients Over Age 50. (See Figure 6.) The rate of Case patients over the age of 50 receiving two or more prescriptions was 1.2 times higher than the rate for the corresponding control patients.

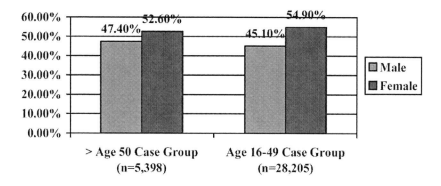

Figure 5. Proprietary Database Demographics

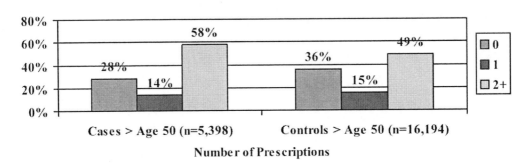

Figure 6. Case and Control Medication Use Frequency Over Age 50

c. Frequently Used Medication Classes

The most frequently used medication classes in the **Over 50 Case Group** and the Over 50 Control Group are listed below, in descending order by frequency of use. (See Table 5). An * identifies drug classes characterized as Potentially Driver-Impairing (PDI) Medication classes.

Approximately one-third of the case patients **Over Age 50** used a drug from one of the drug classes considered inappropriate for use in older individuals (Beers, 1997). Estrogenic drugs represent the most frequently used drug class in both the cases and controls. This class of drugs is used for treatment of menopausal symptoms and should not impair driving. Lipid lowering drugs, hypotensive drugs, and other treatment of cardiovascular conditions were commonly used in both groups. Certain PDI medications appeared to be used more frequently in the Case group than the Control group. For example, narcotic analgesics were used by 13.4 percent of the **Over Age 50 Case Group** compared to only 6 percent of the **Over Age 50 Control Group**. Similarly, the skeletal muscle relaxants were used by 4.7 percent of the **Over Age 50 Case Group** compared to slightly over 1 percent of the **Over Age 50 Control Group**. Anti-anxiety agents were used by 7.1 percent of the **Over Age 50 Case Group** in contrast to 3.7 percent of the **Over Age 50 Control Group**.

Though not required within the scope of this study, a brief analysis of the characteristics of medication use within individuals ages 16-49 was carried out. The number of prescriptions received during the Event Window for the **Age 16-49 Case Group** ranged between zero and 37 prescriptions per person. Fifty-two percent of the **Age 16-49 Case Group** received no prescriptions, 16 percent received one prescription and 32 percent received two or more prescriptions. (See Figure 7). Thirty-nine percent of females used two or more prescriptions, while 24 percent of males received one or more prescriptions.

The number of prescriptions in the **Age 16-49 Control Group** ranged from zero to 34 prescriptions. Within this group 61 percent received no prescriptions, 17 percent received one prescription, and 22 percent received two or more prescriptions. Twenty-six percent of female patients received one or more prescriptions in contrast to 18 percent of males.

The most frequently used medication classes in the **Age 16-49 Case Group** and the **Age 16-49 Control Group** are listed below, in descending order by frequency of use. (See Table 6). An * identifies the Potentially Driver-Impairing (PDI) drug classes.

Table 5. Frequency of Use by MedicationClass for Cases and Controls Over Age 50

Medication Classes	> Age 50 Case Group (n=5,398)	> Age 50 Control Group (n=16,194)
ESTROGENIC AGENS	15%	13.3%
*NARCOTIC ANALGESICS	13.4%	--
LIPID LOWERING DRUGS	13.1%	13%
NSAIDS AND COX INHIBITORS	12.4%	--
*HYPOTENSIVES, ACE INHIBITORS	11.7%	9.8%
*GASTRIC AND SECRETION REDUCERS	11%	7.5%
*CALCIUM CHANNEL BLOCKERS	9%	7.4%
*SSRI ANTIDEPRESSANTS	8.3%	5.5%
*BETA-ADRENERGIC BLOCKING AGENTS	7.8%	--
*ANTIHISTIMINES	7.7%	5.3%
PENICILLINS	--	4%
*ANTIANXIETY AGENTS	7.1%	3.7%
THYROID HORMONES	6.7%	--
HYPOGLYCEMICS, INSULIN-RELEASE	5.3%	--
SKELETAL MUSCLE RELAXANTS	4.7%	--
*GLUCOCORTICOIDS	4.3%	3.2%
MACROLIDES	--	2.8%

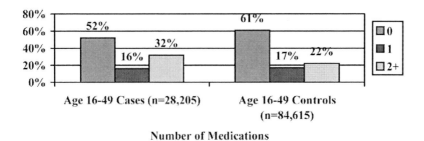

Figure 7. Case and Control Medication Use Frequency Ages 16-49

Table 6. Frequency of Use by Medication Class for Cases and Controls Ages 16-49

Medication Class	Ages 16-49 Case Group	Medication Class	Ages 16-49 Control Group
*ANAGELSICS, NARCOTIS	10.2%	CONTRACEPTIVES	7%
*NSAIDS, COX2 INHIBITORS	7.3%	*ANTIHISTIMINES	4.3%
CONTRACEPTIVES, ORAL	5.7%	PENICILLINS	4.1%
*SSRIs	6.2%	*ANALGESICS,NARCOTICS	4.0%
*ANTIHISTIMINES	5.6%	*SSRIs	3.9%
PENICILLINS	5.4%	*NSAIDS, COX 2 INHIB	3.2%

Table 6. (Continued)

Medication Class	Ages 16-49 Case Group	Medication Class	Ages 16-49 Control Group
MACROLIDES	4.2%	MACROLIDES	2.9%
*SKELETAL MUSC RELAX	4.1%	*GI ACID SECR REDUCERS	2.1%
*GI ACID SECRETION REDUCERS	3.5%	*BETA-ADRENERGIC	1.9%
*BETA BLOCKING AGENTS	2.9%	TETRACYCLINES	1.9%
EXPECTORANTS	2.7%	NASAL STEROIDS	1.7%
*GLUCOCORTICOIDS	4.3%	*GLUCOCORTICOIDS	1.7%
*ANTICONVULSANTS	2.6%	EXPECTORANTS	1.5%
CEPHALOSORINS – 1ST gen	2.0%	*ANTI-ANXIETY AGENTS	1.5%
THYROID HORMONES	1.9%	*THYROID HORMONES	1.2%

Oral Contraceptives were frequently used drugs in both the Ages 16-49 cases and controls. Other drug classes frequently used in both groups included antihistamines, antibiotics, beta-adrenergic anti-asthma agents, glucocorticoids, and expectorants. PDI medications appeared to be used more frequently in the Case group than the Control group. For example, the narcotic analgesic class was used by 10 percent of the Ages 16-49 Case Group compared to 4 percent of the Ages 16-49 Control Group. Similarly, the skeletal muscle relaxant class was used by 4.1 percent of the Ages 16-49 Case Group compared to less than 1 percent of the Ages 16-49 Control Group. SSRI antidepressants were used by 6.2 percent of the Case Group while only 3.9 percent of the Control Group used this class.

Individuals Ages 16-49 involved in a crash were more likely to be taking medications than non-crash-involved individuals (48% versus 39%). Ages 16-49 Case patients had more than two prescriptions by a factor of 1.5 times more than the control patients (See Figures 8 and 9) did.

Comparing Ages 16-49 Cases and Ages 16-49 Controls to the Over Age 50 Cases and Controls reinforces the observation that older individuals in general use more prescriptions than younger individuals do. (See Figures 8 and 9). Almost twice as many younger individuals versus older individuals received no prescriptions (cases 52% versus 28% and controls 61% versus 36%), while a greater percentage of older individuals received multiple prescriptions than younger cases and controls respectively (58% versus 32% and 49% versus 22%). The use of multiple prescriptions greatly increases the potential for driver impairment from medication drug interactions.

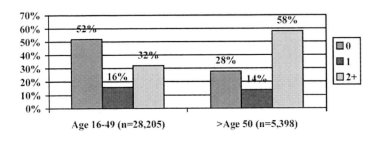

Figure 8. Comparison of Cases Between Age Groups by Number of Medications

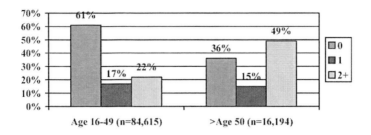

Figure 9. Comparison of Controls Between Age Groups by Number of Medications

d. Most Frequently Appearing Drug Combinations

The most frequently appearing drug combinations in the Over Age 50 Case Group were in descending order of frequency (for full list see Appendix VII, Tables 3a and 3b):

Narcotics and skeletal muscle relaxants and narcotics and anti-anxiety drugs are combinations that result in a potentiating effect causing extreme disorientation. Certain antibiotics and gastric acid secretion reducers inhibit the metabolism of narcotics and other drugs. SSRIs inhibit the metabolism of narcotics and by themselves cause anxiety and disorientation.

The most frequently appearing drug combinations in the Over Age 50 Control Group were in descending order of frequency:

Table 7. Most Frequently Appearing Drug Combinations in Cases Over Age 50

Most Frequently Appearing Drug Combinations in Cases Over Age 50
Narcotics and NSAIDs
Skeletal Muscle Relaxants and NSAIDs
Narcotics and Skeletal Muscle Relaxants
Narcotics and Skeletal Muscle Relaxants and NSAIDs
Narcotics and Antibiotics
Gastric Acid Secretion Reducers and Narcotics
Anti-Anxiety Drugs and Narcotics
Serotonin Reuptake Inhibitor (SSRI) Antidepressants and Narcotics
Narcotics and NSAIDs and Antibiotics

Table 8. Most Frequently Appearing Drug Combinations in Controls Over Age 50

Most Frequently Appearing Drug Combinations in Controls Over Age 50
Estrogens and Progestational Agents
Narcotics and NSAIDs
Expectorants and Macrolides
Beta Adrenergics and Glucocorticoids
Narcotics and Antibiotics
Skeletal Muscle Relaxants and NSAIDs
Nasal Anti-inflammatory Steroids and Antihistamines
Penicillins and Antihistamines

Table 9. Examples of Drug Classes ThatMay Impair Driving

Drug Class	Possible Effects
Anti Diabetic Drugs	Hypoglycemia
Anticholinergics	Blurred vision
Narcotic analgesics	Sedation
Anti-hypertensive drugs	Hypotension
Sedative/Hypnotics	Sedation
Antidepressants	Sedation, dizziness
Allergy drugs	Sedation, dizziness
Anti-arrhythmics	Fainting (syncope)
Anticonvulsants	Ataxia, dizziness, sedation
Skeletal Muscle Relaxants	Dizziness, sedation

e. Use of Driver-Impairing Medications

The data were further analyzed to identify the rate of use of medications that we defined as being potentially driver impairing (PDI). (Refer to Appendix VII, Table 4a and 4b). See Table 9 below for examples of driver impairing drug classes and their possible effects.

Many of the above mentioned driver impairing drug classes have been determined to be potentially inappropriate for use particularly by older adults. These drugs cause excessive sedation, confusion, orthostatic hypotension, cardiac effects, depression, and weakness. Additional types of drugs are risky when used in the older adult with certain underlying medical conditions, such as cardiac conditions, depression, seizure disorders, respiratory disorders, parkinsonism, and cognitive impairment. The use of these potentially inappropriate drugs in older patients with these conditions may exacerbate these conditions or cause CNS side effects (Fick, 2003).

The use of PDI medications is widespread in the both case groups. Approximately 64 percent of the **Over Age 50 Case** patients received potentially driver-impairing medications. In contrast, 54 percent of the **Over Age 50 Control** patients received potentially driver-impairing medications. (See Figure 10). Similarly, 35 percent of the **Under Age 50 Case** patients received potentially driver-impairing medications compared to 24 percent of the **Under Age 50 Control** patients.

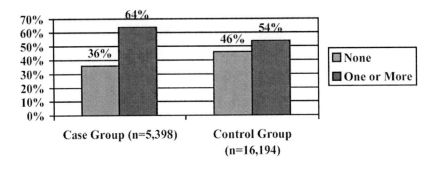

Figure 10. Potential Driver Impairing Medication Use in Over Age 50 Cases and Controls

Table 10. Examples of Medical Conditions That May Impair Driving

Condition	Possible Effects
Diabetes	Hypoglycemia
Arthritis	Stiffness
Epilepsy	Seizures
Depression	Inattentiveness
Insomnia	Daytime Sleepiness
Arrhythmias	Fainting (syncope)
Cardiovascular disease	Stroke, MI,
Alzheimer's	Confusion
Parkinsonism	Stiffness, dementia

Interestingly, 19 percent of the Over Age 50 Case Females who had one or more prescriptions (2,204 patients) had received a prescription for the Narcotic Analgesic Class in the 60 day period preceding the motor vehicle crash. Similarly, 19 percent of the Over Age 50 Case Males who had one or more prescriptions (1,660 patients) had received a prescription for the Narcotic Analgesic Class. Furthermore, 8 percent of prescription-receiving females in the Over Age 50 Case group received prescriptions for Skeletal Muscle Relaxants. And a somewhat fewer number (5%) of prescription-taking males received prescriptions for Skeletal Muscle Relaxants. Both the narcotic analgesic class and the skeletal muscle relaxant class are extremely driver impairing.

Other worrisome PDI medication classes that appeared in frequencies greater than 5 percent of Cases Over Age 50 include Antidepressants (18%), Anti-Diabetic Agents (14%), Anti-anxiety agents (10%), Anticonvulsants (5%), and Anti-hypertensive Agents (38%). (Refer to Appendix VII, Table 4a and 4b).

f. Appearance of PDI Medical Conditions

We performed additional analysis to identify the percentage of individuals in the Case group and the Control group who have been diagnosed with PDI medical conditions. (Appendix VII, Tables 7a and 7b). See Table 10 below for examples of driver impairing medical conditions and their possible effects.

Of considerable note is that nearly 51 percent of the **Over Age 50 Case** patients submitted an insurance claim for a diagnosis for PDI conditions in the Event Window. This is especially important in light of the fact that only 36 percent of the **Over Age 50 Control** patients submitted an insurance claim for a PDI condition. Clearly, a higher percentage of individuals in the crash-involved groups had been diagnosed with one of the PDI conditions (See Figure 11).

The most frequently appearing diagnoses in the **Over Age 50 Case** Group are Cardiovascular Disease (17.9%), Hypertension (16%), Allergies (15%), Diabetes (9.7%), and Respiratory Infections (7.4%). In the **Over Age 50 Control Group** the most frequently appearing diagnoses group are Cardiovascular Diseases (8.9%), Hypertension (8%), Allergies (6%), Diabetes (4%), and Respiratory Infections (4%). Thus, while the top five conditions are basically the same in the cases and controls, the frequency of appearance is about twice the rate in the cases than in the controls.

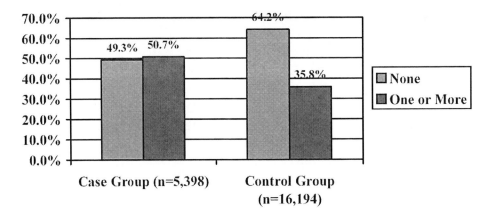

Figure 11. Potential Driver Impairing Disease Appearance in Over Age 50 Cases and Controls

g. Drug Interactions and Drug/Disease Conflicts

We performed further analyses on the prescription and medical data to determine whether the use of multiple medications, which increases the risk of drug/drug interactions and drug/disease conflicts, occurred more frequently among the crash-involved drivers. We looked for three factors that can have driver-impairing effects: drug interactions, disease/drug interactions that aggravate a driver impairing disease, or a disease that can influence the side effects of a driver-impairing drug.

We identified 24 percent of the Over Age 50 Case patients as exhibiting overlapping use of medications that are known to interact. (Appendix VII, Table 5a and 5b). Conversely, only 16 percent of the Over Age 50 Control patients exhibited concomitant use of interacting medications. (See Figure 12). In the Ages 16-49 case group, 8 percent exhibited overlapping drugs know to interact, compared to only four percent (4%) of the Ages 16-49 controls.

Eight percent (8%) of the Over Age 50 Case patients exhibited potential Drug/Disease conflicts compared to only 4 percent in the control group (See Figure 13). (Refer also to Appendix VII, Tables 8a and 8b). Among the Ages 16-49 Cases 2 percent exhibited potential drug/disease conflicts compared to 1 percent of the controls.

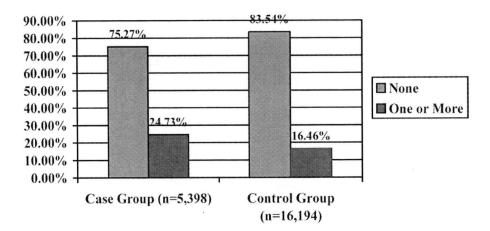

Figure 12. Drug Interaction Conflicts Among Over Age 50 Cases and Controls

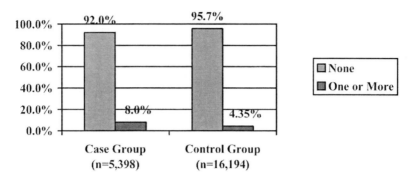

Figure 13. Drug/Disease Conflicts Among Cases and Controls Over Age 50

2. *General Findings: Case Control Analysis*

The odds ratios for driver impairing medications used, driver impairing disease groups present, drug interaction conflicts, and drug-disease conflicts are listed in Appendix VIII Table 1 through Table 4.

a. Driver Impairing Medications

As indicated by Appendix VIII, Table 1, 39 of the 90 driver impairing drug pharmacologic classes had point estimate odds ratios over 1.2, with the lower bound also over 1.1 (indicating $p<.05$). Of these 35 pharmacologic classes, 27 have specific warnings about sedation, dizziness, drowsiness, and the need for caution when driving especially until the effects of the drug on driving are known.

Over age 50 drivers taking specific driver-impairing medications seem more likely to be involved in motor vehicle crashes than those not taking these medications (See Table 11). For example, the likelihood of being involved in an MVC for people taking barbiturates is 7.50 times greater than that for people not taking barbiturates. People taking antihistamines were three times more likely to have an MVC than people not taking antihistamines. Non-narcotic antitussives (also available as a common nonprescription medicine) appear to increase MVC risk by 123 percent.

This study did not consider the possible influence of maturation bias or survivor effects. We were not able to determine *de novo* exposure or prolonged exposure to prescribed medications. These are useful variables to evaluate because certain side effects are more prominent at the initiation of therapy and with continued use the body adapts to these side effects. Further research is needed to assess MVC risks when comparing initial medication use with longer-term medication use.

Seven of the fifteen medication classes in our analysis with highest odds ratios are drug classes that have been reported to be especially problematic in older patients (Beers MH, 1997). Medications classes such as barbiturates, belladonna alkaloids, antihistamines, long half-life anti-anxiety agents, antiemetic/antivertigo agents, certain narcotic analgesics, skeletal muscle relaxants, certain platelet aggregation inhibitors, fluoxetine, certain hypotensives, and certain antipsychotic agents are considered potentially inappropriate for use in older adults (Curtis et al., 2004).

Table 11. Top 15 Medication classeswith Highest Odds Ratios (p ≤ .05)[2]

Drug Class	Odds Ratio (OR) with 95% C.I.	Possible Effects	Indication for Use
BARBITURATES	7.50 (2.35, 23.91)	Drowsiness	Nervousness, Seizures
ANTIHISTAMINES	3.00 (1.05, 8.55)	Dizziness, bronchospasm. Avoid alcohol and other medicines that affect the CNS	Asthma, Allergies
ANTITUSSIVES, NON-NARCOTIC	2.23 (1.30, 3.82)	Dizziness, drowsiness, depression	Cough
ANALGESICS, NARCOTICS	2.22 (1.98, 2.49)	Dizziness, drowsiness, blurred vision	Pain
ANTIPSYCHOTICS, ATYPICAL, DOPAMINE, & SEROTONIN ANTAG	2.20 (1.37, 3.52)	Drowsiness	Schizophrenia
SKELETALMUSCLE RELAXANTS	2.09 (1.71, 2.55)	Dizziness, drowsiness, lightheadedness	MuscleSpasms
ANTI-ANXIETY DRUGS	2.00 (1.72, 2.31)	Drowsiness	Anxiety
ANTICONVUL-SANTS	1.97 (1.64, 2.38)	Drowsiness	Seizures
SEROTONIN-2 ANTAGONIST/REUPTAKE INHIBITORS (SARIS)	1.90 (1.49, 2.44)	Dizziness, drowsiness, headache, confusion	Depression
BELLADONNA ALKALOIDS	1.85 (1.08, 3.19)	Dizziness, drowsiness, confusion	GIsymptoms
INSULINS	1.80 (1.45, 2.22)	Hypoglycemia	Diabetes Mellitus
HYPOTENSIVES, SYMPATHOLYTIC	1.79 (1.17, 2.74)	Hypotension, drowsiness, blurred vision	Hypertension
SEROTONIN-NOREPINEPHRINE REUPTAKE INHIB (e.g., VENLAFAXINE)	1.78 (1.19, 2.66)	Dizziness, drowsiness, hypertension, seizures	Depression
PLATELET AGGREGATION INHIBITORS	1.69 (1.17, 2.43)	Headache, weakness, shakes, aches	Stroke prevention
ANTIEMETIC/ANTI VERTIGO AGENTS	1.63 (1.17, 2.28)	Drowsiness, dizziness	Nausea, vomiting, vertigo

A review of the literature identified a number of articles that assessed the relationship between medications and automobile crashes in the older adult. An article published by McGwin in 2000 found that drivers over age 65 in Alabama had elevated odds ratios (OR) at the 95 percent confidence interval for involvement in at-fault automobile crashes for the following medication classes:

NSAIDs   **OR=1.7 (CI: 1.0, 2.6);**
ACE Inhibitor hypotensives   **OR=1.6 (CI: 1.0, 2.7);**
Anticoagulants   **OR=2.6 (CI: 1.0, 73)**
Benzodiazepine use   **OR=5.2 (CI: 0.9, 30).**

And in 2000, Sims reported:

Hypnotic medications   **RR=2.9; 95% CI:1.3, 6.6; p=0.01 (Sims, et al, 2000)**

The results of our analyses were remarkably similar:

NSAIDs   **OR=1.58 (CI: 1.41, 1.76)**
ACE Inhibitors   **OR=1.23 (CI: 1.11, 1.37);**
Oral Anticoagulants   **OR=1.31 (CI: 1.01, 1.70), and**
Benzodiazepine anti-anxiety   **OR=2.0 (CI: 1.72, 2.31).**

In each of these cases, the Odds Ratios (or relative risk in the case of the Sims study) identified were similar in magnitude to those of the cited studies.

Additional studies published in years 1992-2000, report associations among medication usage, the older adult, and motor vehicle crashes (Foley, 1995, Leveille, 1994, Ray, 1992, Hemmelgam, 1997, Hu, 1998, and Koepsell, 1994).

b. Driver Impairing Disease Groups

Study subjects with driver-impairing diseases appeared more likely to have a MVC than subjects that present without these disorders. For example, the Odds Ratio for head trauma is 36, suggesting that subjects with a history of that condition[3] were 36 times more likely to be involved in a MVC than people without that history. Acidosis had the second highest Odds Ratio of 15. The study design methodology attempted to rule out head trauma as a result of a MVC by employing temporal sequence and date of service screens. The resulting risk was a measure of subjects with existing head trauma who subsequently experienced an MVC.

As indicated by Appendix VIII, Table 2, 79 of the 200 driver impairing disease classes (40%) had statistically significant odds ratios over 1.4. Thefifteen disease groups with highest odds ratios are shown below in Table 12. Note that many of these disease groups have either a small number of cases with diseases or small number of controls with diseases or both, and although the p values were less than or equal to .05, caution must be taken when using these estimated values for Odds Ratios. For example, the disease group "acidosis" had only five cases and one control with the disease; disease group "neurotic disorder" had four cases and one control with the disease; disease group "delirium, acute" had four cases and one control with the disease; disease group "consciousness alteration" had 12 cases and four controls with the disease.

Conversely, the following disease groups had more than 50 cases and elevated Odds Ratios (p<.05): Depression, Ankylosing Spondylitis, Anxiety Disorders, CNS Excitation (nervousness, confusion), Back Pain, Congestive Heart Failure, Asthma, Diabetes Mellitus, Abdominal Pain, COPD, Ischemic Heart Disease, Cardiovascular Disease, GI Hemorrhage, Hypertension, Respiratory Infections, Arthritis, Bleeding, Arrhythmias, and Thyroid Disease.

The conditions that we identified with elevated Odds Ratios can be grouped by Disorder Type as follows:

CNS Disorders: Depression, Anxiety Disorders, Nervousness and Confusion, Neurotic Disorders, Delirium, Drowsiness, personality Disorders, Alcoholism, Insomnia, Extrapyramidal Reactions, Anxiety Disorders, and Bipolar Disorders

Previous studies have shown some association between depression and crashes (Sims, 2000). Patients who suffer from depression may be at higher risk for motor vehicle crashes. They have impaired attention and concentration, anxiety, irritability, agitation, fatigue, insomnia, and weakness. The depressed patient may also take risks, make suicidal gestures, or consume alcohol. Similarly, side effects of antidepressants may adversely affect cognitive and psychomotor function. Crashes may also result from the tricyclic anti-depressant drug-induced postural hypotension, cardiac arrhythmias, and convulsions (Edwards, 1995). Alcoholism and alcohol use have definitively been associated with motor vehicle crashes by numerous studies, both in the U.S. and worldwide. In our study we found an increased risk of automobile crashes in patients with the conditions below showing elevated significant risks.

Depression,	OR=3.99; CI:3.19, 4.99; p=.000.
Alcoholism	OR=5.44; CI:2.95-10.01, p=.000;
Stress disorders	OR=5.4; CI:1.81-16.11, p=.002;
Psychoses	OR=3.27; CI:1.44-7.42, p=.005;
Insomnia	OR=3.16; CI:1.69-5.92, p=.000;
Anxiety disorders	OR=2.87; CI:2.03-4.04, p=.000;
Drowsiness	OR=9.0; CI:2.9-27.91, p=.000;
Extrapyramidal disorders	OR=3.6; CI:1.56-8.33, p=.003; and
CNS excitation	OR=2.55; CI:1.94-3.35, p=.000

Joint and Muscle Disorders: Ankylosing Spondylitis, Arthritis, Osteoarthritis, Back Pain, and Muscle Spasms

Arthritis, history of falls, back pain and other impairments of physical function have been associated with increased crash involvement among older adults (Lyman, 2001 and Sims, 2001). In our analysis, we found increased risks in patients with:

Ankylosing spondylitis,	OR=3.33; CI:2.23-4.96, p=.000;
Back pain,	OR=2.42; CI:2.03-2.88, p=.000;
Fractures and injuries,	OR=2.34; CI:2.04-2.69, p=.000;
Muscle spasms,	OR=2.15; CI:1.33-3.5, p=.002; and
Arthritis,	OR=1.54; CI:1.12-2.11, p=.008.

Endocrine Disorders: Diabetes Mellitusand Thyroid Disorder

The impact of diabetes mellitus on older drivers has been questioned. Although McGwin et al. (1999) reported an adjusted OR of 2.5 (CI: 0.9-7.2) among drivers over age 65 who had been involved in crashes in the 4-year study period, he concludes that there is no evidence that older drivers with diabetes are at increased risk for automobile crashes. He does state that there remains the possibility that those with more severe diabetes or have had multiple crashes are at increased risk (McGwin, 1999). Conversely, Koepsell et al. found injury risk 2.6 times higher in older diabetic drivers (95% CI:1.4-4.7) and especially those treated with insulin (OR=5.8; CI:1.2-28.7) or oral hypoglycemic agents (OR=3.1; CI:0.9-11.0) (Koepsell, 1994). Drivers with medical conditions that can change abruptly, such as diabetes, are at increased risk for crashes (Carr, 2000). Our analysis showed an association of:

Diabetes mellitus,	OR=2.07; CI:1.81-2.37, p=.000.
Diabetic ketoacidosis,	OR=5.44; CI:1.81-16.11, p=.002.

Cardiovascular Disorders: Congestive Heart Failure, Ischemic Heart Disease, Cardiovascular Disease, Hypertension, Arrhythmias, Hypotension, Syncope, Angina, and Edema

McGwin (2000) found that older drivers with heart disease OR=1.5 (CI:1.0-2.2) or stroke OR=1.9 (CI: 0.9-3.9) were more likely to be involved in at-fault automobile crashes. Sims et al. (2000) noted increased risk with self-reported stroke or transient ischemic attacks (RR=2.7; CI:1.1-6.6 p=.03). Gresset et al. (1994) reported that arrhythmias were associated with a significant increased risk of road crashes (OR=1.63, CI:1.0-2.65). Koepsell et al. (1994) found increases in injury risk in older drivers with coronary artery disease OR=1.4. Our analysis similarly showed an increase in risk for motor vehicle crashes and various cardiovascular disorders.

Angina,	OR=2.18; CI:1.15-4.15, p=.018;
Congestive heart failure,	OR=2.1; CI:1.53-2.89, p=.000;
CVA,	OR=1.97; CI:1.2-3.25, p=.008;
Ischemic heart disease,	OR=1.83; CI:1.48-2.27, p=.000;
Stroke,	OR=1.69; CI:1.07-2.67, p=.025;
Hypertension,	OR=1.65; CI:1.48-1.84, p=.000; and
Arrhythmias,	OR=1.5; CI:1.16-1.94, p=.002.

Respiratory Disorders: Asthma, COPD, Respiratory Infections, Bronchopneumonia, and pulmonary edema.

Respiratory disorders are not specifically associated with increased risk for driver impairment. However, individuals with respiratory disorders often suffer from reduced sleep quality associated with breathing difficulties. Sleep apnea has been associated with increased risk of motor vehicle crashes (Masa et al., 2000). In our analysis we did find increased risk in patients with:

Asthma,	OR=2.08; CI:1.55-2.8, p=.000;
COPD,	OR=1.89; CI:1.47-2.43, p=.000;
Respiratory Infections,	OR=1.56; CI:1.35-1.82, p=.000;
Sleep apnea,	OR=1.83; CI:1.26-2.67, p=.002; and

Pulmonary edema, OR=2.63; CI:1.28-5.38, p=.008.

Head trauma and some other disease groups such as hemorrhage and alteration of consciousness could be both causes and results of MVCs. Due to the limitations of claims data, it is difficult to determine with assurance the true temporal relationship that existed.

c. Drug Interaction Conflicts and Drug-Disease Conflicts

Drug interaction conflicts and drug-disease conflicts that result in increased driver impairing effects were also analyzed.[4] Odds ratios of each conflict are displayed in Appendix VIII, Tables 3 and 4. Most conflicts have either a small number of cases, a small number of controls, or both, which makes the full assessment of their effects problematic without further analysis.

Table 13 listed 10 drug-drug (interaction) conflicts with highest statistically significant odds ratios, and Table 14 shows the 10 drug-disease conflicts with the highest statistically significant odds ratios.

Table 12. Top 15 Disease groupswith Highest Odds Ratios (p≤ .05)

Disease Groups	Odds Ratio with 95% C.I.	Driver Impairing Effects
HEAD TRAUMA	36.00 (11.09, 116.90)	Confusion, dizziness, drowsiness
ACIDOSIS	15.00 (1.75, 128.40)	
NEUROTIC DISORDER	12.00 (1.34, 107.37)	Confusion
DELIRIUM, ACUTE	**10.50 (2.18, 50.55)**	**Confusion, seizures**
CONSCIOUSNESS ALTERATION	9.00 (2.90, 27.91)	Drowsiness,
PERSONALITY DISORDERS	9.00 (1.82, 44.59)	Confusion, impaired judgment
HEMORRHAGE, UNSPEC	6.00 (1.10, 32.76)	Dizziness
ALCOHOLISM	5.44 (2.95, 10.01)	Confusion, dizziness, drowsiness, impaired judgment
DIABETIC KETOACIDOSIS	5.40 (1.81, 16.11)	Confusion, dizziness, Impaired judgment
STRESS DISORDERS	5.40 (1.81, 16.11)	Impaired judgment
VISUAL DISTURBANCES	4.71 (1.83, 12.16)	Impaired vision
DEPRESSION	3.99 (3.19, 4.99)	Confusion, drowsiness, Impaired judgment
PSYCHIATRIC DISORDERS	3.72 (2.99, 4.63)	Confusion, anxiety, drowsiness, impaired judgment
PLEURAL EFFUSION	3.69 (1.78, 7.68)	Breathing difficulties
EXTRAPYRAMIDAL REACTIONS	3.60 (1.56, 8.33)	Tremors, muscle difficulties

Table 13. Drug Interaction Conflictswith Highest Odds Ratios (p≤.05)

Drug 1	Drug 2	Odds Ratio with 95% C.I.
ANTICONVULSANTS	ANTIFUNGALAGENTS	21.00 (2.58, 170.69)
SEROTONIN-NOREPINEPHRINE REUPTAKE-INHIB (SNRIS)	QUINOLONES	21.00 (2.58, 170.69)
SKELETAL MUSCLE RELAXANTS	ANTIPSYCHOTICS, ATYPICAL, DOPAMINE, & SEROTONIN ANTAG	18.00 (2.17, 149.52)
HYPOGLYCEMICS, INSULIN-RELEASE STIMULANT TYPE	ABSORBABLE SULFONAMIDES	15.00 (1.75, 128.40)
SEROTONIN SPECIFIC REUPTAKE INHIBITOR (SSRIS)	ALPHA-2 RECEPTOR ANTAGONIST ANTIDEPRESSANTS	15.00 (1.75, 128.40)
ANTICONVULSANTS	BELLADONNAALKALOIDS	12.00 (1.34, 107.37)
TRICYCLIC ANTIDEPRESSANTS & REL. NON-SEL. RU-INHIB	ANTIPSYCHOTICS, ATYPICAL, DOPAMINE,& SEROTONIN ANTAG	10.50 (2.18, 50.55)
ANTI-ANXIETY DRUGS	LINCOSAMIDES	7.50 (1.46, 38.66)
SEROTONIN SPECIFIC REUPTAKE INHIBITOR (SSRIS)	SEROTONIN-NOREPINEPHRINE REUPTAKE- INHIB (SNRIS)	7.50 (1.46, 38.66)
BARBITURATES	ANTICONVULSANTS	6.00 (1.50, 23.99)

The study results suggest that interacting medicines had higher Odds Ratios than when the same medicines were taken alone. For example, Odds Ratios for insulin-release stimulant type hypoglycemics and for tricyclic antidepressants were 1.50 and 1.41 respectively, while Odds Ratio for subjects taking both was 4.50.[5] The magnitude that the Odds Ratio is increased due to the presence of an interacting drug varies among drug-drug pairs. The Odds Ratio for serotonin-norepinephrine reuptake-inhibitors (SNRIs) antidepressants itself is 1.78 and for non-barbiturate sedative-hypnotics is 1.48. If each were used together with anticonvulsants, the Odds Ratios became 3.67 and 3.92 respectively. It is interesting to note that the Odds Ratios for certain drugs alone were higher than together with other drugs. For example, the Odds Ratio for barbiturates itself is 7.50 but is 6.00 when taken with anticonvulsants.[6] Due to small sample sizes (there were ten cases and four controls taking barbiturates and six cases and three controls taking both barbiturates and anticonvulsants), extra caution needs to be taken when examining the risk shift for these conflicts.

Most drug-disease conflicts had higher Odds Ratios than the drugs and diseases alone. Narcotic analgesics had an Odds Ratio of 2.22 while the Odds Ratio of the conflict of narcotic analgesics and Chronic Hepatitis C without coma is 12.00. The Odds Ratio of alpha/beta-adrenergic blocking agents itself is 1 compared to 7.5 for the conflict of alpha/beta-adrenergic blocking agents and other primary cardiomyopathies.

As indicated in Appendix VIII, Table 3 and Table 4, only a small number of cases and controls experienced drug-drug conflicts and drug-disease conflicts. The estimated Odds Ratios and their 95 percent confidence interval are questionable. It is also premature to come to any conclusion about the increase and decrease of Odds Ratios for the conflicts compared to those for the drugs and diseases alone.

d. Odds Ratios for Categorical Variables

Number of medications used, number of driver-impairing medications used, number of driver-impairing disease groups, number of drug-drug conflicts, and number of drug-disease conflicts have been converted into categorical variables. The unadjusted Odds Ratios are shown in Table 15.

Study subjects taking any medications are 1.43 times more likely to be involved in a MVC than people taking no medications.

Table 14. Drug Disease Conflictswith Highest Odds Ratios (p≤.05)

Drug	Disease	Odds Ratio with 95% C.I.
GLUCOCORTICOIDS	ANXIETYSTATE UNSPEC	15.00 (1.75, 128.40)
ANALGESICS, NARCOTICS	CHR HEPATITIS C WOCOMA	12.00 (1.34, 107.37)
ANTI-NARCOLEPSY/ANTI-HYPERKINESIS, STIMULANT-TYPE	UNS HYPERTENSION	12.00 (1.34, 107.37)
ALPHA/BETA-ADRENERGIC BLOCKING AGENTS	OTH PRIMARY CARDIOMYOPATHIES	7.50 (1.46, 38.66)
CALCIUM CHANNEL BLOCKING AGENTS	SYNCOPE/COLLAPSE	7.00 (1.81, 27.07)
HYPOTENSIVES, ACE INHIBITORS	SYNCOPE/COLLAPSE	6.75 (2.08, 21.92)
ORAL ANTICOAGULANTS, COUMARIN TYPE	OTH PRIMARY CARDIOMYOPATHIES	6.00 (1.10, 32.76)
HYPOTENSIVES, SYMPATHOLYTIC	DIABETES UNCOMPL TYPE II	4.50 (1.60, 12.64)
BETA-ADRENERGIC BLOCKING AGENTS	DIABETES UNCOMPL TYPE I	3.67 (1.52, 8.85)
BETA-ADRENERGIC AGENTS	BENIGN HYPERTENSION	3.20 (1.58, 6.47)

Table 15. Odds Ratios of Categorical Variables

Group	Odds Ratio with 95% C.I.
1 or more medications	1.43 (1.32, 1.54)
1 – 2 PDI medications	1.29 (1.19, 1.41)
3 or more PDI medications	1.87 (1.70, 2.06)
1 – 2 PDI diseases	1.49 (1.37, 1.63)
3 or more PDI diseases	2.20 (2.01, 2.42)
1 – 2 drug-drug conflicts	1.47 (1.33, 1.63)
3 or more drug-drugconflicts	1.92 (1.67, 2.21)
1 or more drug-diseaseconflicts	2.18 (1.89, 2.52)

Compared with study subjects taking no driver-impairing medications, those taking one or two driver-impairing medications are 1.29 times more likely to be involved in a MVC, while the Odds Ratio for people taking three or more is 1.87. Clearly, study subjects taking driver-impairing medications have higher MVC risk. The more driver-impairing medications study subjects use the higher the MVC risk.

A similar relationship is observed for driver-impairing disease and drug-drug interactions. The risk for study subjects with one or two driver-impairing diseases is 1.49 times higher for people without any driver-impairing diseases, while the Odds Ratios for those with three or more driver-impairing diseases increases to 2.20. Drug-drug conflicts appear to increase the risk of being involved in MVCs. One or two drug-drug conflicts increase the odds by 47 percent while three or more drug-drug interactions increase the MVC odds by 92 percent.

The risk of experiencing a MVC for study subjects with at least one drug-disease conflict is 1.2 times higher than for people without any drug-disease conflicts.

e. Logistic Regression Analysis

A conditional logistic regression was performed using categorical variables for number of medications used, number of driver-impairing medications used, number of driver-impairing disease groups, number of drug interaction conflicts, and number of drug-disease conflicts. Most of the variables left in the model by Forward selection and their Odds Ratios are shown in Table 16. The residual chi-square, which indicates the goodness-of-fit, is 182.18 with a degree of freedom of 193 and p-value of 0.70. The model fits adequately. The same model was tested using unconditional logistic regression by adding the two matching variables: age and sex. The result is quite similar. The Hosmer and Lemeshow Goodness-of-Fit test[7] indicates again the model fits adequately (p-value=0.3234).

Although variables for Hypersensitivity Pneumonitis (Yes/No), Tuberculosis (Yes/No), Radiation Therapy ICD (Yes/No), Contraceptive Measures (Yes/No), Electrolyte Disorders (Yes/No), and Sickle Cell Anemia (Yes/No) were also left in the model, the p-values indicated that none of these Odds Ratios were significantly different from 1. Only one case had Hypersensitivity Pneumonitis. Five cases had Tuberculosis. Three cases had Contraceptive Measures. Six cases had Electrolyte Disorders. And one case had Sickle Cell Anemia.

The adjusted Odd Ratios differ from the unadjusted ones. For example, people taking one or two driver-impairing medications had an Odds Ratio of 1.17 after adjusting for other variables compared to the unadjusted 1.29. Every Odds Ratio except that for Hepatic Dysfunction was smaller than the unadjusted correspondents. Compared to the unadjusted 2.73, people with HEPATIC DYSFUNCTION had Odds Ratio of 3.0. GI Ulcer, Hepatitis, and Lipid Abnormalities had Odds Ratios of 1.20, 1.36, and 1.12 when computed directly, while their Odds Ratios became 0.53, 0.29, and 0.76 in the regression model.

The regression model showed an increase in risk among patients receiving one or more PDI medications (OR=1.17; CI:1.08-1.28) and one or more PDI diagnoses (OR=1.15; CI:1.04-1.27). Alcoholism, Asthma, Cardiovascular Disease, Depression, Hepatic Dysfunction, Hyperthyroidism, Anaphylactic shock, Diabetes Mellitus, Head trauma, Ketoacidosis, Syncope, Gastroenteritis, CNS Excitation, Pleural Effusion, GERD, Fractures and Injuries, Psychoses, Visual Disturbances, and Back Pain continued to demonstrate an association among older drivers and motor vehicle crashes. The medications used to treat these conditions, like a double-edged sword, ameliorate the underlying condition but also exacerbate other conditions and cause new symptoms with unwanted side effects.

Conditions such as heart disease, insomnia, parkinsonism, cognitive impairment, seizure disorders, COPD, syncope, falls, and diabetes can be negatively impacted by many drugs that are considered inappropriate in the older adult. Our analysis found that many of the potentially inappropriate medications for use by older adults (Beers, 1997) were used by our study patients and many resulted in increased risk for motor vehicle crashes.

Table 16. Adjusted Odds Ratios from the Regression Model

Variable	Odds Ratio with 95% C.I.
1 – 2 PDI medications (Yes/No)	1.17 (1.08, 1.28)
3 or more PDI medications (Yes/No)	1.38 (1.25, 1.52)
1 – 2 PDI diseases (Yes/No)	1.15 (1.04, 1.27)
3 or more PDI diseases (Yes/No)	1.27 (1.09, 1.47)
Alcoholism (Yes/No)	2.44 (1.23, 4.85)
Asthma (Yes/No)	1.48 (1.07, 2.04)
Cardiovascular Disease(Yes/No)	1.16 (1.01, 1.32)
Depression (Yes/No)	2.02 (1.50, 2.73)
Encephalopathic Syndrome (Yes/No)	0.10 (0.01, 0.92)
GI Ulcer (Yes/No)	0.53 (0.30, 0.91)
Hepatic Dysfunction (Yes/No)	3.00 (1.61, 5.61)
Hepatitis (Yes/No)	0.29 (0.10, 0.82)
Hyperthyroidism (Yes/No)	2.50 (1.03, 6.09)
Anaphylactic Shock (Yes/No)	2.01 (1.23, 3.28)
Lipid Abnormalities (Yes/No)	0.76 (0.65, 0.88)
Lymphadenopathy (Yes/No)	0.10 (0.01, 0.76)
Diabetes Mellitus I and II (Yes/No)	1.49 (1.27, 1.75)
HeadTrauma (Yes/No)	16.87 (5.00, 56.91)
Ketoacidosis(Yes/No)	3.45 (1.05, 11.41)
Syncope (Yes/No)	2.04 (1.16, 3.61)
Diarrhea, Gastroenteritis (Yes/No)	1.45 (1.17, 1.80)
CNS Excitation (Yes/No)	1.62 (1.21, 2.18)
Pleural Effusion-D (Yes/No)	2.34 (1.06, 5.14)
Surgery (Yes/No)	2.32 (1.04, 5.17)
Colon, Irritable (Yes/No)	0.39 (0.18, 0.85)
Gerd(Yes/No)	1.53 (1.14, 2.05)
Cancer (Yes/No)	0.61 (0.47, 0.79)
Fractures and Injuries (Yes/No)	1.67 (1.43, 1.95)
Ankylosing Spondylitis (Yes/No)	1.87 (1.22, 2.88)
Psychoses, Drug Induced (Yes/No)	1.69 (1.25, 2.28)
Visual Disturbances (Yes/No)	2.93 (1.05, 8.18)
Back Pain (Yes/No)	1.73 (1.43, 2.09)

IV. CONCLUSIONS

The results of this analysis suggest that both the kinds and number of medication exposures and the characteristics of diseases/disorders present among study subjects may predict an increase in risk for MVCs among older adults. Sample size and claims data constraints place limits on the strength of some of the associations observed. However, from a public policy perspective, these observations provide ample foundation for both further study and targeted consumer and provide educational interventions directed at pre-empting some of the MVC risk through more selective prescription and use of medications concomitant with driving.

It should be noted that the utility of administrative claim data for the purpose of estimating risk of MVC is not conclusively established by this analysis. Historically, claims data has proven to be useful in analysis of medical events relating to the provision of physician, hospital, and pharmaceutical services. Methods can be employed to mitigate the common sources of error in claims databases. However, in this study the use of claims data may require careful design and validation strategies. The use of ICD9 'E' codes for the specification of 'driver' and 'non-driver' status has not been subject to rigorous validation. Because the influence of a PDI disorder or medication is only relevant to the driver involved in a crash, variability in the integrity of coding specificity with respect to driver/non-driver designation could render any attribution of causality moot. Though analysis of administrative claims data remains a relatively inexpensive mechanism for examining the relationship between PDI and MVC among elderly drivers, future studies using these data must include a validation component to elucidate the extent to which driver misidentificationmay influence results.

From a public policy perspective, the general observations from this analysis are particularly timely given the changes in Medicare to implement drug reimbursement in 2006. This legislation will significantly reduce the cost of medications for Medicare beneficiaries. From an economic perspective, financial barriers to medications act as a governor on excessive and volitional pharmaceutical use, particularly among those with significant budget constraints (e.g., fixed/low income older adults). However, as those financial barriers are lowered, consumers exhibit 'pent up' demand for medications. As has been reported in many studies involving the new implementation of pharmaceutical benefit programs for employers who had previously offered no subsidy for pharmaceuticals, the 'pent-up' demand results in a near- and medium-term surge in medication requests to physicians and subsequent medication usage by beneficiaries. As our results suggest, the numbers of different medications used by study subjects may predict higher risk for MVCs. Thus, a possible unexpected collateral outcome of making pharmaceuticals more affordable for older adults may be an increase in motor vehicle crashes for this population.

As the population continues to age, an increasingly complex interplay of factors will impact driving safety. Older adults will develop chronic diseases that have driver impairing characteristics such as heart disease and the potential for arrhythmias and syncope; diabetes and the potential for ketoacidosis, hypoglycemia and retinal deterioration; depression and the potential for cognitive disturbances; back pain, arthritis, physical mobility impairment and distracting pain. Layered on to the underlying chronic diseases are the medications used to treat those conditions along with their potential to exacerbate other co-existing conditions, induce side effects, and promote dangerous drug interactions. By demonstrating the potential link between multiple drug therapies and MVCs, this study serves to highlight the need for further examination of the relationships between drugs, diseases and the older driver and the subsequent development of educational programs to increase consumer and healthcare provider awareness of this potential safety issue.

APPENDIX I. POTENTIALLY DRIVER IMPAIRING (PDI) DRUG CLASSES

Potential driving impairing drug classes include 409, 500-508, 510, 512-635, 800, 874, 878, 912, 1036-1037, 1300, 1371-1374, 1500, 1566-1570, 1671, 1700, 1720-1728, 1864, 1940, 1943-1945

C. List of National Drug Code Directory Drug Classes, 1995

CODE	DRUG CLASS
0100	**ANESTHETIC DRUGS**
0117	Anesthetics, Local (Injectable)
0118	Anesthetics, General
0119	Adjuncts to Anesthesia / Analeptics
0120	Medicinal Gases
0121	Anesthetics, Topical
0122	Anesthetics, Ophthalmic
0123	Anesthetics, Rectal
0200	**ANTIDOTES**
0281	Antidotes, Specific
0283	Antidotes, General
0285	Antitoxins / Antivenins
0286	Anaphylaxis Treatment Kit
0300	**ANTIMICROBIAL AGENTS**
0346	Penicillins
0347	Cephalosporins
0348	Erythromycins/Lincosamides/Macrolides
0349	Polymyxins
0350	Tetracyclines
0351	Chloramphenicol/Derivatives
0352	Aminoglycosides
0353	Sulfonamides and Trimethoprim
0354	Urinary Tract Antiseptics
0355	Miscellaneous Antibacterial Agents
0356	Antimycobacterial/Anti-Leprosy Agents
0357	Quinolones/Derivatives
0358	Antifungals
0388	Antiviral Agents
0400	**HEMATOLOGIC AGENTS**
0408	Deficiency Anemias
0409	Anticoagulants/Thrombolytics
0410	Blood Components/Substitutes
0411	Hemostatics/Antihemophelics
0500	**CARDIOVASCULAR-RENAL DRUGS**
0501	Cardiac Glycosides
0502	Antiarrhythmic Agents
0503	Antianginal Agents
0504	Vascular Disorders, Cerebral/Peripheral
0505	Agents Used to Treat Shock/Hypotension
0506	Antihypertensive Agents
0507	Diuretics
0508	Coronary Vasodilators
0509	Relaxants/Stimulants, Urinary Tract
0510	Calcium Channel Blockers
0511	Carbonic Anhydrase Inhibitors
0512	Beta Blockers
0513	Alpha Agonist/Alpha Blockers

CODE	DRUG CLASS
0514	ACE Inhibitors
0600	**CENTRAL NERVOUS SYSTEM**
0626	Sedatives and Hypnotics
0627	Antianxiety Agents
0628	Antipsychotic/Antimanics
0630	Antidepressants
0631	Anorexiants/CNS Stimulants
0632	CNS, Miscellaneous
0633	Alzheimer-Type Dementia
0634	Sleep Aid Products-OTC
0635	Antiemetics
0700	**CONTRAST MEDIA/RADIOPHARMACEUT.**
0789	Diagnostics, Radiopaque & Nonradioactive
0790	Diagnostics - Radiopharmaceuticals
0791	Therapeutics - Radiopharmaceuticals
0792	Miscellaneous
0800	**GASTROINTESTINAL AGENTS**
0874	Disorders, Acid/Peptic
0875	Antidiarrheals
0876	Laxatives
0877	Miscellaneous Gastrointestinals
0878	Antispasmodics/Anticholinergics
0879	Antacids
0900	**METABOLIC/NUTRIENTS**
0912	Hyperlipidemia
0913	Vitamins/Minerals
0914	Nutrition, Enteral/Parenteral
0915	Repl/Regs of Electrolytes/Water Balance
0916	Calcium Metabolism
0917	Hematopoietic Growth Factor
1000	**HORMONES/HORMONAL MECHANISMS**
1032	Adrenal Corticosteroids
1033	Androgens/Anabolic Steroids
1034	Estrogens/Progestins
1035	Anterior Pituitary/Hypothalamic Function
1036	Blood Glucose Regulators
1037	Thyroid/Antithyroid
1038	Antidiuretics
1039	Relaxants/Stimulants, Uterine
1040	Contraceptives
1041	Infertility
1042	Growth Hormone Secretion Disorder

1100	IMMUNOLOGICS	1600	OTOLOGICS
1180	Vaccines/Antisera	1670	Otic, Topical (Misc)
1181	Immunomodulators	1671	Vertigo/Motion Sickness/Vomiting
1182	Allergenic extracts		
1183	Immune serums	1700	RELIEF OF PAIN
		1720	Analgesics/General
1200	SKIN/MUCOUS MEMBRANE	1721	Analgesics, Narcotic
1264	Antiseptics/Disinfectants	1722	Analgesics, Non-Narcotic
1265	Dermatologics, Misc.	1723	Antimigraine/Other Headaches
1266	Keratolytics	1724	Antiarthritics
1267	Antiperspirants	1725	Antigout
1268	Topical Steroids	1726	Central Pain Syndrome
1269	Burn/Sunburn, Sunscreen/Suntan Products	1727	NSAID
1270	Acne Products	1728	Antipyretics
1271	Topical Anti-infectives	1729	Menstrual Products
1272	Anorectal Products		
1273	Personal Care (Vaginal) Products	1800	ANTIPARASITICS
1274	Dermatitis/Antipruritics	1860	Antiprotozoals
1275	Topical Analgesics	1862	Anthelmintics
		1863	Scabicides/Pediculicides
1300	NEUROLOGIC DRUGS	1864	Antimalarials
1371	Extrapyramidal Movement Disorders		
1372	Myasthenia Gravis	1900	RESPIRATORY TRACT
1373	Skeletal Muscle Hyperactivity	1940	Antiasthmatics/Bronchodilators
1374	Anticonvulsants	1941	Nasal Decongestants
		1943	Antitussives/Expectorants/Mucolytics
1400	ONCOLYTICS	1944	Antihistamines
1479	Antineoplastics, Miscellaneous	1945	Cold Remedies
1480	Hormonal/Biological Response Mod.	1946	Lozenge Products
1481	Antimetabolites	1947	Corticosteroid-Inhalation/Nasal
1482	Antibiotics,Alkaloids,Enzymes		
1483	DNA Damaging Drugs	2000	UNCLASSIFIED/MISCELLANEOUS
		2087	Unclassified
1500	OPHTHALMICS	2095	Pharmaceutical Aids
1566	Glaucoma	2096	Surgical Aids
1567	Cycloplegics/Mydriatics	2097	Dental Preparation
1568	Ocular Anti-infective/Anti-inflammatory	2098	Dentrifice/Denture Products
1569	Miscellaneous Ophthalmics	2099	Mouth Pine, Cold Sore, Canker
1570	Decongestants/Antiallergy Agents		
1571	Contact Lens Products	2100	HOMEOPATHIC PRODUCTS

APPENDIX II. POTENTIALLY DRIVER IMPAIRING (PDI) MEDICAL CONDITIONS

ICD Group	Potentially Driver Impairing Diagnoses
1566	ABUSE- DRUG
1986	ALCOHOLIC LIVER DISEASE
262	ALCOHOLISM
2646	ALZHEIMER
360	ANAPHYLACTIC SHOCK
268	ANGINA, PECTORIS
269	ANGINA, UNSTABLE
361	ANGIONEUROTIC EDEMA
2658	ANKYLOSING SPONDYLITIS
1562	ANXIETY DISORDERS

(Continued)

ICD Group	Potentially Driver Impairing Diagnoses
273	ARRHYTHMIAS
2602	ARTHRITIS, OSTEOARTHRITIS
2657	ARTHRITIS, PSORIATIC
2601	ARTHRITIS, RHEUMATOID
2603	ARTHROPATHIES, OTHER
274	ASTHMA
275	ATRIAL FIBRILLATION
276	AV BLOCK II TO III
315	BIPOLAR DISORDER
277	BLEPHARASPASM
281	BRADYCARDIA
1203	BRAIN HEMORRHAGE
286	CARDIAC ARREST
287	CARDIOVASCULAR DISEASE
300	CEREBRAL ARTERIOSCLEROSIS
301	CEREBRAL PALSY
306	CIRRHOSIS
307	CNS DEMYELINATING DIS
1409	CNS EXCITATION
102	CONGESTIVE HEART FAILURE
309	COPD
312	DEHYDRATION
1702	DELIRIUM
313	DEMENTIA
314	DEPRESSION
422	DIABETES MELLITUS I AND II
1567	DRUG INDUCED PSYCH DISORDERS
317	DYSKINESIAS
1461	ELECTROLYTE DISORDERS
319	ENCEPHALOPATHIC SYNDROME
320	EPILEPSY
397	EXTRAPYRAMIDAL REACTIONS
2624	FRACTURES AND INJURIES
385	GLAUCOMA,NARROW ANGLE
330	HALLUCINATIONS
424	HEAD TRAUMA
331	HEART BLOCK
347	HYPERTENSION
348	HYPERTHYROIDISM
351	HYPOTENSION
352	HYPOTHYROIDISM
1381	ISCHEMIC HEART DISEASE

(Continued)

ICD Group	Potentially Driver Impairing Diagnoses
367	KIDNEY STONES
421	MALIGNANT NEOPLASM, CNS
379	MYASTHENIA GRAVIS
380	MYELODYSPLASTIC SYNDROME
378	MYOCARDIAL ISCHEMIA
364	MYOCARDITIS
383	MYOPATHY
387	NEUROLEPTIC MALIGNANT SYNDROME
2513	NEUROPATHIES
1671	NUTRITIONAL/ NEURO DEFICIENCY
392	OPTIC NEURITIS
2650	OSTEOGENESIS IMPERFECTA
393	OSTEOMALACIA
2652	OSTEOSARCOMA
394	PANCREATITIS
2461	PANIC DISORDERS
395	PARKINSONISM,PRIMARY
396	PARKINSONISM,SECONDARY
400	PERIPHERAL NEUROPATHY
404	PSEUDOTUMOR CEREBRI
1561	PSYCHOSES
2662	PSYCHOSES, DRUG INDUCED
407	PULMONARY EDEMA
408	PULMONARY EMBOLUS
2653	RENAL OSTEODYSTROPHY
363	RHABDOMYOLYSIS
1977	SEROTONIN SYNDROME SYMPTOMS
1564	STRESS DISORDERS
2648	STROKE
1101	SUBARACHNOID HEMORRHAGE
1894	SUICIDAL BEHAVIOR
919	SYMPTOMS OF DIG-TOXICITY
2581	SYMPTOMS OF ERGOTISM
949	SYNCOPE
1102	VENTRICULAR ARRHYTHMIA
1460	VOLUME DEPLETION

APPENDIX III. DRUG INTERACTION CONFLICTS

DRUG CLASS	DRUG CLASS
SKELETAL MUSCLE RELAXANTS	ANTIPSYCHOTICS,ATYPICAL,DOPAMINE, & SEROTONIN ANTAG
ANTICONVULSANTS	BELLADONNA ALKALOIDS
HYPOGLYCEMICS, BIGUANIDE TYPE (NON- SULFONYLUREAS)	LINCOSAMIDES
SEROTONIN-NOREPINEPHRINE REUPTAKE-INHIB (SNRIS)	QUINOLONES
TRICYCLICANTIDEPRESSANTS & REL. NON-SEL. RU-INHIB	ANTIPSYCHOTICS,ATYPICAL,DOPAMINE, & SEROTONIN ANTAG
ANTICONVULSANTS	ANTIFUNGALAGENTS
HYPOTENSIVES, ACE INHIBITORS	ACE INHIBITOR/CALCIUM CHANNEL BLOCKER COMBINATION
INSULINS	LINCOSAMIDES
HYPOGLYCEMICS,ALPHA-GLUCOSIDASE INHIB TYPE (N-S)	GASTRIC ACID SECRETION REDUCERS
EYE ANTIINFLAMMATORY AGENTS	MACROLIDES
HYPOGLYCEMICS, INSULIN-RELEASE STIMULANT TYPE	ABSORBABLE SULFONAMIDES
SEROTONIN SPECIFIC REUPTAKE	ALPHA-2 RECEPTOR ANTAGONIST
INHIBITOR (SSRIS)	ANTIDEPRESSANTS
SEROTONIN SPECIFIC REUPTAKE	SEROTONIN-NOREPINEPHRINE
INHIBITOR (SSRIS)	REUPTAKE-INHIB (SNRIS)
ANTI-ANXIETY DRUGS	LINCOSAMIDES
DIGITALIS GLYCOSIDES	TETRACYCLINES
EXPECTORANTS	ANTI-NARCOLEPSY/ANTI-HYPERKINESIS, STIMULANT-TYPE
INSULINS	SEROTONIN-NOREPINEPHRINE REUPTAKE-INHIB (SNRIS)
HYPOGLYCEMICS, INSULIN-RESPONSE ENHANCER (N-S)	SEROTONIN-NOREPINEPHRINE REUPTAKE-INHIB (SNRIS)
BARBITURATES	ANALGESICS,NARCOTICS
SEDATIVE-HYPNOTICS,NON-BARBITURATE	BELLADONNA ALKALOIDS
ANTI-ANXIETY DRUGS	ANTIFUNGAL ANTIBIOTICS
ANTI-NARCOLEPSY/ANTI-HYPERKINESIS, STIMULANT-TYPE	QUINOLONES
ANALGESIC/ANTIPYRETICS,SALICYLATES	ORALANTICOAGULANTS,COUMARIN TYPE
ANTICONVULSANTS	ANTIFUNGALANTIBIOTICS
ANTIEMETIC/ANTIVERTIGO AGENTS	ANTIPSYCHOTICS,ATYPICAL,DOPAMINE, & SEROTONIN ANTAG
BELLADONNA ALKALOIDS	NITROFURAN DERIVATIVES

(Continued)

DRUG CLASS	DRUG CLASS
ORAL ANTICOAGULANTS, COUMARIN TYPE	LINCOSAMIDES
LIPOTROPICS	LINCOSAMIDES
SKELETAL MUSCLE RELAXANTS	MACROLIDES
SEROTONIN SPECIFIC REUPTAKE INHIBITOR (SSRIS)	LINCOSAMIDES
EXPECTORANTS	ANTIPSYCHOTICS,ATYPICAL,DOPAMINE, & SEROTONIN ANTAG
EXPECTORANTS	ANTIVIRALS,GENERAL
INSULINS	ANALGESIC/ANTIPYRETICS,NON-SALICYLATE
HYPOGLYCEMICS, INSULIN-RELEASE	ANALGESIC/ANTIPYRETICS,NON-
STIMULANT TYPE	SALICYLATE
BARBITURATES	ANTICONVULSANTS
SEROTONIN-NOREPINEPHRINE REUPTAKE-INHIB (SNRIS)	ANTIVIRALS, GENERAL
ANTIPSYCHOTICS,ATYPICAL,DOPA MINE,& SEROTONIN ANTAG	MACROLIDES
BETA-ADRENERGIC AGENTS	NITROFURAN DERIVATIVES
EYE ANTIHISTAMINES	LOOP DIURETICS
HYPOGLYCEMICS, INSULIN-RESPONSE ENHANCER (N-S)	ALPHA/BETA-ADRENERGIC BLOCKING AGENTS
SEDATIVE-HYPNOTICS,NON-BARBITURATE	ANTICONVULSANTS
ANTICONVULSANTS	SEROTONIN-NOREPINEPHRINE REUPTAKE-INHIB (SNRIS)
GLUCOCORTICOIDS	LINCOSAMIDES
THIAZIDE AND RELATED DIURETICS	LEUKOTRIENE RECEPTOR ANTAGONISTS
SKELETAL MUSCLE RELAXANTS	QUINOLONES
ANTIPSYCHOTICS,ATYPICAL,DOPA MINE,& SEROTONIN ANTAG	BETA-ADRENERGIC BLOCKING AGENTS
BETA-ADRENERGIC AGENTS	LINCOSAMIDES
DIGITALIS GLYCOSIDES	ANTI-ANXIETY DRUGS
SEROTONIN SPECIFIC REUPTAKE INHIBITOR (SSRIS)	ANALGESICS,NARCOTICS
SEROTONIN SPECIFIC REUPTAKE INHIBITOR (SSRIS)	QUINOLONES
BETA-ADRENERGIC AGENTS	MAST CELL STABILIZERS
ANTIPSYCHOTICS,ATYPICAL,DOPA MINE,& SEROTONIN ANTAG	ANTIHISTAMINES

(Continued)

DRUG CLASS	DRUG CLASS
HYPOGLYCEMICS, INSULIN-RESPONSE ENHANCER (N-S)	SEROTONIN SPECIFIC REUPTAKE INHIBITOR (SSRIS)
ANTI-ANXIETY DRUGS	SEROTONIN-NOREPINEPHRINE REUPTAKE-INHIB (SNRIS)
ANTI-ANXIETY DRUGS	TRICYCLICANTIDEPRESSANTS & REL. NON-SEL. RU-INHIB
ORAL ANTICOAGULANTS, COUMARIN TYPE	NSAIDS, CYCLOOXYGENASE INHIBITOR - TYPE
DIGITALIS GLYCOSIDES	THIAZIDE AND RELATED DIURETICS
DIGITALIS GLYCOSIDES	ANTIFUNGAL AGENTS
ANTIARRHYTHMICS	QUINOLONES
ACE INHIBITOR/CALCIUM CHANNEL BLOCKER COMBINATION	ALPHA/BETA-ADRENERGIC BLOCKING AGENTS
CALCIUM CHANNEL BLOCKING AGENTS	ANTIFUNGALANTIBIOTICS
INSULINS	ALPHA/BETA-ADRENERGIC BLOCKING AGENTS
INSULINS	MACROLIDES
INSULINS	NITROFURANDERIVATIVES
HYPOGLYCEMICS, INSULIN-RELEASE STIMULANT TYPE	TRICYCLIC ANTIDEPRESSANT/ PHENOTHIAZINE COMBINATNS
HYPOGLYCEMICS, INSULIN-RELEASE STIMULANT TYPE	ANALGESIC/ANTIPYRETICS, SALICYLATES
HYPOGLYCEMICS, INSULIN-RELEASE STIMULANT TYPE	LINCOSAMIDES
HYPOGLYCEMICS, BIGUANIDE TYPE (NON- SULFONYLUREAS)	ANALGESIC/ANTIPYRETICS, SALICYLATES
HYPOGLYCEMICS, INSULIN-RESPONSE ENHANCER (N-S)	ORAL ANTICOAGULANTS,COUMARIN TYPE
HYPOGLYCEMICS, INSULIN-RESPONSE ENHANCER (N-S)	LINCOSAMIDES
HYPERURICEMIA TX - PURINE INHIBITORS	MACROLIDES
HYPERURICEMIA TX - PURINE INHIBITORS	QUINOLONES
HYPERURICEMIA TX - PURINE INHIBITORS	ANTIVIRALS,GENERAL
SEDATIVE-HYPNOTICS,NON-BARBITURATE	ANTIFUNGALANTIBIOTICS
ANTI-ANXIETY DRUGS	ALPHA-2 RECEPTOR ANTAGONIST ANTIDEPRESSANTS
ANTI-ANXIETY DRUGS	MAOIS - NON-SELECTIVE & IRREVERSIBLE
ANTI-ANXIETY DRUGS	ANTIFUNGAL AGENTS

(Continued)

DRUG CLASS	DRUG CLASS
ANTI-ANXIETY DRUGS	IMMUNOSUPPRESSIVES
ANTI-PSYCHOTICS, PHENOTHIAZINES	SEROTONIN SPECIFIC REUPTAKE INHIBITOR (SSRIS)
ANTI-PSYCHOTICS, PHENOTHIAZINES	MACROLIDES
SEROTONIN SPECIFIC REUPTAKE INHIBITOR (SSRIS)	TRICYCLIC ANTIDEPRESSANT/ BENZODIAZEPINE COMBINATNS
SEROTONIN SPECIFIC REUPTAKE INHIBITOR (SSRIS)	ANTIPSYCHOTICS,ATYPICAL,DOPAMINE, & SEROTONIN ANTAG
TRICYCLICANTIDEPRESSANTS & REL. NON-SEL. RU-INHIB	SEROTONIN-NOREPINEPHRINE REUPTAKE-INHIB (SNRIS)
TRICYCLICANTIDEPRESSANTS & REL. NON-SEL. RU-INHIB	ANTIPSYCHOTICS,DOPAMINE ANTAGONISTS, THIOXANTHENES
TRICYCLICANTIDEPRESSANTS & REL. NON-SEL. RU-INHIB	LINCOSAMIDES
TRICYCLICANTIDEPRESSANTS & REL. NON-SEL. RU-INHIB	ANTIFUNGAL ANTIBIOTICS
TRICYCLICANTIDEPRESSANTS & REL. NON-SEL. RU-INHIB	ANTIFUNGAL AGENTS
ANTI-NARCOLEPSY/ANTI-HYPERKINESIS, STIMULANT-TYPE	MACROLIDES
ANALGESICS,NARCOTICS	ANTIPSYCHOTICS,DOPAMINE ANTAGONISTS,BUTYROPHENONES
ANALGESICS,NARCOTICS	ANTIPSYCHOTICS,ATYPICAL,DOPAMINE, & SEROTONIN ANTAG
ANALGESIC/ANTIPYRETICS,SALICYLATES	PLATELET AGGREGATION INHIBITORS
ANTIMIGRAINE PREPARATIONS	SEROTONIN-NOREPINEPHRINE REUPTAKE-INHIB (SNRIS)
ANTICONVULSANTS	LINCOSAMIDES
ANTITUSSIVES,NON-NARCOTIC	ANTIVIRALS, GENERAL
SKELETAL MUSCLE RELAXANTS	ALPHA-2 RECEPTOR ANTAGONIST ANTIDEPRESSANTS
SKELETAL MUSCLE RELAXANTS	SEROTONIN-NOREPINEPHRINE REUPTAKE-INHIB (SNRIS)
ANTIEMETIC/ANTIVERTIGO AGENTS	SEROTONIN-NOREPINEPHRINE REUPTAKE-INHIB (SNRIS)
ALPHA-2 RECEPTOR ANTAGONIST ANTIDEPRESSANTS	ANTIPSYCHOTICS,ATYPICAL,DOPAMINE, & SEROTONIN ANTAG
SEROTONIN-NOREPINEPHRINE REUPTAKE-INHIB (SNRIS)	MACROLIDES
SEROTONIN-NOREPINEPHRINE REUPTAKE-INHIB (SNRIS)	ANTIFUNGAL AGENTS
NOREPINEPHRINE AND DOPAMINE REUPTAKE INHIB (NDRIS)	ALPHA/BETA-ADRENERGIC BLOCKING AGENTS

(Continued)

DRUG CLASS	DRUG CLASS
ANTIPSYCHOTICS,ATYPICAL,DOPA MINE,& SEROTONIN ANTAG	QUINOLONES
ANTIPSYCHOTICS,ATYPICAL,DOPA MINE,& SEROTONIN ANTAG	ANTIMALARIAL DRUGS
ANTIPSYCHOTICS,ATYPICAL,DOPA MINE,& SEROTONIN ANTAG	ANTIVIRALS, GENERAL
BELLADONNA ALKALOIDS	ORAL ANTICOAGULANTS,COUMARIN TYPE
HEPARIN AND RELATED PREPARATIONS	CEPHALOSPORINS - 1ST GENERATION
ORAL ANTICOAGULANTS, COUMARIN TYPE	PLATELET AGGREGATION INHIBITORS
ORAL ANTICOAGULANTS, COUMARIN TYPE	IMMUNOSUPPRESSIVES
EYE ANTIHISTAMINES	MACROLIDES
EYE ANTIHISTAMINES	QUINOLONES
LOOP DIURETICS	MAST CELL STABILIZERS
LOOP DIURETICS	LEUKOTRIENE RECEPTOR ANTAGONISTS
COLCHICINE	QUINOLONES
ANTIVIRALS, GENERAL	ANTIVIRALS, HIV-SPECIFIC, NUCLEOSIDE ANALOG, RTI
ANTIVIRALS, GENERAL	ANTIVIRALS, HIV-SPECIFIC, NON-NUCLEOSIDE, RTI
ANTIVIRALS, HIV-SPECIFIC, NUCLEOSIDE ANALOG, RTI	ANTIVIRALS, HIV-SPECIFIC, NON-NUCLEOSIDE, RTI
MAST CELL STABILIZERS	LEUKOTRIENE RECEPTOR ANTAGONISTS
CALCIUM CHANNEL BLOCKING AGENTS	SEROTONIN-2 ANTAGONIST/REUPTAKE INHIBITORS (SARIS)
TRICYCLICANTIDEPRESSANTS & REL. NON-SEL. RU-INHIB	MACROLIDES
ANTI-ANXIETY DRUGS	MACROLIDES
TRICYCLICANTIDEPRESSANTS & REL. NON-SEL. RU-INHIB	QUINOLONES
SEROTONIN-NOREPINEPHRINE REUPTAKE-INHIB (SNRIS)	LIPOTROPICS
HYPOGLYCEMICS, INSULIN-RELEASE STIMULANT TYPE	TRICYCLICANTIDEPRESSANTS & REL. NON-SEL. RU-INHIB
ANTIARRHYTHMICS	CALCIUMCHANNEL BLOCKING AGENTS
ANTICONVULSANTS	ORALANTICOAGULANTS,COUMARIN TYPE
ANTI-ANXIETY DRUGS	SEROTONIN SPECIFIC REUPTAKE INHIBITOR (SSRIS)
SEDATIVE-HYPNOTICS,NON-BARBITURATE	ANALGESICS,NARCOTICS
DIGITALIS GLYCOSIDES	MACROLIDES

(Continued)

DRUG CLASS	DRUG CLASS
EXPECTORANTS	SEROTONIN SPECIFIC REUPTAKE INHIBITOR (SSRIS)
SEROTONIN SPECIFIC REUPTAKE INHIBITOR (SSRIS)	ORAL ANTICOAGULANTS,COUMARIN TYPE
DIGITALIS GLYCOSIDES	ANTIARRHYTHMICS
TRICYCLICANTIDEPRESSANTS & REL. NON-SEL. RU-INHIB	ANALGESICS,NARCOTICS
HYPOGLYCEMICS, BIGUANIDE TYPE (NON- SULFONYLUREAS)	SEROTONIN SPECIFIC REUPTAKE INHIBITOR (SSRIS)
ANTI-ANXIETY DRUGS	BETA-ADRENERGIC AGENTS
SKELETAL MUSCLE RELAXANTS	NITROFURAN DERIVATIVES
INSULINS	PLATELET AGGREGATION INHIBITORS
ANTICONVULSANTS	MACROLIDES
HYPOGLYCEMICS, INSULIN-RELEASE STIMULANT TYPE	ANTIFUNGAL AGENTS
ANTICONVULSANTS	NITROFURANDERIVATIVES
SEROTONIN-NOREPINEPHRINE REUPTAKE-INHIB (SNRIS)	ANTIPSYCHOTICS,ATYPICAL,DOPAMINE, & SEROTONIN ANTAG
SEROTONIN-NOREPINEPHRINE REUPTAKE-INHIB (SNRIS)	BETA-ADRENERGIC BLOCKING AGENTS
POTASSIUM SPARING DIURETICS IN COMBINATION	LEUKOTRIENERECEPTOR ANTAGONISTS
ANTI-ANXIETY DRUGS	QUINOLONES
HYPERURICEMIA TX - PURINE INHIBITORS	GASTRIC ACID SECRETION REDUCERS
HYPOGLYCEMICS, INSULIN-RELEASE STIMULANT TYPE	SEROTONIN SPECIFIC REUPTAKE INHIBITOR (SSRIS)
ACE INHIBITOR/CALCIUM CHANNEL BLOCKER COMBINATION	BETA-ADRENERGIC BLOCKING AGENTS
SEDATIVE-HYPNOTICS,NON-BARBITURATE	ANTIFUNGALAGENTS
HYPOGLYCEMICS, INSULIN-RELEASE STIMULANT TYPE	MACROLIDES
INSULINS	GASTRIC ACID SECRETION REDUCERS
GLUCOCORTICOIDS	MACROLIDES
SKELETAL MUSCLE RELAXANTS	BETA-ADRENERGIC BLOCKING AGENTS
ANTIARRHYTHMICS	GASTRIC ACID SECRETION REDUCERS
CALCIUM CHANNEL BLOCKING AGENTS	LINCOSAMIDES
ANTI-PSYCHOTICS, PHENOTHIAZINES	TRICYCLICANTIDEPRESSANTS & REL. NON-SEL. RU-INHIB
SEROTONIN SPECIFIC REUPTAKE INHIBITOR (SSRIS)	ANTIVIRALS, GENERAL

(Continued)

DRUG CLASS	DRUG CLASS
TRICYCLICANTIDEPRESSANTS & REL. NON-SEL. RU-INHIB	ANTI-NARCOLEPSY/ANTI-HYPERKINESIS, STIMULANT-TYPE
TRICYCLICANTIDEPRESSANTS & REL. NON-SEL. RU-INHIB	ANTIVIRALS, GENERAL
ANTICONVULSANTS	ALPHA-2 RECEPTOR ANTAGONIST ANTIDEPRESSANTS
ORAL ANTICOAGULANTS, COUMARIN TYPE	CEPHALOSPORINS - 1ST GENERATION
SEROTONIN SPECIFIC REUPTAKE INHIBITOR (SSRIS)	ANTIMIGRAINE PREPARATIONS
ANTI-ANXIETY DRUGS	LEUKOTRIENE RECEPTOR ANTAGONISTS
ANTITUSSIVES,NON-NARCOTIC	ANTIHISTAMINES
CALCIUM CHANNEL BLOCKING AGENTS	SEROTONIN-NOREPINEPHRINE REUPTAKE-INHIB (SNRIS)
SEROTONIN SPECIFIC REUPTAKE INHIBITOR (SSRIS)	NITROFURANDERIVATIVES
SEROTONIN-2 ANTAGONIST/ REUPTAKE INHIBITORS (SARIS)	BETA-ADRENERGIC BLOCKING AGENTS
NOREPINEPHRINE AND DOPAMINE REUPTAKE INHIB (NDRIS)	BETA-ADRENERGIC BLOCKING AGENTS
HYPOGLYCEMICS, BIGUANIDE TYPE (NON- SULFONYLUREAS)	TRICYCLICANTIDEPRESSANTS & REL. NON-SEL. RU-INHIB
SEROTONIN SPECIFIC REUPTAKE INHIBITOR (SSRIS)	ANTIPARKINSONISM DRUGS,ANTICHOLINERGIC
SEROTONIN SPECIFIC REUPTAKE INHIBITOR (SSRIS)	LIPOTROPICS
CALCIUM CHANNEL BLOCKING AGENTS	GASTRIC ACID SECRETION REDUCERS
HYPOGLYCEMICS, BIGUANIDE TYPE (NON- SULFONYLUREAS)	MACROLIDES
CALCIUM CHANNEL BLOCKING AGENTS	MACROLIDES
ANTICONVULSANTS	PLATELETAGGREGATION INHIBITORS
TRICYCLICANTIDEPRESSANTS & REL. NON-SEL. RU-INHIB	ORAL ANTICOAGULANTS,COUMARIN TYPE
BETA-ADRENERGIC BLOCKING AGENTS	ANTIMALARIAL DRUGS
EXPECTORANTS	ANTIHISTAMINES
INSULINS	SEROTONIN SPECIFIC REUPTAKE INHIBITOR (SSRIS)
INSULINS	ANTIFUNGALAGENTS
PLATELET AGGREGATION INHIBITORS	NSAIDS, CYCLOOXYGENASE INHIBITOR - TYPE
SEROTONIN SPECIFIC REUPTAKE INHIBITOR (SSRIS)	MACROLIDES

(Continued)

DRUG CLASS	DRUG CLASS
PLATELET AGGREGATION INHIBITORS	THYROIDHORMONES
HYPOGLYCEMICS, INSULIN-RELEASE STIMULANT TYPE	GASTRIC ACID SECRETION REDUCERS
INSULINS	BETA-ADRENERGIC BLOCKING AGENTS
INSULINS	LIPOTROPICS
CALCIUM CHANNEL BLOCKING AGENTS	ALPHA-ADRENERGIC BLOCKING AGENTS
BETA-ADRENERGIC AGENTS	MACROLIDES
DIGITALIS GLYCOSIDES	CALCIUM CHANNEL BLOCKING AGENTS
DIGITALIS GLYCOSIDES	ALPHA/BETA-ADRENERGIC BLOCKING AGENTS
ACE INHIBITOR/CALCIUM CHANNEL BLOCKER COMBINATION	CALCIUMCHANNEL BLOCKING AGENTS
ACE INHIBITOR/CALCIUM CHANNEL BLOCKER COMBINATION	ALPHA-ADRENERGIC BLOCKING AGENTS
CALCIUM CHANNEL BLOCKING AGENTS	ANTI-ULCERPREPARATIONS
EXPECTORANTS	TRICYCLICANTIDEPRESSANTS & REL. NON-SEL. RU-INHIB
EXPECTORANTS	SEROTONIN-NOREPINEPHRINE REUPTAKE-INHIB (SNRIS)
INSULINS	TRICYCLICANTIDEPRESSANTS & REL. NON-SEL. RU-INHIB
INSULINS	ANTIVIRALS,GENERAL
HYPOGLYCEMICS, INSULIN-RELEASE STIMULANT TYPE	HYPOGLYCEMICS,ALPHA-GLUCOSIDASE INHIB TYPE (N-S)
HYPOGLYCEMICS, INSULIN-RELEASE STIMULANT TYPE	HYPOGLYCEMICS, INSULIN-RESPONSE ENHANCER (N-S)
HYPOGLYCEMICS, BIGUANIDE TYPE (NON- SULFONYLUREAS)	SEROTONIN-NOREPINEPHRINE REUPTAKE-INHIB (SNRIS)
HYPOGLYCEMICS, BIGUANIDE TYPE (NON- SULFONYLUREAS)	PLATELET AGGREGATION INHIBITORS
HYPOGLYCEMICS, BIGUANIDE TYPE (NON- SULFONYLUREAS)	ABSORBABLE SULFONAMIDES
HYPOGLYCEMICS, BIGUANIDE TYPE (NON- SULFONYLUREAS)	NITROFURAN DERIVATIVES
HYPOGLYCEMICS, INSULIN-RESPONSE ENHANCER (N-S)	PLATELETAGGREGATION INHIBITORS
ANTI-ANXIETY DRUGS	NITROFURAN DERIVATIVES
SEROTONIN SPECIFIC REUPTAKE INHIBITOR (SSRIS)	ANTIPARKINSONISM DRUGS,OTHER

(Continued)

DRUG CLASS	DRUG CLASS
SEROTONIN SPECIFIC REUPTAKE INHIBITOR (SSRIS)	ANTIFUNGAL AGENTS
ANTI-NARCOLEPSY/ANTI-HYPERKINESIS, STIMULANT-TYPE	ANTIVIRALS,GENERAL
ANTICONVULSANTS	IMMUNOSUPPRESSIVES
SKELETAL MUSCLE RELAXANTS	LINCOSAMIDES
SEROTONIN-NOREPINEPHRINE REUPTAKE-INHIB (SNRIS)	ORAL ANTICOAGULANTS,COUMARIN TYPE
BELLADONNA ALKALOIDS	ANTIFUNGAL AGENTS
BETA-ADRENERGIC AGENTS	BETA-ADRENERGICS AND GLUCOCORTICOIDS COMBINATION
BETA-ADRENERGICS AND GLUCOCORTICOIDS COMBINATION	BETA-ADRENERGIC BLOCKING AGENTS
BETA-ADRENERGICS AND GLUCOCORTICOIDS COMBINATION	LEUKOTRIENE RECEPTOR ANTAGONISTS
LIPOTROPICS	MACROLIDES
LIPOTROPICS	ANTIFUNGALANTIBIOTICS
HEPARIN AND RELATED PREPARATIONS	ORAL ANTICOAGULANTS,COUMARIN TYPE
ORAL ANTICOAGULANTS, COUMARIN TYPE	QUINOLONES
ORAL ANTICOAGULANTS, COUMARIN TYPE	CEPHALOSPORINS - 2ND GENERATION
EYE ANTIINFLAMMATORY AGENTS	POTASSIUM SPARING DIURETICS
EYE ANTIHISTAMINES	POTASSIUM SPARING DIURETICS IN COMBINATION
ANTIMALARIAL DRUGS	ANTIVIRALS, GENERAL
HYPOGLYCEMICS, BIGUANIDE TYPE (NON- SULFONYLUREAS)	GASTRIC ACID SECRETION REDUCERS
LIPOTROPICS	QUINOLONES
SEROTONIN SPECIFIC REUPTAKE INHIBITOR (SSRIS)	TRICYCLICANTIDEPRESSANTS & REL. NON-SEL. RU-INHIB
HYPOGLYCEMICS, INSULIN-RELEASE STIMULANT TYPE	ORAL ANTICOAGULANTS,COUMARIN TYPE
INSULINS	HYPOGLYCEMICS, INSULIN-RELEASE STIMULANT TYPE
HYPOGLYCEMICS, BIGUANIDE TYPE (NON- SULFONYLUREAS)	QUINOLONES
INSULINS	HYPOGLYCEMICS, INSULIN-RESPONSE ENHANCER (N-S)
CALCIUM CHANNEL BLOCKING AGENTS	NOREPINEPHRINE AND DOPAMINE REUPTAKE INHIB (NDRIS)
HYPOGLYCEMICS, INSULIN-RELEASE STIMULANT TYPE	HYPOGLYCEMICS, BIGUANIDE TYPE (NON- SULFONYLUREAS)
INSULINS	QUINOLONES

(Continued)

DRUG CLASS	DRUG CLASS
GLUCOCORTICOIDS	IMMUNOSUPPRESSIVES
DIGITALIS GLYCOSIDES	LOOP DIURETICS
SKELETAL MUSCLE RELAXANTS	ORAL ANTICOAGULANTS,COUMARIN TYPE
HYPOTENSIVES, ACE INHIBITORS	CALCIUM CHANNEL BLOCKING AGENTS
ACE INHIBITOR/CALCIUM CHANNEL BLOCKERCOMBINATION	GASTRIC ACID SECRETION REDUCERS
HYPOGLYCEMICS, BIGUANIDE TYPE (NON- SULFONYLUREAS)	ORALANTICOAGULANTS,COUMARIN TYPE
HYPOGLYCEMICS,ALPHA-GLUCOSIDASE INHIB TYPE (N-S)	LIPOTROPICS
SEROTONIN SPECIFIC REUPTAKE INHIBITOR (SSRIS)	ANTI-NARCOLEPSY/ANTI-HYPERKINESIS, STIMULANT-TYPE
PLATELET AGGREGATION INHIBITORS	QUINOLONES
HYPOTENSIVES, ACE INHIBITORS	POTASSIUM SPARING DIURETICS IN COMBINATION
INSULINS	ABSORBABLE SULFONAMIDES
LIPOTROPICS	NITROFURANDERIVATIVES
LIPOTROPICS	ANTIFUNGALAGENTS
HYPOGLYCEMICS, BIGUANIDE TYPE (NON- SULFONYLUREAS)	HYPOGLYCEMICS, INSULIN-RESPONSE ENHANCER (N-S)
POTASSIUM SPARING DIURETICS	LOOP DIURETICS
HYPOGLYCEMICS, INSULIN-RESPONSE ENHANCER (N-S)	ANTIFUNGAL AGENTS
SKELETAL MUSCLE RELAXANTS	PLATELET AGGREGATION INHIBITORS
BELLADONNA ALKALOIDS	MACROLIDES
BETA-ADRENERGIC AGENTS	BETA-ADRENERGIC BLOCKING AGENTS
ORAL ANTICOAGULANTS, COUMARIN TYPE	THYROID HORMONES
INSULINS	HYPOGLYCEMICS, BIGUANIDE TYPE (NON- SULFONYLUREAS)
ANTIMIGRAINE PREPARATIONS	BETA-ADRENERGIC BLOCKING AGENTS
TRICYCLICANTIDEPRESSANTS & REL. NON-SEL. RU-INHIB	LIPOTROPICS
HYPOGLYCEMICS, BIGUANIDE TYPE (NON- SULFONYLUREAS)	LIPOTROPICS
ACE INHIBITOR/CALCIUM CHANNEL BLOCKER COMBINATION	THIAZIDEAND RELATEDDIURETICS
TRICYCLICANTIDEPRESSANTS & REL. NON-SEL. RU-INHIB	ANTIMIGRAINE PREPARATIONS
ORAL ANTICOAGULANTS, COUMARIN TYPE	MACROLIDES

(Continued)

DRUG CLASS	DRUG CLASS
HYPOTENSIVES, ACE INHIBITORS	LOOP DIURETICS
BETA-ADRENERGIC AGENTS	LEUKOTRIENE RECEPTOR ANTAGONISTS
DIGITALIS GLYCOSIDES	POTASSIUM SPARING DIURETICS IN COMBINATION
LIPOTROPICS	IMMUNOSUPPRESSIVES
CALCIUM CHANNEL BLOCKING AGENTS	BETA-ADRENERGIC BLOCKING AGENTS
HYPOGLYCEMICS, INSULIN-RESPONSE ENHANCER (N-S)	BETA-ADRENERGIC BLOCKING AGENTS
HYPOGLYCEMICS, INSULIN-RELEASE STIMULANT TYPE	QUINOLONES
HYPOTENSIVES, ACE INHIBITORS	THIAZIDE AND RELATED DIURETICS
HYPOGLYCEMICS, INSULIN-RESPONSE ENHANCER (N-S)	LIPOTROPICS
HYPOGLYCEMICS, INSULIN-RELEASE STIMULANT TYPE	LIPOTROPICS
ACE INHIBITOR/CALCIUM CHANNEL BLOCKER COMBINATION	LOOP DIURETICS
CALCIUM CHANNEL BLOCKING AGENTS	CHOLINESTERASEINHIBITORS
HYPOGLYCEMICS, INSULIN-RELEASE STIMULANT TYPE	NITROFURAN DERIVATIVES
HYPOGLYCEMICS, BIGUANIDE TYPE (NON- SULFONYLUREAS)	ANTIFUNGAL AGENTS
HYPOGLYCEMICS, BIGUANIDE TYPE (NON- SULFONYLUREAS)	ANTIVIRALS, GENERAL
HYPOGLYCEMICS, INSULIN-RESPONSE ENHANCER (N-S)	ANALGESIC/ANTIPYRETICS, SALICYLATES
HYPOGLYCEMICS, INSULIN-RESPONSE ENHANCER (N-S)	MACROLIDES
HYPOGLYCEMICS, INSULIN-RESPONSE ENHANCER (N-S)	NITROFURAN DERIVATIVES
TRICYCLICANTIDEPRESSANTS & REL. NON-SEL. RU-INHIB	ANTIPARKINSONISM DRUGS,OTHER
ANALGESIC/ANTIPYRETICS,NON-SALICYLATE	PLATELET AGGREGATION INHIBITORS
ANTIPSYCHOTICS,ATYPICAL,DOPA MINE,& SEROTONIN ANTAG	BETA-ADRENERGIC AGENTS
ALPHA/BETA-ADRENERGIC BLOCKING AGENTS	BETA-ADRENERGIC BLOCKING AGENTS
PLATELET AGGREGATION INHIBITORS	CEPHALOSPORINS - 1ST GENERATION
GLUCOCORTICOIDS	NITROFURANDERIVATIVES
EYE ANTIINFLAMMATORY AGENTS	QUINOLONES

(Continued)

DRUG CLASS	DRUG CLASS
THIAZIDE AND RELATED DIURETICS	POTASSIUM SPARING DIURETICS IN COMBINATION
COLCHICINE	MACROLIDES
ANTIVIRALS, HIV-SPECIFIC, PROTEASE INHIBITORS	ANTIVIRALS, HIV-SPECIFIC, NUCLEOSIDE ANALOG, RTI
HYPOGLYCEMICS, BIGUANIDE TYPE (NON- SULFONYLUREAS)	BETA-ADRENERGIC BLOCKING AGENTS
CALCIUM CHANNEL BLOCKING AGENTS	ANTIFUNGALAGENTS
HYPOGLYCEMICS, INSULIN-RESPONSE ENHANCER (N-S)	GASTRIC ACID SECRETION REDUCERS
CALCIUM CHANNEL BLOCKING AGENTS	IMMUNOSUPPRESSIVES
HYPOGLYCEMICS, BIGUANIDE TYPE (NON- SULFONYLUREAS)	HYPOGLYCEMICS,ALPHA-GLUCOSIDASE INHIB TYPE (N-S)
ANTI-ANXIETY DRUGS	ANTIVIRALS, GENERAL
HYPOGLYCEMICS, INSULIN-RELEASE STIMULANT TYPE	BETA-ADRENERGIC BLOCKING AGENTS
DIGITALIS GLYCOSIDES	BETA-ADRENERGIC BLOCKING AGENTS
DIGITALIS GLYCOSIDES	HYPOTENSIVES,SYMPATHOLYTIC
DIGITALIS GLYCOSIDES	HYPOTENSIVES,ANGIOTENSIN RECEPTOR ANTAGONIST
DIGITALIS GLYCOSIDES	POTASSIUM SPARING DIURETICS
CALCIUM CHANNEL BLOCKING AGENTS	ALPHA/BETA-ADRENERGIC BLOCKING AGENTS
HYPOGLYCEMICS, INSULIN-RELEASE STIMULANT TYPE	SEROTONIN-NOREPINEPHRINE REUPTAKE-INHIB (SNRIS)
HYPOGLYCEMICS, INSULIN-RELEASE STIMULANT TYPE	PLATELET AGGREGATION INHIBITORS
HYPOGLYCEMICS,ALPHA-GLUCOSIDASE INHIB TYPE (N-S)	HYPOGLYCEMICS, INSULIN-RESPONSE ENHANCER (N-S)
HYPOTENSIVES, ACE INHIBITORS	POTASSIUM SPARING DIURETICS
LIPOTROPICS	ANTIVIRALS,GENERAL
SEROTONIN SPECIFIC REUPTAKE INHIBITOR (SSRIS)	PLATELET AGGREGATION INHIBITORS
GLUCOCORTICOIDS	ANTIFUNGAL AGENTS
ALPHA-ADRENERGIC BLOCKING AGENTS	BETA-ADRENERGIC BLOCKING AGENTS
THIAZIDE AND RELATED DIURETICS	LOOP DIURETICS
ACE INHIBITOR/CALCIUM CHANNEL BLOCKER COMBINATION	POTASSIUM SPARING DIURETICS IN COMBINATION

(Continued)

DRUG CLASS	DRUG CLASS
HYPOGLYCEMICS, INSULIN-RELEASE STIMULANT TYPE	ANTIVIRALS, GENERAL
HYPOGLYCEMICS, INSULIN-RESPONSE ENHANCER (N-S)	TRICYCLICANTIDEPRESSANTS & REL. NON-SEL. RU-INHIB
ORAL ANTICOAGULANTS, COUMARIN TYPE	ABSORBABLE SULFONAMIDES
GLUCOCORTICOIDS	ANTIFUNGAL ANTIBIOTICS
CHOLINESTERASE INHIBITORS	BETA-ADRENERGIC BLOCKING AGENTS
INSULINS	ORALANTICOAGULANTS,COUMARIN TYPE
HYPOGLYCEMICS, INSULIN-RELEASE STIMULANT TYPE	ALPHA/BETA-ADRENERGIC BLOCKING AGENTS
TRICYCLICANTIDEPRESSANTS & REL. NON-SEL. RU-INHIB	PLATELET AGGREGATION INHIBITORS
POTASSIUM SPARING DIURETICS IN COMBINATION	LOOPDIURETICS
HYPOGLYCEMICS, INSULIN-RESPONSE ENHANCER (N-S)	QUINOLONES
ANTIARRHYTHMICS	LIPOTROPICS
SKELETAL MUSCLE RELAXANTS	ANTIPSYCHOTICS,ATYPICAL,DOPAMINE, & SEROTONIN ANTAG

APPENDIX IV. DRUG-DISEASE CONFLICT

DRUG CLASS	DISEASE CONFLICT
GLUCOCORTICOIDS	ANXIETY STATE UNSPEC
ANTI-NARCOLEPSY/ANTI-HYPERKINESIS, STIMULANT-TYPE	UNSHYPERTENSION
ANALGESICS,NARCOTICS	CHR HEPATITIS C WOCOMA
LOOP DIURETICS	AC/UNSHEPATITIS C WOCOMA
BETA-ADRENERGIC AGENTS	PRIMARY PULMONARY HYPERTENSION
ANALGESICS,NARCOTICS	CIRRHOSIS LIVER WO ALCOHOL
CALCIUM CHANNEL BLOCKING AGENTS	SYNCOPE/COLLAPSE
HYPOGLYCEMICS, BIGUANIDE TYPE (NON- SULFONYLUREAS)	SYNCOPE/COLLAPSE
SEROTONIN SPECIFIC REUPTAKE INHIBITOR (SSRIS)	CHRHEPATITIS C WOCOMA
BETA-ADRENERGIC BLOCKING AGENTS	DIABETES RENAL MANIF TYPE II
LOOP DIURETICS	DIABETES RENAL MANIF TYPE II
GLUCOCORTICOIDS	DEPRESSIVE TYPE PSYCHOSIS
GLUCOCORTICOIDS	MAJ DEPRESS DIS SGL EPI MODERATE

(Continued)

DRUG CLASS	DISEASE CONFLICT
ANTIHISTAMINES	UNS AFFECTIVE PSYCHOSIS
ANTIHISTAMINES	GRANDMALY WO INTRACT EPILEPSY
BETA-ADRENERGICS AND GLUCOCORTICOIDS COMBINATION	BENIGN HYPERTENSION
NSAIDS, CYCLOOXYGENASE INHIBITOR - TYPE	HYPERTENSIVE HEART DIS UNSPEC
BETA-ADRENERGIC BLOCKING AGENTS	UNS HEARTFAILURE
INSULINS	CIRRHOSIS LIVER WO ALCOHOL
SEROTONIN SPECIFIC REUPTAKE INHIBITOR (SSRIS)	OTH CHRONIC NONALCOHOLIC LIVER DIS
ANTICONVULSANTS	CHRONICRENALFAILURE
DIGITALIS GLYCOSIDES	SYNCOPE/COLLAPSE
ALPHA/BETA-ADRENERGIC BLOCKING AGENTS	OTH PRIMARY CARDIOMYOPATHIES
INSULINS	DIABETES RENAL MANIF TYPE II
SEROTONIN SPECIFIC REUPTAKE INHIBITOR (SSRIS)	CHRONIC RENALFAILURE
QUINOLONES	CHRONICRENALFAILURE
HYPOTENSIVES, ACE INHIBITORS	SYNCOPE/COLLAPSE
ORAL ANTICOAGULANTS,COUMARIN TYPE	OTH PRIMARY CARDIOMYOPATHIES
HYPOTENSIVES,SYMPATHOLYTIC	DIABETES UNCOMPL TYPE II
BETA-ADRENERGIC AGENTS	BENIGN HYPERTENSION
ANALGESICS,NARCOTICS	HEPATITIS B WO COMA AC/UNS WODELTA
ANALGESICS,NARCOTICS	CHR HEPATITIS C W COMA
POTASSIUM SPARING DIURETICS	AC/UNSHEPATITIS C WOCOMA
ANTICONVULSANTS	CHR HEPATITIS C WOCOMA
HYPOTENSIVES,SYMPATHOLYTIC	DIABETES UNCOMP TYPE II UNCONTRD
HYPOTENSIVES,ANGIOTENSIN RECEPTOR ANTAGONIST	DIABETES RENAL MANIF TYPE II
HYPOTENSIVES, ACE INHIBITORS	DIABETES RENAL MANIF TYPE I
THIAZIDE AND RELATED DIURETICS	DIABETES RENAL MANIF TYPE I
QUINOLONES	DIABETES RENAL MANIF TYPE I
INSULINS	DIABETES RENAL MANIF TYPE II UNC
HYPOTENSIVES,ANGIOTENSIN RECEPTOR ANTAGONIST	DIABETES EYE MANIF TYPE II
HYPOTENSIVES,ANGIOTENSIN RECEPTOR ANTAGONIST	DIABETES NEURO MANIF TYPE II
BETA-ADRENERGIC BLOCKING AGENTS	DIABETES NEUR MANIF TYPE II UNCN

(Continued)

DRUG CLASS	DISEASE CONFLICT
ANTI-ANXIETY DRUGS	ACUTEDELIRIUM
ANTI-MANIA DRUGS	BIPOLAR AFFECT DIS DEPRESS UNS
ANTI-MANIA DRUGS	UNS MANICDEPRESSIVE PSYCHOSIS
SEDATIVE-HYPNOTICS,NON-BARBITURATE	UNS AFFECTIVE PSYCHOSIS
SEROTONIN SPECIFIC REUPTAKE INHIBITOR(SSRIS)	UNS AFFECTIVE PSYCHOSIS
ANTICONVULSANTS	UNS AFFECTIVE PSYCHOSIS
SEROTONIN SPECIFIC REUPTAKE INHIBITOR(SSRIS)	OTHER AFFECTIVE PSYCHOSES
GLUCOCORTICOIDS	NEUROTIC DEPRESSION
GLUCOCORTICOIDS	ADJUST REAC BRIEF DEPRESSIVE
GLUCOCORTICOIDS	PETITMAL WO INTRACT EPILEPSY
ANTIHISTAMINES	PETITMAL WO INTRACT EPILEPSY
SEROTONIN SPECIFIC REUPTAKE INHIBITOR(SSRIS)	GRAND MALY WO INTRACT EPILEPSY
GLUCOCORTICOIDS	GRANDMALY WO INTRACT EPILEPSY
LOOP DIURETICS	UNS EPILEPSY WO INTRACT EPILEPSY
NSAIDS, CYCLOOXYGENASE INHIBITOR - TYPE	MALIGNANTHYPERTENSION
BETA-ADRENERGIC BLOCKING AGENTS	HYPERTEN HEART DIS WCHF
INSULINS	RENALHYPERTUNSPEC/FAILURE
SEDATIVE-HYPNOTICS,NON BARBITURATE	RENALHYPERTUNSPEC/FAILURE
ANTICONVULSANTS	RENALHYPERTUNSPEC/FAILURE
LOOP DIURETICS	RENALHYPERT UNSPEC/FAILURE
BETA-ADRENERGIC AGENTS	OTH PRIMARY CARDIOMYOPATHIES
ALPHA/BETA-ADRENERGIC BLOCKING AGENTS	CONGESTIVE HEART FAILURE
DIGITALIS GLYCOSIDES	LEFT HEART FAILURE
INSULINS	LEFT HEART FAILURE
ORAL ANTICOAGULANTS,COUMARIN TYPE	LEFT HEART FAILURE
BETA-ADRENERGIC AGENTS	CARDIOMEGALY
SEDATIVE-HYPNOTICS,NON-BARBITURATE	OBSTRUCTCHRON BRONCHITIS W EXAC
BETA-ADRENERGIC BLOCKING AGENTS	OTH EMPHYSEMA
ANALGESIC/ANTIPYRETICS,NON-SALICYLATE	UNS ASTHMA WOSTATUS ASTHMATICUS

(Continued)

DRUG CLASS	DISEASE CONFLICT
POTASSIUM SPARING DIURETICS	ALCOHOLICCIRRHOSIS LIVER
ANALGESICS,NARCOTICS	BILIARY CIRRHOSIS
GLUCOCORTICOIDS	BILIARY CIRRHOSIS
ANTI-ANXIETY DRUGS	OTHCHRONIC NONALCOHOLIC LIVER DIS
LIPOTROPICS	OTHCHRONIC NONALCOHOLIC LIVER DIS
ANALGESICS,NARCOTICS	OTHSEQUELAE CHRONIC LIVER DISEASE
ANALGESICS,NARCOTICS	UNSHEPATITIS
LIPOTROPICS	UNSHEPATITIS
NSAIDS, CYCLOOXYGENASE INHIBITOR - TYPE	UNS HEPATITIS
CALCIUM CHANNEL BLOCKING AGENTS	OTHER DISORDERS LIVER
HYPOTENSIVES,ANGIOTENSIN RECEPTOR ANTAGONIST	UNS DISORDER LIVER
BETA-ADRENERGIC BLOCKING AGENTS	UNS DISORDER LIVER
GLUCOCORTICOIDS	UNS DISORDER LIVER
LOOP DIURETICS	UNS DISORDER LIVER
HYPOTENSIVES, ACE INHIBITORS	UNS ACUTE RENAL FAILURE
POTASSIUM SPARING DIURETICS IN COMBINATION	UNS ACUTERENAL FAILURE
HYPOGLYCEMICS, BIGUANIDE TYPE (NON- SULFONYLUREAS)	CHRONICRENALFAILURE
SEDATIVE-HYPNOTICS,NON-BARBITURATE	CHRONICRENALFAILURE
ANALGESIC/ANTIPYRETICS,NON-SALICYLATE	CHRONIC RENALFAILURE
DIGITALIS GLYCOSIDES	UNS RENALFAILURE
HYPOTENSIVES, ACE INHIBITORS	UNS RENALFAILURE
SEDATIVE-HYPNOTICS,NON-BARBITURATE	SYNCOPE/COLLAPSE
SEROTONIN SPECIFIC REUPTAKE INHIBITOR (SSRIS)	SYNCOPE/COLLAPSE
ANTIPSYCHOTICS,ATYPICAL,DOPAMINE,& SEROTONIN ANTAG	SYNCOPE/COLLAPSE
INSULINS	KIDNEYREPLACED BY TRANSPLANT
INSULINS	RENALDIALYSISSTATUS
ANALGESICS,NARCOTICS	RENALDIALYSISSTATUS
NSAIDS, CYCLOOXYGENASE INHIBITOR - TYPE	BENIGNHYPERTENSION
BETA-ADRENERGIC BLOCKING AGENTS	DIABETES UNCOMPL TYPE I

(Continued)

DRUG CLASS	DISEASE CONFLICT
NSAIDS, CYCLOOXYGENASE INHIBITOR - TYPE	UNSHYPERTENSION
GLUCOCORTICOIDS	DEPRESSIVE DISORDER NEC
BETA-ADRENERGIC BLOCKING AGENTS	UNS ASTHMA WOSTATUS ASTHMATICUS
LOOP DIURETICS	CIRRHOSIS LIVER WO ALCOHOL
ANALGESICS,NARCOTICS	UNSRENALFAILURE
HYPOTENSIVES, ACE INHIBITORS	DIABETES RENAL MANIF TYPE II
LEUKOTRIENE RECEPTOR ANTAGONISTS	BENIGNHYPERTENSION
NSAIDS, CYCLOOXYGENASE INHIBITOR - TYPE	CONGESTIVE HEART FAILURE
HYPOTENSIVES, ACE INHIBITORS	CHRONICRENALFAILURE
HYPOTENSIVES,ANGIOTENSIN RECEPTOR ANTAGONIST	DIABETES UNCOMPL TYPE II
HYPOGLYCEMICS, INSULIN-RELEASE STIMULANT TYPE	CONGESTIVE HEART FAILURE
SEROTONIN SPECIFIC REUPTAKE INHIBITOR (SSRIS)	CONGESTIVE HEART FAILURE
BETA-ADRENERGIC AGENTS	UNS HYPERTENSION
HYPOGLYCEMICS, INSULIN-RESPONSE ENHANCER (N-S)	CONGESTIVE HEART FAILURE
BETA-ADRENERGIC BLOCKING AGENTS	CHRONICRENAL FAILURE
LOOP DIURETICS	CHRONICRENAL FAILURE
HYPOTENSIVES,ANGIOTENSIN RECEPTOR ANTAGONIST	DIABETES UNCOMPL TYPE I
BETA-ADRENERGIC BLOCKING AGENTS	DIABETES UNCOMP TYPE II UNCONTRD
HYPOTENSIVES,MISCELLANEOUS	DIABETES UNCOMPL TYPE II
ALPHA/BETA-ADRENERGIC BLOCKING AGENTS	DIABETES UNCOMPL TYPE II
ALPHA/BETA-ADRENERGIC BLOCKING AGENTS	DIABETES UNCOMPL TYPE I
HYPOTENSIVES,ANGIOTENSIN RECEPTOR ANTAGONIST	DIABETES UNCOMP TYPE II UNCONTRD
BETA-ADRENERGIC BLOCKING AGENTS	DIABETES NEURO MANIF TYPE I
GLUCOCORTICOIDS	PANIC DISORDER
LEUKOTRIENE RECEPTOR ANTAGONISTS	UNSHYPERTENSION
NSAIDS, CYCLOOXYGENASE INHIBITOR - TYPE	BENIGN HYPERTEN HEART DIS UNSPEC
BETA-ADRENERGIC AGENTS	HYPERTENHEARTDIS W CHF
DIGITALIS GLYCOSIDES	OTH PRIMARY CARDIOMYOPATHIES
LEUKOTRIENE RECEPTOR ANTAGONISTS	CONGESTIVE HEART FAILURE

(Continued)

DRUG CLASS	DISEASE CONFLICT
SEROTONIN SPECIFIC REUPTAKE INHIBITOR(SSRIS)	UNS CARDIOVASCULAR DISEASE
CALCIUM CHANNEL BLOCKING AGENTS	UNS HEPATITIS
ANALGESICS,NARCOTICS	UNS DISORDER LIVER
ANALGESICS,NARCOTICS	UNS ACUTERENAL FAILURE
HYPOGLYCEMICS, INSULIN-RELEASE STIMULANT TYPE	CHRONICRENAL FAILURE
HYPOGLYCEMICS, INSULIN-RESPONSE ENHANCER (N-S)	CHRONICRENAL FAILURE
ANALGESICS,NARCOTICS	CHRONICRENALFAILURE
INSULINS	UNSRENALFAILURE
HYPOGLYCEMICS, INSULIN-RELEASE STIMULANT TYPE	UNS RENALFAILURE
INSULINS	SYNCOPE/COLLAPSE
BETA-ADRENERGIC BLOCKING AGENTS	KIDNEY REPLACED BY TRANSPLANT
BETA-ADRENERGIC BLOCKING AGENTS	DIABETES UNCOMPL TYPE II
ORAL ANTICOAGULANTS, COUMARINTYPE	CONGESTIVE HEART FAILURE
BETA-ADRENERGIC AGENTS	CONGESTIVE HEART FAILURE
INSULINS	CHRONICRENALFAILURE
DIGITALIS GLYCOSIDES	CONGESTIVE HEART FAILURE
NSAIDS, CYCLOOXYGENASE INHIBITOR - TYPE	VOLUMEDEPLETIONDISORDER
HYPOGLYCEMICS, INSULIN-RELEASE STIMULANT TYPE	OTH PRIMARY CARDIOMYOPATHIES
BETA-ADRENERGIC BLOCKING AGENTS	SYNCOPE/COLLAPSE
SEDATIVE-HYPNOTICS,NON-BARBITURATE	AC/UNSHEPATITIS C WOCOMA
ANALGESICS,NARCOTICS	AC/UNSHEPATITIS C WOCOMA
HYPOGLYCEMICS, INSULIN-RELEASE STIMULANT TYPE	DIABETES RENAL MANIF TYPE II
INSULINS	DIABETES RENAL MANIF TYPE I
DIGITALIS GLYCOSIDES	UNS HEARTFAILURE
BETA-ADRENERGIC BLOCKING AGENTS	OBSTRUCTCHRON BRONCHITIS W EXAC
ANALGESIC/ANTIPYRETICS, SALICYLATES	UNS ASTHMA WOSTATUS ASTHMATICUS
SEDATIVE-HYPNOTICS,NON-BARBITURATE	CHRONIC AIRWAY OBSTRUCTION NEC
LOOP DIURETICS	UNS RENALFAILURE
VASODILATORS,CORONARY	SYNCOPE/COLLAPSE
BETA-ADRENERGIC BLOCKING AGENTS	CHRONIC AIRWAY OBSTRUCTION NEC

(Continued)

DRUG CLASS	DISEASE CONFLICT
BETA-ADRENERGIC BLOCKING AGENTS	OTH PRIMARY CARDIOMYOPATHIES
TRICYCLICANTIDEPRESSANTS & REL. NON-SEL. RU-INHIB	CONGESTIVE HEART FAILURE
HYPOGLYCEMICS, BIGUANIDE TYPE (NON- SULFONYLUREAS)	DIABETES RENAL MANIF TYPE II
INSULINS	OTH PRIMARY CARDIOMYOPATHIES
INSULINS	CONGESTIVE HEART FAILURE
HYPOGLYCEMICS, BIGUANIDE TYPE (NON- SULFONYLUREAS)	CONGESTIVE HEART FAILURE
PLATELET AGGREGATION INHIBITORS	CONGESTIVE HEART FAILURE
BETA-ADRENERGIC BLOCKING AGENTS	DIABETES EYE MANIF TYPE II
POTASSIUM SPARING DIURETICS	CIRRHOSIS LIVER WO ALCOHOL
BETA-ADRENERGIC BLOCKING AGENTS	CONGESTIVE HEART FAILURE
BETA-ADRENERGIC BLOCKING AGENTS	DIABETES NEURO MANIF TYPE II
GLUCOCORTICOIDS	ANXIETY STATE UNSPEC

APPENDIX V. ICD-9-CM CODES FOR MOTOR VEHICLE ACCIDENTS

Definitions and Examples Related to Transport Accidents

Transport Accident (ES800-E848)

Any accident involving device designed primarily for, or being used at the time primarily for conveying persons or goods from one place to another.

Includes: accidents involving: aircraft and spacecraft (E840-E845); watercraft (E830-E838); motor vehicle (E810-E825); railway (E800-E807); other road vehicles (E826-E829)

Motor Vehicle Accident (ES800-E848)

A transport accident involving a motor vehicle. It is defined as a motor vehicle traffic accident or as a motor vehicle nontraffic accident according to whether the accident occurs on a public highway or elsewhere.

Excludes: injury or damage due to cataclysm
injury or damage while a motor vehicle, not under its own power; is being loaded on, or unloaded from, another conveyance.

Motor Vehicle Traffic Accident

Any motor vehicle accident occurring on a public highway (i.e., originating, terminating, or involving a vehicle partially on the highway). A motor vehicle accidentis assumed to have occurred on the highway unless another place is specified, except in the case of accidents involving only off-read motor vehicles which are classified as nontraffic accidents unless the contrary is stated.

Motor Vehicle Nontraffic Accident

Any motor vehicle accident which occurs entirely in any place other than a public highway.

Public Highway (Trafficway) or Street

The entire width between property lines (or other boundary lines) of every way or place, of which any part is open to the use of the public for purposes of vehicular traffic as a matter of right or custom. A roadway is that party of the public highway designed, improved, or ordinarily used, for vehicular travel.

Includes: approaches(public) to: docks, publicbuilding, station

Excludes: *driveway (private); parking lot; ramp*
roads in: airfield; farm; industrial premises; mine; private grounds; quarry.

Motor Vehicle

Any mechanically or electrically powered device not operated on rails, upon which any person or property may be transported or drawn upon a highway. Any object such as a trailer, coaster, sled, or wagon being towed by a motor vehicle is considered a part of the motor vehicle.

Includes: automobile (any type) bus; construction machinery, farm and industrial machinery, steam roller, tractor, army tank, highway grader, or similar vehicle on wheels or treads, while in transport under own power; fire engine (motorized); motorcycle; motorized bicycle (moped) or scoter; trolley bus not operating on rails; truck; van.

Excludes: devices used solely to move persons or material within the confines of a building and its premises, such as: building elevator; coal car in mine; electric baggage or mail truck used solely within a railroad station; electric truck used solely within an industrial plant; moving overhead crane.

Motorcycle

A two-wheeled motor vehicle having one or two riding saddles and sometimes having a third when for the support of a sidecar. The sidecar is consideredpart of the motorcycle.

Includes: motorized: bicycle (moped); scooter; tricycle.

Off-Road Motor Vehicle

A motor vehicle of special design, to enable it to negotiate rough or soft terrain or snow. Examples of special design are high construction, special wheels and tires, drives by treads, or support on a cushion of air.

Includes: all terrain vehicle (ATV); army tank; hovercraft, on land or swamp; snowmobile.

Driver

A driver of a motor vehicle is the occupant of the motor vehicle operating it or intending to operate it. A motorcyclist is the driver of a motorcycle. Other authorized occupants of a motor vehicle are passengers.

Other Road Vehicle

Any device, except a motor vehicle in, on, or by which any person or property may be transportedon a highway.

Includes: animal carrying a person or goods; animal-drawn vehicles; animal harnessed to conveyance; bicycle (pedal cycle); streetcar; tricycle (pedal).
Excludes: pedestrian conveyance (definition (q))

Note: For definitions of motor vehicle traffic accident, and related terms, see definitions (e) to (k).

Excludes: accidents involving motor vehicle and aircraft

The following fourth-digit subdivisions are for use with categories E810-E819 to identify the injured person:

.0 Driver of motor vehicle other than motorcycle
(See definition (1).
.1 Passenger in motor vehicle other than motorcycle

(See definition (1).

.2 Motorcyclist
See definition (1)

.3 Passenger on motorcycle
See definition (1).

.4 Occupant of streetcar

.5 Rider of animal; occupant of animal-drawn vehicle

.6 Pedal cyclist
See definition (p)

.7 Pedestrian
See definition (r)

.8 Other specified person
Occupant of vehicle other than above; Person in railway train involved in accident; Unauthorized rider of motor vehicle.

.9 Unspecified person

Motor Vehicle Traffic Accidents (E810-E819)

- Note: For definitions of motor vehicle traffic accident, and related terms, see definitions (e) to (k).
  - Excludes: accidents involving motor vehicle and aircraft (E840.0-E845.9)
- The following fourth-digit subdivisions are for use with categories E810-E819 to identify the injured person:
  .0 Driver of motor vehicle other than motorcycle
       See definition (l)
  .1 Passenger in motor vehicle other than motorcycle
       See definition (l)
  .2 Motorcyclist
       See definition (l)
  .3 Passenger on motorcycle
       See definition (l)
  .4 Occupant of streetcar
  .5 Rider of animal; occupant of animal-drawn vehicle
  .6 Pedal cyclist
       See definition (p)
  .7 Pedestrian
       See definition (r)
  .8 Other specified person
       Occupant of vehicle other than above
       Person in railway train involved in accident
       Unauthorized rider of motor vehicle
  .9 Unspecified person

- **E810 Motor vehicle traffic accident involving collision with train**

- Requires fourth digit. See beginning of section E800-E845 for codes and definitions.
- Excludes: motor vehicle collision with object set in motion by railway train (E815.0-E815.9)
  - railway train hit by object set in motion by motor vehicle (E818.0-E818.9)
- **E811 Motor vehicle traffic accident involving re-entrant collision with another motor vehicle**
  Includes: collision between motor vehicle, which accidentally leaves the roadway then reenters the same roadway, or the opposite roadway on a divided highway, and another motor vehicle
  Excludes: collision on the same roadway when none of the motor vehicles involved have left and re-entered the roadway (E812.0-E812.9)
- **E812 Other motor vehicle traffic accident involving collision with motor vehicle**
  Includes: collision with another motor vehicle parked, stopped, stalled, disabled, or abandoned on the highway
      motor vehicle collision NOS
  Excludes: collision with object set in motion by another motor vehicle (E815.0-E815.9)
      re-entrant collision with another motor vehicle (E811.0-E811.9)
- **E813 Motor vehicle traffic accident involving collision with other vehicle**
  Includes: collision between motor vehicle, any kind,and:
      other road (nonmotor transport) vehicle, such as:
          animal carrying a person
          animal-drawn vehicle
          pedal cycle
          streetcar
  Excludes: collision with:
      object set in motion by nonmotor road vehicle (E815.0-E815.9)
      pedestrian (E814.0-E814.9)
      nonmotor road vehicle hit by object set in motion by motor vehicle (E818.0-E818.9)
- **E814 Motor vehicle traffic accident involving collision with pedestrian**
  Includes: collision between motor vehicle, any kind,and
      pedestrian pedestrian dragged, hit, orrun over by motor vehicle, any kind
  Excludes: pedestrian hit by object set in motion by motor vehicle (E818.0-E818.9)
- **E815 Other motor vehicle traffic accident involving collision on the highway**
  Includes: collision (due toloss of control) (on highway)between motor vehicle, any kind,
      and:
          abutment (bridge) (overpass)
          animal (herded) (unattended)
          fallen stone, traffic sign, tree, utility pole
          guard rail or boundary fence
          inter-highway divider
          landslide (not moving)

Multiple Medications and Vehicle Crashes: Analysis of Databases 71

object set in motion by railway train or road vehicle (motor) (nonmotor)
object thrown in front of motor vehicle
safety island
temporary traffic sign or marker
wall of cut made for road
other object, fixed, movable, or moving

Excludes: collision with:

any object off the highway (resulting from loss of control) (E816.0-E816.9)

any object which normally would have been off the highway and is not stated to have been on it (E816.0-E816.9)

motor vehicle parked, stopped, stalled, disabled, or abandoned on highway (E812.0-E812.9)

moving landslide (E909.2)

motor vehicle hit by object:

set in motionby railway train or road vehicle (motor) (nonmotor) (E818.0-E818.9)

thrown into or on vehicle (E818.0-E818.9)

- **E816 Motor vehicle traffic accident due to loss ofcontrol, without collision on the highway**

  Includes: motor vehicle:

  failing to make curve and:

  colliding with object off the highway

  overturning

  stopping abruptly off the highway

  going out of control (due to)

  blowout and:

  colliding with object off the highway

  overturning

  stopping abruptly off the highway

  burst tire and:

  colliding with object off the highway

  overturning

  stopping abruptly off the highway

  driver falling asleep and:

  colliding with object off the highway

  overturning

  stopping abruptly off the highway

  driver inattention and:

  colliding with object off the highway

  overturning

  stopping abruptly off the highway

  excessive speed and:

  colliding with object off the highway

  overturning

  stopping abruptly off the highway

  failure of mechanical part and:

colliding with object off the highway

overturning

stopping abruptly off the highway

Excludes: collision on highway following loss of control (E810.0-E815.9)

loss of control of motor vehicle following collision on the highway (E810.0-E815.9)

- **E817 Noncollision motor vehicle traffic accident while boarding or alighting**

  Includes: fall down stairs of motor bus while boarding or alighting

  fall from car in street while boarding or alighting

  injured by moving part of the vehicle while boardingor alighting

  trapped by door of motor bus boarding or alighting while boarding or alighting

- **E818 Other noncollision motor vehicle traffic accident**

  Includes: accidental poisoning from exhaust gas generated by motor vehicle while in

motion

breakage of any part of motor vehicle while in motion

explosionofany part of motor vehicle while in motion

fall, jump, or being accidentally pushed from motor vehicle while in motion

fire starting in motor vehicle while in motion

hit by object thrown into or on motor vehicle while in motion

injured by being thrown against some part of, or object in motor vehicle while in
motion

injury from moving part of motor vehicle while in motion

object falling in or on motor vehicle while in motion

object thrown on motor vehicle while in motion

collision of railway train or road vehicle except motor vehicle, with object set in
motion by

motor vehicle motor vehicle hit by object set in motion by railway train or road
vehicle (motor) (nonmotor)

pedestrian, railway train, or road vehicle (motor) (nonmotor) hit by object set in
motion by motor vehicle

Excludes: collision between motor vehicle and:

object set in motion by railway train or road vehicle (motor) (nonmotor)
(E815.0-E815.9)

object thrown towards the motor vehicle (E815.0-E815.9)

person overcome by carbon monoxide generated by stationary motor vehicle off
the roadway with motor running (E868.2)

- **E819 Motor vehicle traffic accident of unspecified nature**

  Includes: motor vehicle traffic accident NOS

  traffic accident NOS

Motor Vehicle Nontraffic Accidents (E820-E825)

- Note: For definitions of motor vehicle nontraffic accident and related terms see
  definition (a) to (k).

- Includes: accidents involving motor vehicles being used in recreational or sporting activities off the highway
  - collision and noncollision motor vehicle accidents occurring entirely off the highway
- Excludes: accidents involving motor vehicle and:
  - aircraft (E840.0-E845.9)
  - watercraft (E830.0-E838.9)
  - accidents, not on the public highway, involving agricultural and construction machinery but not involving another motor vehicle (E919.0, E919.2, E919.7)
- The following fourth-digit subdivisions are for use with categories E820-E825 to identify the injured person:
  - .0 Driver of motor vehicle other than motorcycle
    - See definition (l)
  - .1 Passenger in motor vehicle other than motorcycle
    - See definition (l)
  - .2 Motorcyclist
    - See definition (l)
  - .3 Passenger on motorcycle
    - See definition (l)
  - .4 Occupant of streetcar
  - .5 Rider of animal; occupant of animal-drawn vehicle
  - .6 Pedal cyclist
    - See definition (p)
  - .7 Pedestrian
    - See definition (r)
  - .8 Other specified person
    - Occupant of vehicle other than above
    - erson on railway train involved in accident
    - Unauthorized rider of motor vehicle
  - .9 Unspecified person
- **E820 Nontraffic accident involving motor-driven snow vehicle**

  Includes: breakage of part of motor-driven snow vehicle (not on public highway)

  fall from motor-driven snow vehicle (not on public highway)

  hit by motor-driven snow vehicle (not on public highway)

  overturning of motor-driven snow vehicle (not on public highway)

  run over or dragged by motor-driven snow vehicle (not on public highway)

  collision of motor-driven snow vehicle with:

  animal (being ridden) (-drawn vehicle)

  another off-road motor vehicle

  other motor vehicle, not on public highway

  railway train

  other object, fixed or movable

injury caused by rough landing of motor-driven snow vehicle (after leaving ground on rough terrain)

Excludes: accident on the public highway involving motor driven snow vehicle (E810.0-E819.9)

- **E821 Nontraffic accident involving other off-road motor vehicle**
  - **Includes:** breakage of part of off-road motor vehicle, except snow vehicle (not on public highway)

    fall from off-road motor vehicle, except snow vehicle (not on public highway)

    hit by off-road motor vehicle, except snow vehicle (not on public highway)

    overturning of off-road motor vehicle, except snow vehicle (not on public highway)

    run over or dragged by off-road motor vehicle, except snow vehicle (not on public highway)

    thrown against some part of or object in off-road motor vehicle, except snow vehicle (not on public highway)

    collision with:

    animal (being ridden) (-drawn vehicle)

    another off-road motor vehicle, except snow vehicle

    other motor vehicle, not on public highway

    other object, fixed or movable
  - **Excludes:** accident on public highway involving off-road motor vehicle (E810.0-E819.9)

    collision between motor driven snow vehicle and other off-road motor vehicle (E820.0-E820.9)

    hovercraft accident on water (E830.0-E838.9)
- **E822 Other motor vehicle nontraffic accident involving collision with moving object**

  Includes: collision, not on public highway,between motor vehicle, except off-road motor vehicle and:

  animal

  nonmotor vehicle

  other motor vehicle, except off-road motor vehicle

  pedestrian

  railway train

  other moving object

  Excludes: collision with:

  motor-driven snow vehicle (E820.0-E820.9)

  other off-road motor vehicle (E821.0-E821.9)
- **E823 Other motor vehicle nontraffic accident involving collision with stationary object**

  Includes: collision, not on public highway,between motor vehicle, except off-road motor vehicle, and any object, fixed or movable, but not in motion
- **E824 Other motor vehicle nontraffic accident while boarding and alighting**

  Includes: fall while boarding or alighting from motor vehicle except off-road motor vehicle, not on public highway

injury frommoving part of motor vehicle while boarding or alighting from motor

vehicle except off-road motor vehicle, not on public highway

trapped by door of motor vehicle while boarding or alighting from motor vehicle

except off-road motor vehicle, not on public highway

- **E825 Other motor vehicle nontraffic accident of other and unspecified nature**

Includes: accidental poisoning from carbon monoxidegenerated by motor vehicle while in motion, not on public highway

breakage of any part of motor vehicle while in motion, not on public highway

explosion of any part of motor vehicle while in motion, not on public highway

fall, jump, or being accidentally pushed from motor vehicle while in motion, not on public highway

fire starting in motor vehicle while in motion, notonpublic highway

hit by object thrown into, towards, or on motor vehicle while in motion, not on public highway

injured by being thrown against some part of, or object in motor vehicle while in motion, not on public highway

injury frommoving part of motor vehicle while in motion, not on public highway

object falling in or on motor vehicle while in motion, not on public highway

motor vehicle nontraffic accident NOS

Excludes: fall from or in stationary motor vehicle (E884.9, E885)

overcome by carbon monoxide or exhaust gas generated by stationary motor vehicle

off the roadway with motor running (E868.2)

struck by falling object from or in stationary motor vehicle (E916)

- **E826 Pedal cycle accident**

Includes: breakage of any part of pedal cycle

collision between pedal cycle and:

animal (being ridden) (herded) (unattended)

another pedal cycle

nonmotor road vehicle, any

pedestrian

other object, fixed, movable, or moving,not set in motion by motor vehicle, railway train, or aircraft

entanglement in wheel of pedal cycle

fall from pedal cycle

hit by object falling or thrown on the   pedal cycle

pedal cycle accident NOS

pedal cycle overturned

- **E827 Animal-drawn vehicle accident**

Includes: breakage of any part of vehicle

collision between animal-drawn vehicle and:

animal (being ridden) (herded) (unattended)

nonmotor road vehicle, except

pedal cycle pedestrian, pedestrian conveyance, or pedestrian vehicle

other object, fixed, movable, or moving,not set in motion by motor vehicle,

railway train, or aircraft

fall from animal-drawn vehicle

knocked down by animal-drawn vehicle

overturning of animal-drawn vehicle

run over by animal-drawn vehicle

thrown from animal-drawn vehicle

Excludes: collision of animal-drawn vehicle with pedal cycle (E826.0-E826.9)

- **E828 Accident involvinganimal being ridden**

Includes: collision between animal being ridden and:

another animal

nonmotor road vehicle, except pedal cycle, and animal-drawn vehicle

pedestrian, pedestrian conveyance, or pedestrian vehicle

other object, fixed, movable, or moving,not set in motion by motor vehicle,

railway train, or aircraft

fall from animal being ridden

knocked down by animal being ridden

thrown from animal being ridden

trampled by animal being

ridden ridden animal stumbled and fell

Excludes: collision of animal being ridden with:

animal-drawn vehicle (E827.0-E827.9)

pedal cycle (E826.0-E826.9)

- **E829 Other road vehicle accidents**

Includes: accident while boardingor alighting from

streetcar

nonmotor road vehicle not classifiable to E826-E828

blow from object in

streetcar

nonmotor road vehicle not classifiable to E826-E828

breakage of any part of

streetcar

nonmotor road vehicle not classifiable to E826-E828

caught in door of

streetcar

nonmotor road vehicle not classifiable to E826-E828

derailment of

streetcar

nonmotor road vehicle not classifiable to E826-E828

fall in, on, or from

streetcar

nonmotor road vehicle not classifiable to E826-E828

fire in

streetcar

nonmotor road vehicle not classifiable to E826-E828

collision between streetcar or nonmotor road vehicle, except as in E826-E828, and:

animal (not being ridden)

another nonmotor road vehicle not classifiable to E826-E828

pedestrian

other object, fixed, movable, or moving,not set in motion by motor vehicle, railway train, or aircraft

nonmotor road vehicle accident NOS

streetcar accident NOS

Excludes: collision with:

animal being ridden (E828.0-E828.9)

animal-drawn vehicle (E827.0-E827.9)

pedal cycle (E826.0-E826.9)

- **E830 Accident to watercraft causing submersion**

Requires fourth digit. See beginning of section E800-E845 for codes and definitions.

Includes: submersion and drowning due to:

boat overturning

boat submerging

falling or jumping from burning ship

falling or jumping from crushed watercraft

ship sinking

other accident to watercraft

- **E831 Accident to watercraft causing other injury**

Includes: any injury, except submersion and drowning, as a result of an accident to watercraft

burned while ship on fire

crushed between ships in collision

crushed by lifeboat after abandoning ship

fall due to collision or other accident to watercraft

hit by falling object due to accident to watercraft

injured in watercraft accident involving collision

struck by boat or part thereof after fall or jump from damaged boat

Excludes: burns from localized fire or explosion on board ship (E837.0-E837.9)

- **E832 Other accidental submersion or drowning in water transport accident**

Requires fourth digit. See beginning of section E800-E845 for codes and definitions.

Includes: submersion or drowning as a result of an accident other than accident to the

watercraft, such as:

fall:

from gangplank

from ship

overboard

thrown overboard by motion of ship

washed overboard

Excludes: submersion or drowning of swimmer or diver who voluntarily jumps from boat not involved in an accident (E910.0-E910.9)

APPENDIX VI. NONPROPRIETARY DATABASE, RESTRICT DEFINITION

Table 1a. Number of Physician Visits of MVA Patients by Age and Gender

| | Gender | | | | | |
| | Male | | Female | | Both | |
	N	PCTN	N	PCTN	N	PCTN
Age Group						
Under 50	202	72	201	75	403	74
50+	79	28	66	25	145	26
All Age	281	100	267	100	548	100

Table 1b. Number of Physician Visits MVA Patients by Age and Gender (Weighted)

| | Gender | | | | | |
| | Male | | Female | | Both | |
	N	PCTN	N	PCTN	N	PCTN
Age Group						
Under 50	6,073,420	73	5,969,219	73	12,042,639	73
50+	2,211,212	27	2,246,376	27	4,457,588	27
All Age	8,284,632	100	8,215,595	100	16,500,227	100

Multiple Medications and Vehicle Crashes: Analysis of Databases

Table 2a. Number of Physician Visits of MVA Patients by Age, Gender, and Number of Medications

| | | Gender | | | | Both | |
| | | Male | | Female | | | |
		N	PCTN	N	PCTN	N	PCTN
Age Group	Number of Medications						
Under 50	Recorded						
	0	100	50	111	55	211	52
	1	48	24	38	19	86	21
	2	26	13	35	17	61	15
	3	18	9	10	5	28	7
	4	6	3	3	1	9	2
	5	2	1			2	0
	6	2	1	4	2	6	1
	All	202	100	201	100	403	100
50+	Number of Medications Recorded						
	0	37	47	30	45	67	46
	1	21	27	15	23	36	25
	2	11	14	11	17	22	15
	3	6	8	8	12	14	10
	4			1	2	1	1
	5	1	1			1	1
	6	3	4	1	2	4	3
	All	79	100	66	100	145	100

Table 2a. (Continued)

| | | Gender | | | | Both | |
| | | Male | | Female | | | |
		N	PCTN	N	PCTN	N	PCTN
All Age	Number of Medications Recorded						
	0	137	49	141	53	278	51
	1	69	25	53	20	122	22
	2	37	13	46	17	83	15
	3	24	9	18	7	42	8
	4	6	2	4	1	10	2
	5	3	1			3	1
All Age	Number of Medications Recorded						
	6	5	2	5	2	10	2
	All	281	100	267	100	548	100

Table 2b. Number of Physician Visits of MVA Patients by Age, Gender, and Number of Medications (Weighted)

| | | Gender | | | | Both | |
| | | Male | | Female | | | |
		N	PCTN	N	PCTN	N	PCTN
Age Group	Number of Medications Recorded						
Under 50	Recorded						
	0	2,841,274	47	3,079,362	52	5,920,636	49
	1	1,286,281	21	1,037,349	17	2,323,630	19
	2	998,445	16	1,125,928	19	2,124,373	18
	3	684,345	11	427,516	7	1,111,861	9
	4	157,643	3	119,860	2	277,503	2
	5	66,612	1			66,612	1
	6	38,820	1	179,204	3	218,024	2
	All	6,073,420	100	5,969,219	100	12,042,639	100
50+	Number of Medications Recorded						
	0	919,741	42	814,643	36	1,734,384	39
	1	559,257	25	575,021	26	1,134,278	25
	2	236,868	11	425,836	19	662,704	15
	3	193,142	9	264,325	12	457,467	10
	4			120,767	5	120,767	3
	5	59,983	3			59,983	1
	6	242,221	11	45,784	2	288,005	6
	All	2,211,212	100	2,246,376	100	4,457,588	100

Table 2b. (Continued)

		Gender				Both	
		Male		Female			
		N	PCTN	N	PCTN	N	PCTN
All Age	Number of Medications Recorded						
	0	3,761,015	45	3,894,005	47	7,655,020	46
	1	1,845,538	22	1,612,370	20	3,457,908	21
	2	1,235,313	15	1,551,764	19	2,787,077	17
	3	877,487	11	691,841	8	1,569,328	10
	4	157,643	2	240,627	3	398,270	2
	5	126,595	2			126,595	1
	6	281,041	3	224,988	3	506,029	3
	All	8,284,632	100	8,215,595	100	16,500,227	100

Table 3a. Number of Physician Visits of MVA Patients by Gender, Age Group, and Specific Combinations of Drug Classes

Gender	Age Group	Drug Class 1	Drug Class 2	Drug Class 3	Drug Class 4	Drug Class 5	Drug Class 6	N	PCTN
Male	Under 50	Antiarthritics						13	18
Male	Under 50	NSAID						10	14
Male	Under 50	Antidepressants						7	10
Male	Under 50	Analgesics, narcotic						6	8
Male	Under 50	Analgesics, non-narcotic						6	8
Male	Under 50	Analgesics, narcotic	Antiarthritics					3	4
Male	Under 50	Antiarthritics	Skeletal muscle hyperactivity					3	4
Male	Under 50	Analgesics, non-narcotic	Antiarthritics					2	3
Male	Under 50	Analgesics, non-narcotic	Antidepressants					2	3
Male	Under 50	NSAID	Skeletal muscle hyperactivity					2	3
Male	Under 50	Adrenal corticosteroids	Cephalosporins					1	1
Male	Under 50	Alpha agonist/alpha blockers	Antidepressants	Antidepressants	Antipsychotic/antimanics			1	1
Male	Under 50	Analgesics, narcotic	Analgesics, non-narcotic	Antidepressants	NSAID			1	1
Male	Under 50	Analgesics, narcotic	Analgesics/general					1	1
Male	Under 50	Analgesics, narcotic	Anesthetics, local (injectable)	Topical steroids				1	1
Male	Under 50	Analgesics, narcotic	Antianxiety agents	Antiarthritics				1	1
Male	Under 50	Analgesics, narcotic	Antianxiety agents	Anticonvulsants	Antidepressants			1	1
Male	Under 50	Analgesics, narcotic	Antianxiety agents	Disorders, acid/peptic	Skeletal muscle hyperactivity			1	1
Male	Under 50	Analgesics, narcotic	Antianxiety agents	Skeletal muscle hyperactivity				1	1
Male	Under 50	Analgesics, narcotic	Antiarthritics	Anticonvulsants	Antidepressants	Disorders, acid/peptic	Vitamins/minerals	1	1
Male	Under 50	Analgesics, narcotic	NSAID					1	1

Table 3a. (Continued)

Gender	Age Group	Drug Class 1	Drug Class 2	Drug Class 3	Drug Class 4	Drug Class 5	Drug Class 6	N	PCTN
Male	Under 50	Analgesics, narcotic	Skeletal muscle hyperactivity					1	1
Male	Under 50	Analgesics, non-narcotic	Antidepressants	Antidepressants				1	1
Male	Under 50	Analgesics, non-narcotic	Skeletal muscle hyperactivity					1	1
Male	Under 50	Antiarthritics	Disorders, acid/peptic					1	1
Male	Under 50	Anticonvulsants						1	1
Male	Under 50	Anticonvulsants	Antidepressants					1	1
Male	Under 50	Ocular anti-infective/anti-inflammatory						1	1
Male	Under 50	Unclassified						1	1
Male	50+	Antiarthritics						5	17
Male	50+	Anticonvulsants						3	10
Male	50+	Antidepressants						3	10
Male	50+	NSAID						3	10
Male	50+	NSAID	Skeletal muscle hyperactivity					2	7
Male	50+	Skeletal muscle hyperactivity						2	7
Male	50+	ACE inhibitors	Adrenal corticosteroids	Analgesics, non-narcotic	Antiarrhythmic agents	Topical anti-infectives		1	3
Male	50+	ACE inhibitors	Antiarthritics	Beta blockers				1	3
Male	50+	Adrenal corticosteroids						1	3
Male	50+	Alpha agonist/alpha blockers	Antidiarrheals	Disorders, acid/peptic	Diuretics	Homeopathic products	Repl/regs of electrolytes/water balance	1	3
Male	50+	Analgesics, narcotic						1	3
Male	50+	Analgesics, narcotic	Antianxiety agents	Antidepressants	Antihypertensive agents	Calcium metabolism	Thyroid/antithyroid	1	3

Table 3a. (Continued)

Gender	Age Group	Drug Class 1	Drug Class 2	Drug Class 3	Drug Class 4	Drug Class 5	Drug Class 6	N	PCTN
Male	50+	Analgesics, narcotic	Antiarthritics	Antiarthritics	Disorders, acid/peptic	Hyperlipidemia	Skeletal muscle hyperactivity	1	3
Male	50+	Analgesics, narcotic	NSAID					1	3
Male	50+	Analgesics, non-narcotic						1	3
Male	50+	Analgesics, non-narcotic	Antidepressants	Antidepressants				1	3
Male	50+	Analgesics, non-narcotic	NSAID					1	3
Male	50+	Analgesics, non-narcotic	Skeletal muscle hyperactivity					1	3
Female	Under 50	Antiarthritics						9	13
Female	Under 50	Analgesics, narcotic						7	10
Female	Under 50	NSAID	Skeletal muscle hyperactivity					6	9
Female	Under 50	Analgesics, narcotic	Antiarthritics	Skeletal muscle hyperactivity				5	7
Female	Under 50	NSAID						5	7
Female	Under 50	Antiarthritics	Skeletal muscle hyperactivity					4	6
Female	Under 50	Skeletal muscle hyperactivity						4	6
Female	Under 50	Analgesics, narcotic	Antiarthritics					3	4
Female	Under 50	Analgesics, narcotic	Skeletal muscle hyperactivity					3	4
Female	Under 50	Unclassified						3	4
Female	Under 50	Adrenal corticosteroids						2	3
Female	Under 50	Antiarthritics	Disorders, acid/peptic					2	3
Female	Under 50	Anticonvulsants						2	3
Female	Under 50	Adrenal corticosteroids	Analgesics, non-narcotic					1	1

Gender	Age Group	Drug Class 1	Drug Class 2	Drug Class 3	Drug Class 4	Drug Class 5	Drug Class 6	N	PCTN
Female	Under 50	Adrenal corticosteroids	Anesthetics, local (injectable)					1	1
Female	Under 50	Adrenal corticosteroids	Topical analgesics					1	1
Female	Under 50	Alpha agonist/alpha blockers	Analgesics, narcotic	Anticoagulants/thrombolytics	Antidepressants	Antidepressants	Relaxants/stimulants, urinary tract	1	1
Female	Under 50	Analgesics, narcotic	Analgesics, narcotic	Analgesics, narcotic				1	1
Female	Under 50	Analgesics, narcotic	Analgesics, narcotic	Antidepressants	Antihistamines	CNS, miscellaneous	Skeletal muscle hyperactivity	1	1
Female	Under 50	Analgesics, narcotic	Antianxiety agents	Antiasthmatics/bronch odilators	Calcium channel blockers	Disorders, acid/peptic	Disorders, acid/peptic	1	1
Female	Under 50	Analgesics, narcotic	NSAID					1	1
Female	Under 50	Analgesics, narcotic	NSAID	Skeletal muscle hyperactivity				1	1
Female	Under 50	Analgesics, non-narcotic						1	1
Female	Under 50	Analgesics, non-narcotic	Antiarthritics					1	1
Female	Under 50	Analgesics, non-narcotic	Skeletal muscle hyperactivity					1	1
Female	Under 50	Anticonvulsants	Antidepressants					1	1
Female	Under 50	Antidepressants						1	1
Female	Under 50	Topical steroids						1	1
Female	50+	Analgesics, narcotic						4	18
Female	50+	Antiarthritics						3	14
Female	50+	NSAID						3	14
Female	50+	Analgesics, narcotic	Antiarthritics					2	9
Female	50+	Analgesics, narcotic	NSAID	Skeletal muscle hyperactivity				2	9
Female	50+	ACE inhibitors	Analgesics, narcotic	Antidepressants				1	5

Table 3a. (Continued)

Gender	Age Group	Drug Class 1	Drug Class 2	Drug Class 3	Drug Class 4	Drug Class 5	Drug Class 6	N	PCTN
Female	50+	Adrenal corticosteroids	NSAID					1	5
Female	50+	Analgesics, narcotic	Antianxiety agents	Antiarthritics	Skeletal muscle hyperactivity			1	5
Female	50+	Analgesics, non-narcotic						1	5
Female	50+	Analgesics, non-narcotic	NSAID					1	5
Female	50+	NSAID	Skeletal muscle hyperactivity					1	5
Female	50+	Ocular anti-infective/anti-inflammatory						1	5
Female	50+	Topical steroids						1	5

Table 3b. Number of Physician Visits of MVA Patients by Gender, Age Group, and Specific Combinations of Drug Classes (Weighted)

Gender	Age Group	Drug Class 1	Drug Class 2	Drug Class 3	Drug Class 4	Drug Class 5	Drug Class 6	N	PCTN
Male	Under 50	Antiarthritics						399,959	18
Male	Under 50	NSAID						322,255	14
Male	Under 50	Analgesics, non-narcotic						173,906	8
Male	Under 50	Antidepressants						164,156	7
Male	Under 50	Analgesics, narcotic						128,470	6
Male	Under 50	Analgesics, narcotic	Skeletal muscle hyperactivity					108,225	5
Male	Under 50	Analgesics, non-narcotic	Antidepressants					104,035	5
Male	Under 50	Analgesics, non-narcotic	Skeletal muscle hyperactivity					93,513	4

Table 3b. (Continued)

Gender	Age Group	Drug Class 1	Drug Class 2	Drug Class 3	Drug Class 4	Drug Class 5	Drug Class 6	N	PCTN
Male	Under 50	Analgesics, non-narcotic	Antidepressants	Antidepressants				91,252	4
Male	Under 50	Analgesics, non-narcotic	Antiarthritics					83,037	4
Male	Under 50	Adrenal corticosteroids	Cephalosporins					63,189	3
Male	Under 50	NSAID	Skeletal muscle hyperactivity					59,262	3
Male	Under 50	Analgesics, narcotic	Antiarthritics					58,560	3
Male	Under 50	Analgesics, narcotic	Antianxiety agents	Disorders, acid/peptic	Skeletal muscle hyperactivity			56,544	2
Male	Under 50	Antiarthritics	Skeletal muscle hyperactivity			.		51,483	2
Male	Under 50	Analgesics, narcotic	NSAID					46,793	2
Male	Under 50	Analgesics, narcotic	Antianxiety agents	Antiarthritics				42,024	2
Male	Under 50	Analgesics, narcotic	Analgesics/general					40,954	2
Male	Under 50	Analgesics, narcotic	Anesthetics, local (injectable)	Topical steroids				37,719	2
Male	Under 50	Analgesics, narcotic	Antianxiety agents	Skeletal muscle hyperactivity				31,758	1
Male	Under 50	Anticonvulsants						24,290	1
Male	Under 50	Ocular anti-infective/anti-inflammatory						13,496	1
Male	Under 50	Analgesics, narcotic	Analgesics, non-narcotic	Antidepressants	NSAID			12,870	1
Male	Under 50	Analgesics, narcotic	Antianxiety agents	Anticonvulsants	Antidepressants			12,055	1
Male	Under 50	Alpha agonist/ alpha blockers	Antidepressants	Antidepressants	Antipsychotic/ antima nics			11,055	0
Male	Under 50	Anticonvulsants	Antidepressants					11,055	0
Male	Under 50	Antiarthritics	Disorders, acid/peptic					9,398	0
Male	Under 50	Analgesics, narcotic	Antiarthritics	Anticonvulsants	Antidepressants	acid/peptic	Vitamins/minerals	7,512	0

Gender	Age Group	Drug Class 1	Drug Class 2	Drug Class 3	Drug Class 4	Drug Class 5	Drug Class 6	N	PCTN
Male	Under 50	Unclassified						3,842	0
Male	50+	Antiarthritics						148,489	15
Male	50+	Analgesics, narcotic	Antiarthritics	Antiarthritics	Disorders, acid/peptic	Hyperlipidemia	Skeletal muscle hyperactivity	100,188	10
Male	50+	Antidepressants						98,513	10
Male	50+	Alpha agonist/alpha blockers	Antidiarrheals	Disorders, acid/peptic	Diuretics	Homeopathic products	Repl/regs of electrolytes/water balance	78,876	8
Male	50+	NSAID						63,875	7
Male	50+	Analgesics, narcotic	Antianxiety agents	Antidepressants	Antihypertensive agents	Calcium metabolism	Thyroid/antithyroid	63,157	7
Male	50+	ACE inhibitors	Adrenal corticosteroids	Analgesics, non-narcotic	Antiarrhythmic agents	Topical anti-infectives		59,983	6
Male	50+	Anticonvulsants						58,855	6
Male	50+	ACE inhibitors	Antiarthritics	Beta blockers				55,893	6
Male	50+	NSAID	Skeletal muscle hyperactivity					52,464	5
Male	50+	Analgesics, non-narcotic						46,811	5
Male	50+	Skeletal muscle hyperactivity						42,139	4
Male	50+	Analgesics, non-narcotic	Skeletal muscle hyperactivity					42,024	4
Male	50+	Analgesics, narcotic						20,319	2
Male	50+	Analgesics, narcotic	NSAID					15,935	2
Male	50+	Analgesics, non-narcotic	NSAID					7,512	1
Male	50+	Adrenal corticosteroids						4,765	0
Male	50+	Analgesics, non-narcotic	Antidepressants	Antidepressants				2,893	0
Female	Under 50	NSAID	Skeletal muscle hyperactivity					273,057	12

Table 3b. (Continued)

Gender	Age Group	Drug Class 1	Drug Class 2	Drug Class 3	Drug Class 4	Drug Class 5	Drug Class 6	N	PCTN
Female	Under 50	Analgesics, narcotic	Antiarthritics	Skeletal muscle hyperactivity				268,835	12
Female	Under 50	Antiarthritics						255,117	11
Female	Under 50	NSAID						232,209	10
Female	Under 50	Analgesics, narcotic						150,847	7
Female	Under 50	Antiarthritics	Skeletal muscle hyperactivity					137,185	6
Female	Under 50	Analgesics, narcotic	Antiarthritics					126,808	5
Female	Under 50	Unclassified						121,288	5
Female	Under 50	Skeletal muscle hyperactivity						91,674	4
Female	Under 50	Antiarthritics	Disorders, acid/peptic					84,694	4
Female	Under 50	Analgesics, non-narcotic	Skeletal muscle hyperactivity					72,699	3
Female	Under 50	Analgesics, narcotic	Antianxiety agents	Antiasthmatics/bronc hodilators	Calcium channel blockers	Disorders, acid/peptic	Disorders, acid/peptic	71,982	3
Female	Under 50	Adrenal corticosteroids						67,600	3
Female	Under 50	Analgesics, narcotic	Skeletal muscle hyperactivity					58,557	3
Female	Under 50	Analgesics, narcotic	NSAID	Skeletal muscle hyperactivity				44,394	2
Female	Under 50	Adrenal corticosteroids	Analgesics, non-narcotic					43,023	2
Female	Under 50	Anticonvulsants						35,797	2
Female	Under 50	Alpha agonist/ alpha blockers	Analgesics, narcotic	Anticoagulants/ thro mbolytics	Antidepressants	Antidepressants	Relaxants/ stimulants, urinary tract	31,308	1
Female	Under 50	Analgesics, non-narcotic	Antiarthritics					24,453	1
Female	Under 50	Analgesics, narcotic	NSAID					21,815	1
Female	Under 50	Topical steroids						18,747	1
Female	Under 50	Anticonvulsants	Antidepressants					17,876	1

Gender	Age Group	Drug Class 1	Drug Class 2	Drug Class 3	Drug Class 4	Drug Class 5	Drug Class 6	N	PCTN
Female	Under 50	Adrenal corticosteroids	Anesthetics, local (injectable)					14,663	1
Female	Under 50	Analgesics, narcotic	Analgesics, narcotic	Antidepressants	Antihistamines	CNS, miscellaneous	Skeletal muscle hyperactivity	14,663	1
Female	Under 50	Adrenal corticosteroids	Topical analgesics					12,877	1
Female	Under 50	Analgesics, non-narcotic						11,514	0
Female	Under 50	Antidepressants						7,684	0
Female	Under 50	Analgesics, narcotic	Analgesics, narcotic	Analgesics, narcotic				6,027	0
Female	50+	Analgesics, narcotic	Antianxiety agents	Antiarthritics	Skeletal muscle hyperactivity			120,767	14
Female	50+	NSAID						119,756	14
Female	50+	Antiarthritics						116,216	14
Female	50+	ACE inhibitors	Analgesics, narcotic	Antidepressants				91,242	11
Female	50+	Analgesics, narcotic						83,399	10
Female	50+	Analgesics, non-narcotic						79,797	9
Female	50+	Ocular anti-infective/anti-inflammatory						67,835	8
Female	50+	Analgesics, narcotic	Antiarthritics					35,840	4
Female	50+	Adrenal corticosteroids	NSAID					32,511	4
Female	50+	Topical steroids						30,263	4
Female	50+	Analgesics, narcotic	NSAID	Skeletal muscle hyperactivity				27,300	3
Female	50+	NSAID	Skeletal muscle hyperactivity					22,791	3
Female	50+	Analgesics, non-narcotic	NSAID					18,337	2

Table 4a. Number of Physician Visits of MVA Patients by Age, Gender, and Number of Potential Driver Impairing Medications

| | | Gender | | | | | |
| | | Male | | Female | | Both | |
		N	PCTN	N	PCTN	N	PCTN
Age Group Under 50	Number of Potential Impairing Medications						
	0	106	52	122	61	228	57
	1	48	24	36	18	84	21
	2	29	14	30	15	59	15
	3	11	5	9	4	20	5
	4	5	2	1	0	6	1
	5	2	1	1	0	3	1
	6	1	0	2	1	3	1
	All	202	100	201	100	403	100
50+	Number of Potential Impairing Medications						
	0	41	52	32	48	73	50
	1	20	25	16	24	36	25
	2	10	13	9	14	19	13
	3	6	8	7	11	13	9
	4			1	2	1	1
	5	1	1	1	2	2	1
	6	1	1			1	1
	All	79	100	66	100	145	100
All Age	Number of Potential Impairing Medications						
	0	147	52	154	58	301	55
	1	68	24	52	19	120	22
	2	39	14	39	15	78	14
	3	17	6	16	6	33	6

Multiple Medications and Vehicle Crashes: Analysis of Databases

Table 4a. (Continued)

		Gender				Both	
		Male		Female			
		N	PCTN	N	PCTN	N	PCTN
All Age	Number of Potential Impairing Medications						
	4	5	2	2	1	7	1
	5	3	1	2	1	5	1
	6	2	1	2	1	4	1
	All	281	100	267	100	548	100

Table 4b. Number of Physician Visits of MVA Patients by Age, Gender, and Number of Potential Driver Impairing Medications

		Gender				Both	
		Male		Female			
		N	PCTN	N	PCTN	N	PCTN
Age Group Under 50	Number of Potential Impairing Medications						
	0	2,984,378	49	3,358,017	56	6,342,395	53
	1	1,350,510	22	1,084,545	18	2,435,055	20
	2	1,028,611	17	999,880	17	2,028,491	17
	3	511,965	8	401,945	7	913,910	8
	4	153,775	3	6,879	0	160,654	1
	5	12,873	0	31,308	1	44,181	0
	6	31,308	1	86,645	1	117,953	1
	All	6,073,420	100	5,969,219	100	12,042,639	100

National Highway Traffic Safety Administration

Table 4b. (Continued)

		Gender				Both	
		Male		Female			
		N	PCTN	N	PCTN	N	PCTN
50+	Number of Potential Impairing Medications						
	0	1,008,577	46	872,853	39	1,881,430	42
	1	532,692	24	686,634	31	1,219,326	27
	2	248,612	11	309,768	14	558,380	13
	3	257,986	12	210,570	9	468,556	11
	4			120,767	5	120,767	3
	5	63,157	3	45,784	2	108,941	2
	6	100,188	5			100,188	2
	All	2,211,212	100	2,246,376	100	4,457,588	100
All Age	Number of Potential Impairing Medications						
	0	3,992,955	48	4,230,870	51	8,223,825	50
	1	1,883,202	23	1,771,179	22	3,654,381	22
	2	1,277,223	15	1,309,648	16	2,586,871	16
	3	769,951	9	612,515	7	1,382,466	8
All Age	Number of Potential Impairing Medications						
	4	153,775	2	127,646	2	281,421	2
	5	76,030	1	77,092	1	153,122	1
	6	131,496	2	86,645	1	218,141	1
	All	8,284,632	100	8,215,595	100	16,500,227	100

Multiple Medications and Vehicle Crashes: Analysis of Databases

Table 5a. Number of Physician Visits of MVA Patients by Age, Gender, and Number of Conflict Medications

		Gender					
		Male		Female		Both	
		N	PCTN	N	PCTN	N	PCTN
Age Group Under 50	Number of Drug-Drug Conflicts						
	0	185	92	193	96	378	94
	1	7	3	3	1	10	2
	2	4	2	1	0	5	1
	3	1	0			1	0
	4	2	1			2	0
	5	1	0	1	0	2	0
	6	2	1	1	0	3	1
	7			1	0	1	0
	10			1	0	1	0
	All	202	100	201	100	403	100
50+	Number of Drug-Drug Conflicts						
	0	75	95	57	86	132	91
	1	2	3	8	12	10	7
	2	2	3			2	1
	4			1	2	1	1
	All	79	100	66	100	145	100
All Age	Number of Drug-Drug Conflicts						
	0	260	93	250	94	510	93
	1	9	3	11	4	20	4
	2	6	2	1	0	7	1
	3	1	0			1	0
	4	2	1	1	0	3	1
	5	1	0	1	0	2	0
	6	2	1	1	0	3	1

Table 5a. (Continued)

		Gender				Both	
		Male		Female			
		N	PCTN	N	PCTN	N	PCTN
All Age	Number of Drug-Drug Conflicts						
	7			1	0	1	0
	10			1	0	1	0
	All	281	100	267	100	548	100

Table 5b. Number of Physician Visits of MVA Patients by Age, Gender, and Number of Conflict Medications (Weighted)

		Gender				Both	
		Male		Female			
		N	PCTN	N	PCTN	N	PCTN
Age Group Under 50	Number of Drug-Drug Conflicts						
	0	5,714,275	94	5,750,312	96	11,464,587	95
	1	155,752	3	27,648	0	183,400	2
	2	119,255	2	12,055	0	131,310	1
	3	16,847	0			16,847	0
	4	43,363	1			43,363	0
	5	7,512	0	14,663	0	22,175	0
	6	16,416	0	71,982	1	88,398	1
	7			31,308	1	31,308	0
	10			61,251	1	61,251	1
	All	6,073,420	100	5,969,219	100	12,042,639	100

Multiple Medications and Vehicle Crashes: Analysis of Databases

Table 5b. (Continued)

| | | Gender | | | | | |
| | | Male | | Female | | Both | |
		N	PCTN	N	PCTN	N	PCTN
50+	Number of Drug-Drug Conflicts						
	0	2,026,019	92	1,797,027	80	3,823,046	86
	1	21,848	1	403,565	18	425,413	10
	2	163,345	7			163,345	4
	4			45,784	2	45,784	1
	All	2,211,212	100	2,246,376	100	4,457,588	100
All Age	Number of Drug-Drug Conflicts						
	0	7,740,294	93	7,547,339	92	15,287,633	93
	1	177,600	2	431,213	5	608,813	4
	2	282,600	3	12,055	0	294,655	2
	3	16,847	0			16,847	0
	4	43,363	1	45,784	1	89,147	1
	5	7,512	0	14,663	0	22,175	0
	6	16,416	0	71,982	1	88,398	1
All Age	Number of Drug-Drug Conflicts						
	7			31,308	0	31,308	0
	10			61,251	1	61,251	0
	All	8,284,632	100	8,215,595	100	16,500,227	100

Table 6a. Number of Physician Visits of MVA Patients by Age, Gender, and Potential Driver Impairing Disease Groups

Gender	Age Group	Disease Group	N	PCTN
Male	Under 50	FRACTURES AND INJURIES	89	66
Male	Under 50	CNS EXCITATION	13	10
Male	Under 50	PSYCHOSES, DRUG INDUCED	7	5
Male	Under 50	DEPRESSION	6	4
Male	Under 50	HEAD TRAUMA	3	2
Male	Under 50	ANXIETY DISORDERS	2	1
Male	Under 50	BIPOLAR DISORDER	2	1
Male	Under 50	SEROTONIN SYNDROME SYMPTOMS	2	1
Male	Under 50	ANKYLOSING SPONDYLITIS	1	1
Male	Under 50	ARTHROPATHIES, OTHER	1	1
Male	Under 50	EPILEPSY	1	1
Male	Under 50	HYPERTHYROIDISM	1	1
Male	Under 50	OBESITY	1	1
Male	Under 50	PANIC DISORDERS	1	1
Male	Under 50	PERSONALITY DISORDERS	1	1
Male	Under 50	SUICIDAL BEHAVIOR	1	1
Male	Under 50	THYROID DISEASE	1	1
Male	Under 50	TUBERCULOSIS	1	1
Male	50+	FRACTURES AND INJURIES	28	42
Male	50+	ANEURYSM	3	4
Male	50+	CARDIOVASCULAR DISEASE	3	4
Male	50+	CNS EXCITATION	3	4
Male	50+	HYPERTENSION	3	4
Male	50+	PERIPHERAL NEUROPATHY	3	4
Male	50+	SEROTONIN SYNDROME SYMPTOMS	3	4
Male	50+	STROKE	3	4
Male	50+	ANKYLOSING SPONDYLITIS	2	3
Male	50+	DEPRESSION	2	3
Male	50+	ARRHYTHMIAS	1	1
Male	50+	ARTHRITIS, RHEUMATOID	1	1
Male	50+	ATRIAL FIBRILLATION	1	1
Male	50+	CNS DEMYELINATING DIS	1	1
Male	50+	DIABETES MELLITUS I AND II	1	1
Male	50+	DYSKINESIAS	1	1
Male	50+	GASTRITIS	1	1
Male	50+	GI HEMORRHAGE	1	1
Male	50+	HYPERLIPIDEMIA-2	1	1
Male	50+	LIPID ABNORMALITIES	1	1
Male	50+	LUPUS	1	1
Male	50+	PSYCHOSES, DRUG INDUCED	1	1

Table 6a. (Continued)

Gender	Age Group	Disease Group	N	PCTN
Male	50+	SYMPTOMS OF GI IRRITATION	1	1
Male	50+	TEST	1	1
Female	Under 50	FRACTURES AND INJURIES	95	70
Female	Under 50	CNS EXCITATION	13	10
Female	Under 50	HEAD TRAUMA	4	3
Female	Under 50	GI HEMORRHAGE	2	1
Female	Under 50	GI ULCER	2	1
Female	Under 50	PSYCHOSES, DRUG INDUCED	2	1
Female	Under 50	ALCOHOLISM	1	1
Female	Under 50	ANXIETY DISORDERS	1	1
Female	Under 50	ARTHROPATHIES, OTHER	1	1
Female	Under 50	BIPOLAR DISORDER	1	1
Female	Under 50	BLEEDING	1	1
Female	Under 50	DEEP VEIN THROMBOSIS	1	1
Female	Under 50	DEPRESSION	1	1
Female	Under 50	DIABETES MELLITUS I AND II	1	1
Female	Under 50	HEMOPTYSIS	1	1
Female	Under 50	HIV	1	1
Female	Under 50	HYPOTHYROIDISM	1	1
Female	Under 50	PERIPHERAL NEUROPATHY	1	1
Female	Under 50	RESPIRATORY INFECTIONS	1	1
Female	Under 50	SEROTONIN SYNDROME SYMPTOMS	1	1
Female	Under 50	STRESS DISORDERS	1	1
Female	Under 50	TEST	1	1
Female	Under 50	THYROID DISEASE	1	1
Female	50+	FRACTURES AND INJURIES	26	50
Female	50+	CNS EXCITATION	4	8
Female	50+	PSYCHOSES, DRUG INDUCED	3	6
Female	50+	CARDIOVASCULAR DISEASE	2	4
Female	50+	SEROTONIN SYNDROME SYMPTOMS	2	4
Female	50+	ALCOHOLISM	1	2
Female	50+	ANKYLOSING SPONDYLITIS	1	2
Female	50+	ANXIETY DISORDERS	1	2
Female	50+	BLEEDING	1	2
Female	50+	CONGESTIVE HEART FAILURE	1	2
Female	50+	COPD	1	2
Female	50+	DEPRESSION	1	2
Female	50+	HEMATURIA	1	2
Female	50+	HYPERSENSITIVITY REACTIONS	1	2
Female	50+	HYPERTENSION	1	2
Female	50+	LACTIC ACIDOSIS SYMPTOMS	1	2
Female	50+	PERIPHERAL NEUROPATHY	1	2

Table 6a. (Continued)

Gender	Age Group	Disease Group	N	PCTN
Female	50+	PERSONALITY DISORDERS	1	2
Female	50+	PSYCHOSES	1	2
Female	50+	SUICIDAL BEHAVIOR	1	2

Table 6b. Number of Physician Visits of MVA Patients by Age, Gender, and Potential Driver Impairing Disease Groups (Weighted)

Gender	Age Group	Disease Group	N	PCTN
Male	Under 50	FRACTURES AND INJURIES	2,887,395	72
Male	Under 50	CNS EXCITATION	491,691	12
Male	Under 50	PSYCHOSES, DRUG INDUCED	140,095	3
Male	Under 50	DEPRESSION	106,312	3
Male	Under 50	HEAD TRAUMA	70,387	2
Male	Under 50	OBESITY	46,733	1
Male	Under 50	TUBERCULOSIS	45,075	1
Male	Under 50	SEROTONIN SYNDROME SYMPTOMS	40,236	1
Male	Under 50	ANXIETY DISORDERS	32,471	1
Male	Under 50	BIPOLAR DISORDER	26,755	1
Male	Under 50	PERSONALITY DISORDERS	25,595	1
Male	Under 50	SUICIDAL BEHAVIOR	25,595	1
Male	Under 50	ARTHROPATHIES, OTHER	19,304	0
Male	Under 50	HYPERTHYROIDISM	17,923	0
Male	Under 50	THYROID DISEASE	17,923	0
Male	Under 50	PANIC DISORDERS	11,055	0
Male	Under 50	ANKYLOSING SPONDYLITIS	7,512	0
Male	Under 50	EPILEPSY	3,842	0
Male	50+	FRACTURES AND INJURIES	790,192	33
Male	50+	CARDIOVASCULAR DISEASE	238,285	10
Male	50+	HYPERTENSION	238,285	10
Male	50+	SEROTONIN SYNDROME SYMPTOMS	238,285	10
Male	50+	PERIPHERAL NEUROPATHY	105,465	4
Male	50+	HYPERLIPIDEMIA-2	100,188	4
Male	50+	LIPID ABNORMALITIES	100,188	4
Male	50+	DIABETES MELLITUS I AND II	78,876	3
Male	50+	TEST	78,876	3
Male	50+	DEPRESSION	69,759	3
Male	50+	LUPUS	59,983	3
Male	50+	ANKYLOSING SPONDYLITIS	55,958	2
Male	50+	CNS EXCITATION	44,304	2
Male	50+	ANEURYSM	42,335	2
Male	50+	STROKE	42,335	2
Male	50+	ARTHRITIS, RHEUMATOID	32,511	1
Male	50+	GASTRITIS	17,104	1
Male	50+	GI HEMORRHAGE	17,104	1

Table 6b. (Continued)

Gender	Age Group	Disease Group	N	PCTN
Male	50+	SYMPTOMS OF GI IRRITATION	17,104	1
Male	50+	PSYCHOSES, DRUG INDUCED	10,538	0
Male	50+	CNS DEMYELINATING DIS	5,786	0
Male	50+	DYSKINESIAS	5,786	0
Male	50+	ARRHYTHMIAS	4,765	0
Male	50+	ATRIAL FIBRILLATION	4,765	0
Female	Under 50	FRACTURES AND INJURIES	3,043,102	71
Female	Under 50	CNS EXCITATION	491,104	12
Female	Under 50	GI HEMORRHAGE	84,694	2
Female	Under 50	GI ULCER	84,694	2
Female	Under 50	HEAD TRAUMA	77,613	2
Female	Under 50	RESPIRATORY INFECTIONS	70,634	2
Female	Under 50	HIV	61,251	1
Female	Under 50	HYPOTHYROIDISM	42,347	1
Female	Under 50	THYROID DISEASE	42,347	1
Female	Under 50	PSYCHOSES, DRUG INDUCED	31,954	1
Female	Under 50	BLEEDING	29,145	1
Female	Under 50	HEMOPTYSIS	29,145	1
Female	Under 50	ARTHROPATHIES, OTHER	28,682	1
Female	Under 50	ANXIETY DISORDERS	21,416	1
Female	Under 50	DIABETES MELLITUS I AND II	20,083	0
Female	Under 50	STRESS DISORDERS	20,083	0
Female	Under 50	TEST	20,083	0
Female	Under 50	PERIPHERAL NEUROPATHY	17,155	0
Female	Under 50	SEROTONIN SYNDROME SYMPTOMS	14,663	0
Female	Under 50	ALCOHOLISM	10,538	0
Female	Under 50	BIPOLAR DISORDER	10,538	0
Female	Under 50	DEPRESSION	10,538	0
Female	Under 50	DEEP VEIN THROMBOSIS	6,027	0
Female	50+	FRACTURES AND INJURIES	780,948	39
Female	50+	CNS EXCITATION	258,496	13
Female	50+	SEROTONIN SYNDROME SYMPTOMS	172,885	9
Female	50+	CARDIOVASCULAR DISEASE	170,526	8
Female	50+	HYPERTENSION	106,606	5
Female	50+	PSYCHOSES, DRUG INDUCED	83,874	4
Female	50+	ALCOHOLISM	63,920	3
Female	50+	CONGESTIVE HEART FAILURE	63,920	3
Female	50+	BLEEDING	53,755	3
Female	50+	HEMATURIA	53,755	3
Female	50+	COPD	45,149	2
Female	50+	PSYCHOSES	43,933	2
Female	50+	ANKYLOSING SPONDYLITIS	36,361	2
Female	50+	ANXIETY DISORDERS	21,416	1
Female	50+	PERSONALITY DISORDERS	18,525	1

Table 6b. (Continued)

Gender	Age Group	Disease Group	N	PCTN
Female	50+	SUICIDAL BEHAVIOR	18,525	1
Female	50+	PERIPHERAL NEUROPATHY	11,788	1
Female	50+	HYPERSENSITIVITY REACTIONS	5,626	0
Female	50+	LACTIC ACIDOSIS SYMPTOMS	5,626	0
Female	50+	DEPRESSION	2,893	0

Table 7a. Number of Physician Visits of MVA Patients by Age, Gender, and Number of Potential Driver Impairing Disease Groups

			Gender				Both	
		Male		Female				
		N	PCTN	N	PCTN	N	PCTN
Age Group	Number of Potential						
Under 50	Impairing Disease Groups						
	0	89	44	91	45	180	45
	1	96	48	92	46	188	47
	2	14	7	13	6	27	7
	3	2	1	3	1	5	1
	4	1	0	2	1	3	1
	All	202	100	201	100	403	100
50+	Number of Potential Impairing Disease Groups						
	0	35	44	28	42	63	43
	1	34	43	28	42	62	43
	2	4	5	7	11	11	8
	3	1	1	2	3	3	2
	4	3	4	1	2	4	3
	5	2	3			2	1
	All	79	100	66	100	145	100
All Age	Number of Potential Impairing Disease Groups						
	0	124	44	119	45	243	44
	1	130	46	120	45	250	46
	2	18	6	20	7	38	7
	3	3	1	5	2	8	1
	4	4	1	3	1	7	1
	5	2	1			2	0
	All	281	100	267	100	548	100

Multiple Medications and Vehicle Crashes: Analysis of Databases

Table 7b. Number of Physician Visits of MVA Patients by Age, Gender, and Number of Potential Driver Impairing Disease Groups (Weighted)

| | | Gender | | | | Both | |
| | | Male | | Female | | | |
		N	PCTN	N	PCTN	N	PCTN
Age Group Under 50	Number of Potential Impairing Disease Groups						
	0	2,593,123	43	2,546,055	43	5,139,178	43
	1	3,003,455	49	2,745,844	46	5,749,299	48
	2	429,137	7	540,589	9	969,726	8
	3	36,650	1	106,110	2	142,760	1
	4	11,055	0	30,621	1	41,676	0
	All	6,073,420	100	5,969,219	100	12,042,639	100
50+	Number of Potential Impairing Disease Groups						
	0	919,305	42	989,177	44	1,908,482	43
	1	917,876	42	791,528	35	1,709,404	38
	2	80,410	4	276,620	12	357,030	8
	3	33,467	2	82,445	4	115,912	3
	4	81,090	4	106,606	5	187,696	4
	5	179,064	8			179,064	4
	All	2,211,212	100	2,246,376	100	4,457,588	100
All Age	Number of Potential Impairing Disease Groups						
	0	3,512,428	42	3,535,232	43	7,047,660	43
	1	3,921,331	47	3,537,372	43	7,458,703	45
	2	509,547	6	817,209	10	1,326,756	8
	3	70,117	1	188,555	2	258,672	2
	4	92,145	1	137,227	2	229,372	1
	5	179,064	2			179,064	1
	All	8,284,632	100	8,215,595	100	16,500,227	100

Table 8a. Number of Physician Visits of MVA Patients by Age, Gender, and Number of Disease-Drug Conflicts

| | | | Gender | | | | | |
| | | | Male | | Female | | Both | |
			N	PCTN	N	PCTN	N	PCTN
Age Group Under 50	Number of Disease-Drug Conflicts	0	201	100	201	100	402	100
		1	1	0			1	0
		All	202	100	201	100	403	100
50+	Number of Disease-Drug Conflicts	0	79	100	66	100	145	100
		All	79	100	66	100	145	100
All Age	Number of Disease-Drug Conflicts	0	280	100	267	100	547	100
		1	1	0			1	0
		All	281	100	267	100	548	100

Table 8b. Number of Physician Visits of MVA Patients by Age, Gender, and Number of Disease-Drug Conflicts (Weighted)

| | | | Gender | | | | | |
| | | | Male | | Female | | Both | |
			N	PCTN	N	PCTN	N	PCTN
Age Group Under 50	Number of Disease-Drug Conflicts	0	6,057,720	100	5,969,219	100	12,026,939	100
		1	15,700	0			15,700	0
		All	6,073,420	100	5,969,219	100	12,042,639	100
50+	Number of Disease-Drug Conflicts	0	2,211,212	100	2,246,376	100	4,457,588	100
		All	2,211,212	100	2,246,376	100	4,457,588	100
All Age	Number of Disease-Drug Conflicts	0	8,268,932	100	8,215,595	100	16,484,527	100
		1	15,700	0			15,700	0
		All	8,284,632	100	8,215,595	100	16,500,227	100

Appendix VII. Nonproprietary Database, Restrict Definition

Table 1a. Number of Patients by Age and Gender Case Group

Age Group	Gender				Both	
	Female		Male			
	N	PCTN	N	PCTN	N	PCTN
Under 50	15,479	84	12,728	83	28,207	84
50+	2,842	16	2,556	17	5,398	16
All Age	18,321	100	15,284	100	33,605	100

Table 1b. Number of Patients by Age and Gender Control Group

Age Group	Gender				Both	
	Female		Male			
	N	PCTN	N	PCTN	N	PCTN
Under 50	46,437	84	38,184	83	84,621	84
50+	8,526	16	7,668	17	16,194	16
All Age	54,963	100	45,852	100	100,815	100

Table 2a. Number of Patients by Age, Gender, and Number of Medications Case Group

		Gender					
		Female		Male		Both	
		N	PCTN	N	PCTN	N	PCTN
Age Group	Number of Medications						
Under 50	0	6,652	43	8,034	63	14,686	52
	1	2,790	18	1,715	13	4,505	16
	2	2,013	13	1,224	10	3,237	11
	3	1,286	8	635	5	1,921	7
	4	890	6	402	3	1,292	5
	5	517	3	257	2	774	3
	6	369	2	144	1	513	2
	7	270	2	95	1	365	1
	8	185	1	60	0	245	1
	9	131	1	42	0	173	1
	10	87	1	34	0	121	0
	11	65	0	18	0	83	0
	12	42	0	21	0	63	0
	13	31	0	11	0	42	0
	14	36	0	11	0	47	0
	15	28	0	6	0	34	0
	16	18	0	6	0	24	0
	17	15	0	1	0	16	0
	18	9	0	2	0	11	0
	19	6	0	1	0	7	0
	20	7	0	2	0	9	0
	21	6	0	3	0	9	0
	22	4	0	2	0	6	0
	23	4	0			4	0
	24	3	0			3	0

Table 2a. (Continued)

| | | Gender | | | | Both | |
| | | Female | | Male | | | |
		N	PCTN	N	PCTN	N	PCTN
Age Group	Number of Medications						
Under 50	25	4	0			4	0
	26	2	0			2	0
	27	1	0			1	0
	28	1	0	1	0	2	0
	29	1	0			1	0
	31	1	0			1	0
	32	2	0			2	0
	34	1	0			1	0
	35	1	0			1	0
	36	1	0			1	0
	37			1	0	1	0
	All	15,479	100	12,728	100	28,207	100
50+	Number of Medications						
	0	638	22	896	35	1,534	28
	1	378	13	367	14	745	14
	2	369	13	331	13	700	13
	3	328	12	231	9	559	10
	4	280	10	195	8	475	9
	5	187	7	125	5	312	6
	6	161	6	91	4	252	5
	7	111	4	84	3	195	4
	8	83	3	53	2	136	3
	9	67	2	52	2	119	2
	10	55	2	26	1	81	2

Table 2a. (Continued)

Age Group	Number of Medications	Gender				Both	
		Female		Male			
		N	PCTN	N	PCTN	N	PCTN
50+	11	30	1	34	1	64	1
	12	26	1	20	1	46	1
	13	32	1	9	0	41	1
	14	25	1	16	1	41	1
	15	15	1	7	0	22	0
	16	10	0	2	0	12	0
	17	10	0	7	0	17	0
	18	5	0	3	0	8	0
	19	7	0	1	0	8	0
	20	4	0	1	0	5	0
	21	5	0	2	0	7	0
	22	3	0			3	0
	23	2	0	2	0	4	0
	24	2	0			2	0
	25	2	0			2	0
	26	1	0	1	0	2	0
	27	1	0			1	0
	28	1	0			1	0
	29	1	0			1	0
	30	1	0			1	0
	32	1	0			1	0
	36	1	0			1	0
	All	2,842	100	2,556	100	5,398	100

Table 2a. (Continued)

| | | Gender | | | | | |
| | | Female | | Male | | Both | |
		N	PCTN	N	PCTN	N	PCTN
All Age	Number of Medications						
	0	7,290	40	8,930	58	16,220	48
	1	3,168	17	2,082	14	5,250	16
	2	2,382	13	1,555	10	3,937	12
	3	1,614	9	866	6	2,480	7
	4	1,170	6	597	4	1,767	5
	5	704	4	382	2	1,086	3
	6	530	3	235	2	765	2
	7	381	2	179	1	560	2
	8	268	1	113	1	381	1
	9	198	1	94	1	292	1
	10	142	1	60	0	202	1
	11	95	1	52	0	147	0
	12	68	0	41	0	109	0
	13	63	0	20	0	83	0
	14	61	0	27	0	88	0
	15	43	0	13	0	56	0
	16	28	0	8	0	36	0
	17	25	0	8	0	33	0
	18	14	0	5	0	19	0
	19	13	0	2	0	15	0
	20	11	0	3	0	14	0
	21	11	0	5	0	16	0
	22	7	0	2	0	9	0
	23	6	0	2	0	8	0
	24	5	0			5	0

Table 2a. (Continued)

		Gender					
		Female		Male		Both	
		N	PCTN	N	PCTN	N	PCTN
All Age	Number of Medications						
	25	6	0			6	0
	26	3	0	1	0	4	0
	27	2	0			2	0
	28	2	0	1	0	3	0
	29	2	0			2	0
	30	1	0			1	0
	31	1	0			1	0
	32	3	0			3	0
	34	1	0			1	0
	35	1	0			1	0
	36	2	0			2	0
	37			1	0	1	0
	All	18,321	100	15,284	100	33,605	100

Table 2b. Number of Patients by Age, Gender, and Number of Medications Control Group

		Gender					
		Female		Male		Both	
		N	PCTN	N	PCTN	N	PCTN
Age Group	Number of Medications						
Under 50	0	25,338	55	26,475	69	51,813	61
	1	8,953	19	5,018	13	13,971	17
	2	5,262	11	3,084	8	8,346	10
	3	2,753	6	1,528	4	4,281	5
	4	1,651	4	855	2	2,506	3
	5	919	2	500	1	1,419	2
	6	540	1	279	1	819	1
	7	349	1	153	0	502	1
	8	216	0	97	0	313	0
	9	139	0	65	0	204	0
	10	119	0	48	0	167	0
	11	65	0	24	0	89	0
	12	27	0	13	0	40	0
	13	24	0	11	0	35	0
	14	23	0	11	0	34	0
	15	9	0	3	0	12	0
	16	16	0	6	0	24	0
	17	7	0	1	0	8	0
	18	5	0	4	0	9	0
	19	8	0	1	0	9	0
	20	3	0	3	0	6	0
	21	4	0	1	0	5	0
	22	1	0	1	0	2	0
	23	1	0	1	0	2	0
	24	2	0			2	0

Multiple Medications and Vehicle Crashes: Analysis of Databases

Table 2b. (Continued)

		Gender				Both	
		Female		Male			
		N	PCTN	N	PCTN	N	PCTN
Age Group	Number of Medications						
Under 50	28			1	0	1	0
	29	1	0			1	0
	34			1	0	1	0
	All	46,437	100	38,184	100	84,621	100
50+	Number of Medications						
	0	2,675	31	3,197	42	5,872	36
	1	1,251	15	1,144	15	2,395	15
	2	1,205	14	999	13	2,204	14
	3	888	10	683	9	1,571	10
	4	676	8	481	6	1,157	7
	5	463	5	332	4	795	5
	6	383	4	239	3	622	4
	7	268	3	169	2	437	3
	8	205	2	122	2	327	2
	9	114	1	95	1	209	1
	10	97	1	47	1	144	1
	11	88	1	40	1	128	1
	12	53	1	34	0	87	1
	13	42	0	29	0	71	0
	14	31	0	15	0	46	0
	15	20	0	12	0	32	0
	16	14	0	6	0	20	0
	17	9	0	8	0	17	0
	18	8	0	4	0	12	0

National Highway Traffic Safety Administration

Table 2b. (Continued)

		Gender				Both	
		Female		Male			
		N	PCTN	N	PCTN	N	PCTN
Age Group	Number of Medications						
50+	19	8	0	4	0	12	0
	20	5	0	3	0	8	0
	21	9	0	1	0	10	0
	22			1	0	1	0
	23	6	0			6	0
	24	3	0	1	0	4	0
	25			1	0	1	0
	26	3	0	1	0	4	0
	27	1	0			1	0
	30	1	0			1	0
	All	8,526	100	7,668	100	16,194	100
All Age	Number of Medications						
	0	28,013	51	29,672	65	57,685	57
	1	10,204	19	6,162	13	16,366	16
	2	6,467	12	4,083	9	10,550	10
	3	3,641	7	2,211	5	5,852	6
	4	2,327	4	1,336	3	3,663	4
	5	1,382	3	832	2	2,214	2
	6	923	2	518	1	1,441	1
	7	617	1	322	1	939	1
	8	421	1	219	0	640	1
	9	253	0	160	0	413	0
	10	216	0	95	0	311	0
	11	153	0	64	0	217	0

Multiple Medications and Vehicle Crashes: Analysis of Databases

Table 2b. (Continued)

| | | Gender | | | | Both | |
| | | Female | | Male | | | |
		N	PCTN	N	PCTN	N	PCTN
All Age	Number of Medications						
	12	80	0	47	0	127	0
	13	66	0	40	0	106	0
	14	54	0	26	0	80	0
	15	29	0	15	0	44	0
	16	32	0	12	0	44	0
	17	16	0	9	0	25	0
	18	13	0	8	0	21	0
	19	16	0	5	0	21	0
	20	8	0	6	0	14	0
	21	13	0	2	0	15	0
	22	1	0	2	0	3	0
	23	7	0	1	0	8	0
	24	5	0	1	0	6	0
	25			1	0	1	0
	26	3	0	1	0	4	0
	27	1	0			1	0
	28			1	0	1	0
	29	1	0			1	0
	30	1	0			1	0
	34			1	0	1	0
	All	54,963	100	45,852	100	100815	100

Table 3a. Number of Patients by Gender, Age Group, and Specific Combinations of Drug Classes

Gender	Age Group	Drug Class 1	Drug Class 2	Drug Class 3	N	PCTN
Female	Under 50	CONTRACEPTIVES,ORAL			658	21
Female	Under 50	PRENATAL VITAMIN PREPARATIONS			214	7
Female	Under 50	SEROTONIN SPECIFIC REUPTAKE INHIBITOR (SSRIS)			211	7
Female	Under 50	ANALGESICS,NARCOTICS			192	6
Female	Under 50	NSAIDS, CYCLOOXYGENASE INHIBITOR - TYPE			152	5
Female	Under 50	PENICILLINS			144	5
Female	Under 50	ANTIHISTAMINES			108	3
Female	Under 50	MACROLIDES			103	3
Female	Under 50	THYROID HORMONES			77	2
Female	Under 50	ESTROGENIC AGENTS			72	2
Female	Under 50	SKELETAL MUSCLE RELAXANTS	NSAIDS, CYCLOOXYGENASE INHIBITOR - TYPE		71	2
Female	Under 50	BETA-ADRENERGIC AGENTS			57	2
Female	Under 50	ABSORBABLE SULFONAMIDES			55	2
Female	Under 50	GASTRIC ACID SECRETION REDUCERS			55	2
Female	Under 50	ANALGESICS,NARCOTICS	NSAIDS, CYCLOOXYGENASE INHIBITOR - TYPE		51	2
Female	Under 50	ANALGESICS,NARCOTICS	PENICILLINS		49	2
Female	Under 50	CEPHALOSPORINS - 1ST GENERATION			48	2
Female	Under 50	TETRACYCLINES			44	1
Female	Under 50	ANTICONVULSANTS			42	1
Female	Under 50	TOPICAL ANTI-INFLAMMATORY STEROIDAL			38	1
Female	Under 50	ANALGESICS,NARCOTICS	SKELETAL MUSCLE RELAXANTS	NSAIDS, CYCLOOXYGENASE INHIBITOR - TYPE	36	1
Female	Under 50	ANTI-ANXIETY DRUGS			36	1

Gender	Age Group	Drug Class 1	Drug Class 2	Drug Class 3	N	PCTN
Female	Under 50	CONTRACEPTIVES,ORAL	SEROTONIN SPECIFIC REUPTAKE INHIBITOR (SSRIS)		36	1
Female	Under 50	SKELETAL MUSCLE RELAXANTS			36	1
Female	Under 50	ANTIFUNGAL AGENTS			34	1
Female	Under 50	TOPICAL ANTIBIOTICS			34	1
Female	Under 50	CONTRACEPTIVES,ORAL	ANTIHISTAMINES		32	1
Female	Under 50	ANTIVIRALS, GENERAL			31	1
Female	Under 50	ANTIMIGRAINE PREPARATIONS			29	1
Female	Under 50	ANALGESICS,NARCOTICS	SKELETAL MUSCLE		28	1
Female	Under 50	EXPECTORANTS			26	1
Female	Under 50	EXPECTORANTS	MACROLIDES		26	1
Female	Under 50	COUGH AND/OR COLD PREPARATIONS			24	1
Female	Under 50	NASAL ANTI-INFLAMMATORY STEROIDS			24	1
Female	Under 50	QUINOLONES			24	1
Female	Under 50	BETA-ADRENERGIC BLOCKING AGENTS			21	1
Female	Under 50	EXPECTORANTS	PENICILLINS		21	1
Female	Under 50	OPHTHALMIC ANTIBIOTICS			21	1
Female	Under 50	NSAIDS, CYCLOOXYGENASE INHIBITOR - TYPE	PENICILLINS		20	1
Female	Under 50	PENICILLINS	ANTIHISTAMINES		20	1
Female	Under 50	GLUCOCORTICOIDS			17	1
Female	Under 50	HYPOTENSIVES, ACE INHIBITORS			16	1
Female	Under 50	SEROTONIN-NOREPINEPHRINE REUPTAKE-INHIB (SNRIS)			16	1
Female	Under 50	LIPOTROPICS			14	0
Female	Under 50	NASAL ANTI-INFLAMMATORY STEROIDS	ANTIHISTAMINES		14	0
Female	Under 50	TOPICAL ANTIFUNGALS			13	0

Table 3a. (Continued)

Gender	Age Group	Drug Class 1	Drug Class 2	Drug Class 3	N	PCTN
Female	Under 50	INSULINS			11	0
Female	Under 50	CALCIUM CHANNEL BLOCKING AGENTS			10	0
Female	Under 50	ANALGESICS,NARCOTICS	CEPHALOSPORINS - 1ST GENERATION		8	0
Female	Under 50	ANTI-NARCOLEPSY/ANTI-HYPERKINESIS, STIMULANT-TYPE			6	0
Female	50+	ESTROGENIC AGENTS			94	25
Female	50+	NSAIDS, CYCLOOXYGENASE INHIBITOR - TYPE			23	6
Female	50+	THYROID HORMONES			23	6
Female	50+	ANALGESICS,NARCOTICS			22	6
Female	50+	LIPOTROPICS			21	6
Female	50+	CALCIUM CHANNEL BLOCKING AGENTS			18	5
Female	50+	HYPOTENSIVES, ACE INHIBITORS			17	5
Female	50+	GASTRIC ACID SECRETION REDUCERS			14	4
Female	50+	SEROTONIN SPECIFIC REUPTAKE INHIBITOR (SSRIS)			12	3
Female	50+	ANTIHISTAMINES			9	2
Female	50+	ANALGESICS,NARCOTICS	NSAIDS, CYCLOOXYGENASE INHIBITOR - TYPE		8	2
Female	50+	ANTI-ANXIETY DRUGS			8	2
Female	50+	ANTICONVULSANTS			8	2
Female	50+	ANALGESICS,NARCOTICS	SKELETAL MUSCLE		6	2
Female	50+	ANALGESICS,NARCOTICS	SKELETAL MUSCLE RELAXANTS	NSAIDS, CYCLOOXYGENASE INHIBITOR - TYPE	6	2
Female	50+	EXPECTORANTS			6	2
Female	50+	SKELETAL MUSCLE RELAXANTS			6	2
Female	50+	TOPICAL ANTI-INFLAMMATORY STEROIDAL			6	2

Gender	Age Group	Drug Class 1	Drug Class 2	Drug Class 3	N	PCTN
Female	50+	CEPHALOSPORINS - 1ST GENERATION			5	1
Female	50+	GLUCOCORTICOIDS			5	1
Female	50+	QUINOLONES			5	1
Female	50+	TOPICAL ANTIFUNGALS			5	1
Female	50+	BETA-ADRENERGIC BLOCKING AGENTS			4	1
Female	50+	CONTRACEPTIVES,ORAL			4	1
Female	50+	OPHTHALMIC ANTIBIOTICS			4	1
Female	50+	ANALGESICS,NARCOTICS	CEPHALOSPORINS - 1ST GENERATION		3	1
Female	50+	ANTIFUNGAL AGENTS			3	1
Female	50+	ANTIMIGRAINE PREPARATIONS			3	1
Female	50+	BETA-ADRENERGIC AGENTS			3	1
Female	50+	MACROLIDES			3	1
Female	50+	PENICILLINS			3	1
Female	50+	SKELETAL MUSCLE RELAXANTS	NSAIDS, CYCLOOXYGENASE INHIBITOR - TYPE		3	1
Female	50+	ANTIVIRALS, GENERAL			2	1
Female	50+	COUGH AND/OR COLD PREPARATIONS			2	1
Female	50+	INSULINS			2	1
Female	50+	ABSORBABLE SULFONAMIDES			1	0
Female	50+	ANALGESICS,NARCOTICS	PENICILLINS		1	0
Female	50+	NASAL ANTI-INFLAMMATORY STEROIDS			1	0
Female	50+	NSAIDS, CYCLOOXYGENASE INHIBITOR - TYPE	PENICILLINS		1	0
Female	50+	SEROTONIN-NOREPINEPHRINE REUPTAKE-INHIB (SNRIS)			1	0
Female	50+	TETRACYCLINES			1	0
Male	Under 50	ANALGESICS,NARCOTICS			251	13

Gender	Age Group	Drug Class 1	Drug Class 2	Drug Class 3	N	PCTN
Male	Under 50	NSAIDS, CYCLOOXYGENASE INHIBITOR - TYPE			138	7
Male	Under 50	PENICILLINS			119	6
Male	Under 50	SEROTONIN SPECIFIC REUPTAKE INHIBITOR (SSRIS)			117	6
Male	Under 50	ANTIHISTAMINES			103	5
Male	Under 50	GASTRIC ACID SECRETION REDUCERS			86	4
Male	Under 50	MACROLIDES			75	4
Male	Under 50	ANALGESICS,NARCOTICS	NSAIDS, CYCLOOXYGENASE INHIBITOR - TYPE		63	3
Male	Under 50	CEPHALOSPORINS - 1ST GENERATION			61	3
Male	Under 50	ANTICONVULSANTS			59	3
Male	Under 50	TETRACYCLINES			57	3
Male	Under 50	ANALGESICS,NARCOTICS	PENICILLINS		50	3
Male	Under 50	BETA-ADRENERGIC AGENTS			50	3
Male	Under 50	ANALGESICS,NARCOTICS	SKELETAL MUSCLE		49	2
Male	Under 50	SKELETAL MUSCLE RELAXANTS	NSAIDS, CYCLOOXYGENASE INHIBITOR - TYPE		38	2
Male	Under 50	BETA-ADRENERGIC BLOCKING AGENTS			35	2
Male	Under 50	HYPOTENSIVES, ACE INHIBITORS			34	2
Male	Under 50	SKELETAL MUSCLE RELAXANTS			34	2
Male	Under 50	TOPICAL ANTI-INFLAMMATORY STEROIDAL			34	2
Male	Under 50	ANTI-NARCOLEPSY/ANTI-HYPERKINESIS, STIMULANT-TYPE			32	2
Male	Under 50	LIPOTROPICS			28	1
Male	Under 50	ANALGESICS,NARCOTICS	SKELETAL MUSCLE RELAXANTS	NSAIDS, CYCLOOXYGENASE INHIBITOR - TYPE	27	1
Male	Under 50	ANTI-ANXIETY DRUGS			27	1

Gender	Age Group	Drug Class 1	Drug Class 2	Drug Class 3	N	PCTN
Male	Under 50	TOPICAL ANTIBIOTICS			27	1
Male	Under 50	ANALGESICS,NARCOTICS	CEPHALOSPORINS - 1ST GENERATION		26	1
Male	Under 50	QUINOLONES			26	1
Male	Under 50	THYROID HORMONES			26	1
Male	Under 50	GLUCOCORTICOIDS			25	1
Male	Under 50	EXPECTORANTS			23	1
Male	Under 50	EXPECTORANTS	PENICILLINS		22	1
Male	Under 50	TOPICAL ANTIFUNGALS			22	1
Male	Under 50	EXPECTORANTS	MACROLIDES		21	1
Male	Under 50	ABSORBABLE SULFONAMIDES			19	1
Male	Under 50	ANTIVIRALS, GENERAL			19	1
Male	Under 50	INSULINS			18	1
Male	Under 50	NSAIDS, CYCLOOXYGENASE INHIBITOR - TYPE	PENICILLINS		18	1
Male	Under 50	OPHTHALMIC ANTIBIOTICS			18	1
Male	Under 50	NASAL ANTI-INFLAMMATORY STEROIDS	ANTIHISTAMINES		17	1
Male	Under 50	CALCIUM CHANNEL BLOCKING AGENTS			15	1
Male	Under 50	SEROTONIN-NOREPINEPHRINE REUPTAKE-INHIB (SNRIS)			14	1
Male	Under 50	PENICILLINS	ANTIHISTAMINES		13	1
Male	Under 50	NASAL ANTI-INFLAMMATORY STEROIDS			12	1
Male	Under 50	COUGH AND/OR COLD PREPARATIONS			11	1
Male	Under 50	ANTIFUNGAL AGENTS			10	1
Male	Under 50	ANTIMIGRAINE PREPARATIONS			7	0
Male	Under 50	CONTRACEPTIVES,ORAL			5	0

Gender	Age Group	Drug Class 1	Drug Class 2	Drug Class 3	N	PCTN
Male	Under 50	CONTRACEPTIVES,ORAL	SEROTONIN SPECIFIC REUPTAKE INHIBITOR (SSRIS)		1	0
Male	50+	LIPOTROPICS			45	12
Male	50+	HYPOTENSIVES, ACE INHIBITORS			34	9
Male	50+	ANALGESICS,NARCOTICS			31	8
Male	50+	NSAIDS, CYCLOOXYGENASE INHIBITOR - TYPE			31	8
Male	50+	GASTRIC ACID SECRETION REDUCERS			27	7
Male	50+	SEROTONIN SPECIFIC REUPTAKE INHIBITOR (SSRIS)			17	5
Male	50+	CALCIUM CHANNEL BLOCKING AGENTS			16	4
Male	50+	ANTIHISTAMINES			13	4
Male	50+	BETA-ADRENERGIC BLOCKING AGENTS			12	3
Male	50+	TOPICAL ANTI-INFLAMMATORY STEROIDAL			11	3
Male	50+	ANALGESICS,NARCOTICS	NSAIDS, CYCLOOXYGENASE INHIBITOR - TYPE		8	2
Male	50+	ANALGESICS,NARCOTICS	PENICILLINS		8	2
Male	50+	MACROLIDES			8	2
Male	50+	ANTI-ANXIETY DRUGS			7	2
Male	50+	ANTICONVULSANTS			7	2
Male	50+	GLUCOCORTICOIDS			7	2
Male	50+	INSULINS			7	2
Male	50+	NASAL ANTI-INFLAMMATORY STEROIDS	ANTIHISTAMINES		6	2
Male	50+	PENICILLINS			6	2
Male	50+	TETRACYCLINES			6	2
Male	50+	THYROID HORMONES			6	2

Gender	Age Group	Drug Class 1	Drug Class 2	Drug Class 3	N	PCTN
Male	50+	NASAL ANTI-INFLAMMATORY STEROIDS			5	1
Male	50+	OPHTHALMIC ANTIBIOTICS			5	1
Male	50+	SKELETAL MUSCLE RELAXANTS			5	1
Male	50+	ANALGESICS,NARCOTICS	SKELETAL MUSCLE RELAXANTS	NSAIDS, CYCLOOXYGENASE INHIBITOR - TYPE	4	1
Male	50+	ANTIFUNGAL AGENTS			4	1
Male	50+	SKELETAL MUSCLE RELAXANTS	NSAIDS, CYCLOOXYGENASE INHIBITOR - TYPE		4	1
Male	50+	TOPICAL ANTIFUNGALS			4	1
Male	50+	BETA-ADRENERGIC AGENTS			3	1
Male	50+	EXPECTORANTS			3	1
Male	50+	EXPECTORANTS	MACROLIDES		3	1
Male	50+	QUINOLONES			3	1
Male	50+	SEROTONIN-NOREPINEPHRINE REUPTAKE-INHIB (SNRIS)			3	1
Male	50+	COUGH AND/OR COLD PREPARATIONS			2	1
Male	50+	ESTROGENIC AGENTS			2	1
Male	50+	PENICILLINS	ANTIHISTAMINES		2	1
Male	50+	ABSORBABLE SULFONAMIDES			1	0
Male	50+	ANALGESICS,NARCOTICS	SKELETAL MUSCLE		1	0
Male	50+	ANTIMIGRAINE PREPARATIONS			1	0
Male	50+	ANTIVIRALS, GENERAL			1	0
Male	50+	CEPHALOSPORINS - 1ST GENERATION			1	0
Male	50+	EXPECTORANTS	PENICILLINS		1	0

Table 3b. Number of Patients by Gender, Age Group, and Specific Combinations of Drug Classes

Gender	Age Group	Drug Class 1	Drug Class 2	N	PCTN
Female	Under 50	CONTRACEPTIVES,ORAL		3,011	31
Female	Under 50	SEROTONIN SPECIFIC REUPTAKE INHIBITOR (SSRIS)		626	7
Female	Under 50	PENICILLINS		551	6
Female	Under 50	PRENATAL VITAMIN PREPARATIONS		494	5
Female	Under 50	ANTIHISTAMINES		391	4
Female	Under 50	THYROID HORMONES		309	3
Female	Under 50	NSAIDS, CYCLOOXYGENASE INHIBITOR - TYPE		299	3
Female	Under 50	ANALGESICS,NARCOTICS		293	3
Female	Under 50	MACROLIDES		286	3
Female	Under 50	TETRACYCLINES		192	2
Female	Under 50	ESTROGENIC AGENTS		176	2
Female	Under 50	GASTRIC ACID SECRETION REDUCERS		156	2
Female	Under 50	ABSORBABLE SULFONAMIDES		150	2
Female	Under 50	TOPICAL ANTI-INFLAMMATORY STEROIDAL		141	1
Female	Under 50	TOPICAL ANTIBIOTICS		134	1
Female	Under 50	BETA-ADRENERGIC AGENTS		130	1
Female	Under 50	CEPHALOSPORINS - 1ST GENERATION		119	1
Female	Under 50	CONTRACEPTIVES,ORAL	SEROTONIN SPECIFIC REUPTAKE INHIBITOR	116	1
Female	Under 50	ANALGESICS,NARCOTICS	PENICILLINS	113	1
Female	Under 50	CONTRACEPTIVES,ORAL	ANTIHISTAMINES	106	1
Female	Under 50	ANTIMIGRAINE PREPARATIONS		90	1
Female	Under 50	ANTI-ANXIETY DRUGS		89	1

Gender	Age Group	Drug Class 1	Drug Class 2	N	PCTN
Female	Under 50	BETA-ADRENERGIC BLOCKING AGENTS		86	1
Female	Under 50	ANTIFUNGAL AGENTS		81	1
Female	Under 50	QUINOLONES		81	1
Female	Under 50	NASAL ANTI-INFLAMMATORY STEROIDS	ANTIHISTAMINES	79	1
Female	Under 50	EXPECTORANTS		77	1
Female	Under 50	ANTIVIRALS, GENERAL		76	1
Female	Under 50	NASAL ANTI-INFLAMMATORY STEROIDS		76	1
Female	Under 50	ANTICONVULSANTS		75	1
Female	Under 50	OPHTHALMIC ANTIBIOTICS		72	1
Female	Under 50	EXPECTORANTS	MACROLIDES	71	1
Female	Under 50	NOREPINEPHRINE AND DOPAMINE REUPTAKE INHIB (NDRIS)		64	1
Female	Under 50	GLUCOCORTICOIDS		63	1
Female	Under 50	HYPOTENSIVES, ACE INHIBITORS		63	1
Female	Under 50	ANALGESICS,NARCOTICS	NSAIDS, CYCLOOXYGENASE INHIBITOR - TY	60	1
Female	Under 50	TRICYCLIC ANTIDEPRESSANTS & REL. NON-SEL. RU-INHIB		56	1
Female	Under 50	TOPICAL ANTIFUNGALS		53	1
Female	Under 50	VITAMIN A DERIVATIVES		52	1
Female	Under 50	SKELETAL MUSCLE RELAXANTS		50	1
Female	Under 50	CEPHALOSPORINS - 2ND GENERATION		49	1
Female	Under 50	VITAMIN A DERIVATIVES	TETRACYCLINES	49	1
Female	Under 50	BETA-ADRENERGIC AGENTS	GLUCOCORTICOIDS	47	0
Female	Under 50	CALCIUM CHANNEL BLOCKING AGENTS		45	0
Female	Under 50	EXPECTORANTS	PENICILLINS	45	0

Table 3b. (Continued)

Gender	Age Group	Drug Class 1	Drug Class 2	N	PCTN
Female	Under 50	PENICILLINS	ANTIHISTAMINES	44	0
Female	Under 50	LIPOTROPICS		41	0
Female	Under 50	SKELETAL MUSCLE RELAXANTS	NSAIDS, CYCLOOXYGENASE INHIBITOR - TY	35	0
Female	Under 50	ANTI-NARCOLEPSY/ANTI-HYPERKINESIS, STIMULANT-TYPE		25	0
Female	Under 50	ESTROGENIC AGENTS	PROGESTATIONAL AGENTS	24	0
Female	50+	ESTROGENIC AGENTS		417	32
Female	50+	THYROID HORMONES		79	6
Female	50+	ESTROGENIC AGENTS	PROGESTATIONAL AGENTS	73	6
Female	50+	NSAIDS, CYCLOOXYGENASE INHIBITOR - TYPE		68	5
Female	50+	HYPOTENSIVES, ACE INHIBITORS		59	5
Female	50+	LIPOTROPICS		56	4
Female	50+	SEROTONIN SPECIFIC REUPTAKE INHIBITOR (SSRIS)		56	4
Female	50+	BETA-ADRENERGIC BLOCKING AGENTS		51	4
Female	50+	ANTIHISTAMINES		46	4
Female	50+	PENICILLINS		35	3
Female	50+	CALCIUM CHANNEL BLOCKING AGENTS		33	3
Female	50+	GASTRIC ACID SECRETION REDUCERS		32	2
Female	50+	ANALGESICS,NARCOTICS		26	2
Female	50+	ANTI-ANXIETY DRUGS		18	1
Female	50+	ANTIMIGRAINE PREPARATIONS		17	1
Female	50+	QUINOLONES		17	1
Female	50+	MACROLIDES		16	1
Female	50+	NASAL ANTI-INFLAMMATORY STEROIDS		16	1

Gender	Age Group	Drug Class 1	Drug Class 2	N	PCTN
Female	50+	CONTRACEPTIVES,ORAL		14	1
Female	50+	TOPICAL ANTI-INFLAMMATORY STEROIDAL		14	1
Female	50+	GLUCOCORTICOIDS		12	1
Female	50+	ANTICONVULSANTS		11	1
Female	50+	ABSORBABLE SULFONAMIDES		9	1
Female	50+	BETA-ADRENERGIC AGENTS		9	1
Female	50+	SKELETAL MUSCLE RELAXANTS		9	1
Female	50+	CEPHALOSPORINS - 1ST GENERATION		8	1
Female	50+	EXPECTORANTS	MACROLIDES	8	1
Female	50+	NASAL ANTI-INFLAMMATORY STEROIDS	ANTIHISTAMINES	8	1
Female	50+	BETA-ADRENERGIC AGENTS	GLUCOCORTICOIDS	7	1
Female	50+	ANALGESICS,NARCOTICS	NSAIDS, CYCLOOXYGENASE INHIBITOR - TY	6	0
Female	50+	OPHTHALMIC ANTIBIOTICS		6	0
Female	50+	TOPICAL ANTIFUNGALS		6	0
Female	50+	TRICYCLIC ANTIDEPRESSANTS & REL. NON-SEL. RU-INHIB		6	0
Female	50+	EXPECTORANTS		5	0
Female	50+	NOREPINEPHRINE AND DOPAMINE REUPTAKE INHIB (NDRIS)		5	0
Female	50+	TOPICAL ANTIBIOTICS		5	0
Female	50+	ANTIFUNGAL AGENTS		4	0
Female	50+	PENICILLINS	ANTIHISTAMINES	4	0
Female	50+	SKELETAL MUSCLE RELAXANTS	NSAIDS, CYCLOOXYGENASE INHIBITOR - TY	4	0
Female	50+	TETRACYCLINES		4	0

Gender	Age Group	Drug Class 1	Drug Class 2	N	PCTN
Female	50+	ANTIVIRALS, GENERAL		3	0
Female	50+	CEPHALOSPORINS - 2ND GENERATION		3	0
Female	50+	CONTRACEPTIVES,ORAL	ANTIHISTAMINES	3	0
Female	50+	ANALGESICS,NARCOTICS	PENICILLINS	2	0
Female	50+	EXPECTORANTS	PENICILLINS	2	0
Female	50+	ANTI-NARCOLEPSY/ANTI-HYPERKINESIS, STIMULANT-TYPE		1	0
Male	Under 50	PENICILLINS		451	8
Male	Under 50	ANTIHISTAMINES		377	7
Male	Under 50	ANALGESICS,NARCOTICS		325	6
Male	Under 50	NSAIDS, CYCLOOXYGENASE INHIBITOR - TYPE		302	6
Male	Under 50	SEROTONIN SPECIFIC REUPTAKE INHIBITOR (SSRIS)		282	5
Male	Under 50	GASTRIC ACID SECRETION REDUCERS		270	5
Male	Under 50	TETRACYCLINES		262	5
Male	Under 50	MACROLIDES		236	4
Male	Under 50	LIPOTROPICS		182	3
Male	Under 50	BETA-ADRENERGIC AGENTS		174	3
Male	Under 50	ANTICONVULSANTS		151	3
Male	Under 50	TOPICAL ANTI-INFLAMMATORY STEROIDAL		138	3
Male	Under 50	HYPOTENSIVES, ACE INHIBITORS		123	2
Male	Under 50	CEPHALOSPORINS - 1ST GENERATION		122	2
Male	Under 50	NASAL ANTI-INFLAMMATORY STEROIDS		107	2
Male	Under 50	ANALGESICS,NARCOTICS	PENICILLINS	104	2
Male	Under 50	TOPICAL ANTIBIOTICS		96	2

Gender	Age Group	Drug Class 1	Drug Class 2	N	PCTN
Male	Under 50	BETA-ADRENERGIC BLOCKING AGENTS		95	2
Male	Under 50	TOPICAL ANTIFUNGALS		94	2
Male	Under 50	THYROID HORMONES		90	2
Male	Under 50	NASAL ANTI-INFLAMMATORY STEROIDS	ANTIHISTAMINES	88	2
Male	Under 50	ANTI-NARCOLEPSY/ANTI-HYPERKINESIS, STIMULANT-TYPE		87	2
Male	Under 50	GLUCOCORTICOIDS		79	1
Male	Under 50	NOREPINEPHRINE AND DOPAMINE REUPTAKE INHIB (NDRIS)		78	1
Male	Under 50	VITAMIN A DERIVATIVES	TETRACYCLINES	73	1
Male	Under 50	ANTIVIRALS, GENERAL		72	1
Male	Under 50	ANALGESICS,NARCOTICS	NSAIDS, CYCLOOXYGENASE INHIBITOR - TY	70	1
Male	Under 50	EXPECTORANTS	MACROLIDES	68	1
Male	Under 50	ABSORBABLE SULFONAMIDES		66	1
Male	Under 50	OPHTHALMIC ANTIBIOTICS		66	1
Male	Under 50	QUINOLONES		64	1
Male	Under 50	CALCIUM CHANNEL BLOCKING AGENTS		59	1
Male	Under 50	EXPECTORANTS		55	1
Male	Under 50	BETA-ADRENERGIC AGENTS	GLUCOCORTICOIDS	50	1
Male	Under 50	VITAMIN A DERIVATIVES		49	1
Male	Under 50	ANTIMIGRAINE PREPARATIONS		47	1
Male	Under 50	SKELETAL MUSCLE RELAXANTS	NSAIDS, CYCLOOXYGENASE INHIBITOR - TY	45	1
Male	Under 50	ANTI-ANXIETY DRUGS		42	1
Male	Under 50	CONTRACEPTIVES,ORAL		41	1

Table 3b. (Continued)

Gender	Age Group	Drug Class 1	Drug Class 2	N	PCTN
Male	Under 50	PENICILLINS	ANTIHISTAMINES	39	1
Male	Under 50	EXPECTORANTS	PENICILLINS	38	1
Male	Under 50	ANTIFUNGAL AGENTS		37	1
Male	Under 50	CEPHALOSPORINS - 2ND GENERATION		35	1
Male	Under 50	SKELETAL MUSCLE RELAXANTS		30	1
Male	Under 50	TRICYCLIC ANTIDEPRESSANTS & REL. NON-SEL. RU-INHIB		28	1
Male	Under 50	PRENATAL VITAMIN PREPARATIONS		10	0
Male	Under 50	ESTROGENIC AGENTS		4	0
Male	Under 50	CONTRACEPTIVES,ORAL	ANTIHISTAMINES	2	0
Male	Under 50	CONTRACEPTIVES,ORAL	SEROTONIN SPECIFIC REUPTAKE INHIBITOR	2	0
Male	50+	LIPOTROPICS		169	16
Male	50+	HYPOTENSIVES, ACE INHIBITORS		107	10
Male	50+	GASTRIC ACID SECRETION REDUCERS		79	8
Male	50+	NSAIDS, CYCLOOXYGENASE INHIBITOR - TYPE		71	7
Male	50+	BETA-ADRENERGIC BLOCKING AGENTS		69	7
Male	50+	CALCIUM CHANNEL BLOCKING AGENTS		55	5
Male	50+	PENICILLINS		45	4
Male	50+	ANALGESICS,NARCOTICS		35	3
Male	50+	SEROTONIN SPECIFIC REUPTAKE INHIBITOR (SSRIS)		34	3
Male	50+	TOPICAL ANTI-INFLAMMATORY STEROIDAL		31	3
Male	50+	THYROID HORMONES		30	3
Male	50+	ANTIHISTAMINES		28	3
Male	50+	TOPICAL ANTIFUNGALS		19	2

Gender	Age Group	Drug Class 1	Drug Class 2	N	PCTN
Male	50+	MACROLIDES		18	2
Male	50+	NASAL ANTI-INFLAMMATORY STEROIDS		17	2
Male	50+	ANTICONVULSANTS		16	2
Male	50+	BETA-ADRENERGIC AGENTS		16	2
Male	50+	ANTI-ANXIETY DRUGS		14	1
Male	50+	CEPHALOSPORINS - 1ST GENERATION		13	1
Male	50+	QUINOLONES		13	1
Male	50+	ANALGESICS,NARCOTICS	NSAIDS, CYCLOOXYGENASE INHIBITOR - TY	12	1
Male	50+	ANALGESICS,NARCOTICS	PENICILLINS	11	1
Male	50+	EXPECTORANTS		10	1
Male	50+	EXPECTORANTS	MACROLIDES	10	1
Male	50+	GLUCOCORTICOIDS		10	1
Male	50+	NOREPINEPHRINE AND DOPAMINE REUPTAKE INHIB (NDRIS)		10	1
Male	50+	TRICYCLIC ANTIDEPRESSANTS & REL. NON-SEL. RU-INHIB		10	1
Male	50+	ABSORBABLE SULFONAMIDES		9	1
Male	50+	BETA-ADRENERGIC AGENTS	GLUCOCORTICOIDS	9	1
Male	50+	TETRACYCLINES		9	1
Male	50+	SKELETAL MUSCLE RELAXANTS	NSAIDS, CYCLOOXYGENASE INHIBITOR - TY	8	1
Male	50+	ANTIFUNGAL AGENTS		7	1
Male	50+	ANTIVIRALS, GENERAL		7	1
Male	50+	ESTROGENIC AGENTS		5	0
Male	50+	PENICILLINS	ANTIHISTAMINES	5	0

Table 3b. (Continued)

Gender	Age Group	Drug Class 1	Drug Class 2	N	PCTN
Male	50+	CEPHALOSPORINS - 2ND GENERATION		3	0
Male	50+	NASAL ANTI-INFLAMMATORY STEROIDS	ANTIHISTAMINES	3	0
Male	50+	OPHTHALMIC ANTIBIOTICS		3	0
Male	50+	SKELETAL MUSCLE RELAXANTS		3	0
Male	50+	ANTI-NARCOLEPSY/ANTI-HYPERKINESIS, STIMULANT-TYPE		2	0
Male	50+	ANTIMIGRAINE PREPARATIONS		2	0
Male	50+	ESTROGENIC AGENTS	PROGESTATIONAL AGENTS	2	0
Male	50+	EXPECTORANTS	PENICILLINS	2	0
Male	50+	CONTRACEPTIVES,ORAL		1	0
Male	50+	TOPICAL ANTIBIOTICS		1	0

Table 4a. Number of Patients by Age, Gender, and Number of Driver Impairing Medications Case Group

			Gender				Both	
		Female		Male				
		N	PCTN	N	PCTN	N	PCTN
Age Group	Number of Potential Impairing Medications						
Under 50							
	0	9,244	60	8,966	70	18,210	65
	1	2,872	19	2,015	16	4,887	17
	2	1,555	10	933	7	2,488	9
	3	791	5	411	3	1,202	4
	4	435	3	191	2	626	2
	5	237	2	107	1	344	1
	6	143	1	48	0	191	1
	7	89	1	20	0	109	0
	8	48	0	14	0	62	0
	9	23	0	11	0	34	0
	10	17	0	6	0	23	0
	11	11	0	4	0	15	0
	12	7	0	1	0	8	0
	13	4	0	1	0	5	0
	14	1	0			1	0
	18	1	0			1	0
	19	1	0			1	0
	All	15,479	100	12,728	100	28,207	100
50+	Number of Potential Impairing Medications						
	0	922	32	1,019	40	1,941	36
	1	556	20	515	20	1,071	20
	2	441	16	353	14	794	15

Table 4a. (Continued)

		Gender				Both	
		Female		Male			
		N	PCTN	N	PCTN	N	PCTN
Age Group 50+	Number of Potential Impairing Medications						
	3	333	12	244	10	577	11
	4	221	8	159	6	380	7
	5	149	5	110	4	259	5
	6	77	3	62	2	139	3
	7	63	2	43	2	106	2
	8	25	1	26	1	51	1
	9	24	1	12	0	36	1
	10	13	0	8	0	21	0
	11	6	0	4	0	10	0
	12	5	0			5	0
	13	3	0			3	0
	14	3	0			3	0
	15	1	0			1	0
	18			1	0	1	0
	All	2,842	100	2,556	100	5,398	100
All Age	Number of Potential Impairing Medications						
	0	10,166	55	9,985	65	20,151	60
	1	3,428	19	2,530	17	5,958	18
	2	1,996	11	1,286	8	3,282	10
	3	1,124	6	655	4	1,779	5
	4	656	4	350	2	1,006	3
	5	386	2	217	1	603	2

Table 4a. (Continued)

| | | Gender | | | | | |
| | | Female | | Male | | Both | |
		N	PCTN	N	PCTN	N	PCTN
All Age	Number of Potential Impairing Medications						
	6	220	1	110	1	330	1
	7	152	1	63	0	215	1
	8	73	0	40	0	113	0
	9	47	0	23	0	70	0
	10	30	0	14	0	44	0
	11	17	0	8	0	25	0
	12	12	0	1	0	13	0
	13	7	0	1	0	8	0
	14	4	0			4	0
	15	1	0			1	0
	18	1	0	1	0	2	0
	19	1	0			1	0
	All	18,321	100	15,284	100	33,605	100

Table 4b. Number of Patients by Age, Gender, and Number of Driver Impairing Medications Control Group

| | | Gender | | | | | |
| | | Female | | Male | | Both | |
		N	PCTN	N	PCTN	N	PCTN
Age Group Under 50	Number of Potential Impairing Medications						
	0	34,107	73	29,833	78	63,940	76
	1	7,432	16	5,270	14	12,702	15
	2	2,858	6	1,834	5	4,692	6
	3	1,134	2	754	2	1,888	2
	4	471	1	258	1	729	1
	5	218	0	135	0	353	0
	6	114	0	52	0	166	0
	7	59	0	27	0	86	0
	8	18	0	12	0	30	0
	9	15	0	6	0	21	0
	10	3	0	1	0	4	0
	11	5	0	1	0	6	0
	12	1	0	1	0	2	0
	13	2	0			2	0
	All	46,437	100	38,184	100	84,621	100

Table 4b. (Continued)

		Gender				Both	
		Female		Male			
		N	PCTN	N	PCTN	N	PCTN
50+	Number of Potential Impairing Medications						
	0	3,755	44	3,617	47	7,372	46
	1	1,720	20	1,513	20	3,233	20
	2	1,204	14	1,068	14	2,272	14
	3	783	9	622	8	1,405	9
	4	424	5	382	5	806	5
	5	267	3	210	3	477	3
Age Group 50+	Number of Potential Impairing Medications						
	6	151	2	114	1	265	2
	7	100	1	70	1	170	1
	8	51	1	38	0	89	1
	9	34	0	17	0	51	0
	10	20	0	4	0	24	0
	11	12	0	6	0	18	0
	12	3	0	4	0	7	0
	13	1	0	1	0	2	0
	15	1	0	1	0	2	0
	18			1	0	1	0
	All	8,526	100	7,668	100	16,194	100
All Age	Number of Potential Impairing Medications						
	0	37,862	69	33,450	73	71,312	71
	1	9,152	17	6,783	15	15,935	16
	2	4,062	7	2,902	6	6,964	7
	3	1,917	3	1,376	3	3,293	3
	4	895	2	640	1	1,535	2
	5	485	1	345	1	830	1
	6	265	0	166	0	431	0
	7	159	0	97	0	256	0
	8	69	0	50	0	119	0
	9	49	0	23	0	72	0

Table 4b. (Continued)

		Gender					
		Female		Male		Both	
		N	PCTN	N	PCTN	N	PCTN
All Age	Number of Potential Impairing Medications						
	10	23	0	5	0	28	0
	11	17	0	7	0	24	0
	12	4	0	5	0	9	0
	13	3	0	1	0	4	0
	15	1	0	1	0	2	0
	18			1	0	1	0
	All	54,963	100	45,852	100	100815	100

Table 5a. Number of Patients by Age, Gender, and Number of Drug-Drug Conflicts
Case Group

		Gender					
		Female		Male		Both	
		N	PCTN	N	PCTN	N	PCTN
Age Group	Number of Drug Drug Conflicts						
Under 50	0	13,900	90	11,992	94	25,892	92
	1	833	5	452	4	1,285	5
	2	274	2	120	1	394	1
	3	192	1	68	1	260	1
	4	80	1	27	0	107	0
	5	61	0	20	0	81	0
	6	42	0	16	0	58	0
	7	24	0	10	0	34	0
	8	16	0	5	0	21	0
	9	13	0	5	0	18	0
	10	10	0	2	0	12	0
	11	6	0	2	0	8	0
	12	7	0	1	0	8	0
	13	3	0			3	0
	14			1	0	1	0
	15	5	0	1	0	6	0
	16	2	0	2	0	4	0
	17	2	0			2	0
	18	1	0	2	0	3	0
	19	4	0			4	0
	21			1	0	1	0
	23	2	0	1	0	3	0
	24	1	0			1	0
	50	1	0			1	0
	All	15,479	100	12,728	100	28,207	100

Table 5a. (Continued)

		Gender				Both	
		Female		Male			
		N	PCTN	N	PCTN	N	PCTN
Age Group	Number of Drug Drug Conflicts						
50+	0	2,126	75	2,000	78	4,126	76
	1	365	13	280	11	645	12
	2	119	4	77	3	196	4
	3	79	3	78	3	157	3
	4	33	1	35	1	68	1
	5	22	1	24	1	46	1
	6	25	1	20	1	45	1
	7	16	1	9	0	25	0
	8	10	0	10	0	20	0
	9	16	1	6	0	22	0
	10	6	0	3	0	9	0
	11	8	0	6	0	14	0
	12	1	0	3	0	4	0
	13	3	0	2	0	5	0
	14	5	0	1	0	6	0
	17	3	0			3	0
	19	1	0			1	0
	22	1	0			1	0
	23	1	0	1	0	2	0
	24	1	0			1	0
	27	1	0			1	0
	31			1	0	1	0
	All	2,842	100	2,556	100	5,398	100

Table 5a. (Continued)

| | | Gender | | | | | |
| | | Female | | Male | | Both | |
		N	PCTN	N	PCTN	N	PCTN
All Age	Number of Drug Drug Conflicts						
	0	16,026	87	13,992	92	30,018	89
	1	1,198	7	732	5	1,930	6
	2	393	2	197	1	590	2
	3	271	1	146	1	417	1
	4	113	1	62	0	175	1
	5	83	0	44	0	127	0
	6	67	0	36	0	103	0
	7	40	0	19	0	59	0
	8	26	0	15	0	41	0
	9	29	0	11	0	40	0
	10	16	0	5	0	21	0
	11	14	0	8	0	22	0
	12	8	0	4	0	12	0
	13	6	0	2	0	8	0
	14	5	0	2	0	7	0
	15	5	0	1	0	6	0
	16	2	0	2	0	4	0
	17	5	0			5	0
	18	1	0	2	0	3	0
	19	5	0			5	0
	21			1	0	1	0
	22	1	0			1	0
	23	3	0	2	0	5	0
	24	2	0			2	0
	27	1	0			1	0

National Highway Traffic Safety Administration

Table 5a. (Continued)

| | | Gender | | | | | |
| | | Female | | Male | | Both | |
		N	PCTN	N	PCTN	N	PCTN
All Age	Number of Drug Drug Conflicts						
	31			1	0	1	0
	50	1	0			1	0
	All	18,321	100	15,284	100	33,605	100

Table 5b. Number of Patients by Age, Gender, and Number of Drug-Drug Conflicts
Control Group

| | | Gender | | | | | |
| | | Female | | Male | | Both | |
		N	PCTN	N	PCTN	N	PCTN
Age Group	Number of Drug Drug Conflicts						
Under 50							
	0	44,354	96	36,901	97	81,255	96
	1	1,363	3	869	2	2,232	3
	2	331	1	191	1	522	1
	3	212	0	113	0	325	0
	4	77	0	38	0	115	0
	5	34	0	18	0	52	0
	6	22	0	25	0	47	0
	7	19	0	8	0	27	0
	8	7	0	8	0	15	0
	9	4	0	5	0	9	0
	10	4	0			4	0
	11	2	0	1	0	3	0
	12	3	0	1	0	4	0
	13			3	0	3	0
	15	1	0			1	0
	16			2	0	2	0
	17	1	0			1	0
	18	2	0			2	0
	29	1	0			1	0
	33			1	0	1	0
	All	46,437	100	38,184	100	84,621	100
50+	Number of Drug Drug Conflicts						
	0	7,124	84	6,424	84	13,548	84
	1	749	9	667	9	1,416	9

Multiple Medications and Vehicle Crashes: Analysis of Databases

Table 5b. (Continued)

Age Group	Number of Drug Drug Conflicts	Female		Male		Both	
		N	PCTN	N	PCTN	N	PCTN
50+	2	263	3	204	3	467	3
	3	161	2	149	2	310	2
	4	57	1	66	1	123	1
	5	42	0	46	1	88	1
	6	45	1	42	1	87	1
	7	20	0	13	0	33	0
	8	21	0	13	0	34	0
	9	9	0	8	0	17	0
	10	10	0	7	0	17	0
	11	7	0	7	0	14	0
	12	3	0	4	0	7	0
	13	3	0	6	0	9	0
	14	6	0			6	0
	15	1	0	4	0	5	0
	16			2	0	2	0
	17	2	0	1	0	3	0
	18	1	0	1	0	2	0
	19	1	0			1	0
	20			2	0	2	0
	22			1	0	1	0
	25	1	0			1	0
	32			1	0	1	0
	All	8,526	100	7,668	100	16,194	100

Table 5b. (Continued)

		Gender				Both	
		Female		Male			
		N	PCTN	N	PCTN	N	PCTN
All Age	Number of Drug Drug Conflicts						
	0	51,478	94	43,325	94	94,803	94
	1	2,112	4	1,536	3	3,648	4
	2	594	1	395	1	989	1
	3	373	1	262	1	635	1
	4	134	0	104	0	238	0
	5	76	0	64	0	140	0
	6	67	0	67	0	134	0
	7	39	0	21	0	60	0
	8	28	0	21	0	49	0
	9	13	0	13	0	26	0
	10	14	0	7	0	21	0
	11	9	0	8	0	17	0
	12	6	0	5	0	11	0
	13	3	0	9	0	12	0
	14	6	0			6	0
	15	2	0	4	0	6	0
	16			4	0	4	0
	17	3	0	1	0	4	0
	18	3	0	1	0	4	0
	19	1	0			1	0
	20			2	0	2	0
	22			1	0	1	0
	25	1	0			1	0
	29	1	0			1	0
	32			1	0	1	0

Table 5b. (Continued)

		Gender				Both	
		Female		Male			
		N	PCTN	N	PCTN	N	PCTN
All Age	Number of Drug Drug Conflicts						
	33			1	0	1	0
	All	54,963	100	45,852	100	100815	100

Table 6a. Number of Case Patients by Age, Gender, and Potential Driver Impairing Disease Groups

Gender	Age Group	Disease Group	N
Female	Under 50	HYPERSENSITIVITY REACTIONS	1,815
Female	Under 50	RESPIRATORY INFECTIONS	1,620
Female	Under 50	FRACTURES AND INJURIES	1,453
Female	Under 50	PREGNANCY	902
Female	Under 50	DEPRESSION	868
Female	Under 50	PSYCHOSES, DRUG INDUCED	758
Female	Under 50	DIARRHEA, GASTROENTERITIS	655
Female	Under 50	CONTRACEPTIVE MEASURES	533
Female	Under 50	CNS EXCITATION	468
Female	Under 50	ORAL CONTRACEPTION	442
Female	Under 50	ABDOMINAL PAIN	390
Female	Under 50	LACTIC ACIDOSIS SYMPTOMS	346
Female	Under 50	ASTHMA	316
Female	Under 50	SYMPTOMS OF DIG-TOXICITY	294
Female	Under 50	CARDIOVASCULAR DISEASE	285
Female	Under 50	ABNL PREG TERMINATED OR DELIV	269
Female	Under 50	ANXIETY DISORDERS	261
Female	Under 50	HYPERTENSION	261
Female	Under 50	SYMPTOMS OF GI IRRITATION	246
Female	Under 50	COND- REYE SYNDROME RELATED	236
Female	Under 50	THYROID DISEASE	228
Female	Under 50	HEMATOLOGIC DISORDERS	214
Female	Under 50	DIABETES MELLITUS I AND II	188
Female	Under 50	TUBERCULOSIS	186
Female	Under 50	SYMPTOMS OF ERGOTISM	181
Female	Under 50	LIPID ABNORMALITIES	178
Female	Under 50	HIV	176
Female	Under 50	COUGH	174
Female	Under 50	CONTRACEPTION- IMPLANTS	164

Table 6a. (Continued)

Gender	Age Group	Disease Group	N
Female	Under 50	GERD	148
Female	Under 50	CONTRACEPTION- INJECTION (D)	146
Female	Under 50	CHRONIC OTITIS MEDIA	144
Female	Under 50	PANCYTOPENIA	136
Female	Under 50	ANEMIAS, OTHER	123
Female	Under 50	NORMAL PREG TERMINATED	122
Female	Under 50	NORMAL PREGNANCT TERMINATED	122
Female	Under 50	GI HEMORRHAGE	107
Female	Under 50	ANAPHYLACTIC SHOCK	100
Female	Under 50	HEAD TRAUMA	98
Female	Under 50	HEPATIC DYSFUNCTION	98
Female	Under 50	BLEEDING	96
Female	Under 50	OBESITY	95
Female	Under 50	VIRAL ILLNESSES	91
Female	Under 50	MILD FUNGAL INFECTIONS	86
Female	Under 50	BIPOLAR DISORDER	85
Female	Under 50	SYNCOPE	81
Female	Under 50	DIARRHEA	78
Female	Under 50	GASTRITIS	74
Female	Under 50	HEPATITIS	73
Female	Under 50	HEMATURIA	68
Female	Under 50	ALCOHOLISM	67
Female	Under 50	ARRHYTHMIAS	64
Female	Under 50	CANCER	55
Female	Under 50	EDEMA	51
Female	Under 50	ANKYLOSING SPONDYLITIS	49
Female	Under 50	ANEMIA,DEF.FE,OTH	48
Female	Under 50	COLON, IRRITABLE	47
Female	Under 50	ACUTE OTITIS MEDIA	45
Female	Under 50	BRONCHOPNEUMONIA	45
Female	Under 50	PANIC DISORDERS	44
Female	Under 50	PERSONALITY DISORDERS	42
Female	Under 50	ARTHRITIS, RHEUMATOID	39
Female	Under 50	DEHYDRATION	39
Female	Under 50	DERMATITIS,MACULOPAPULAR	39
Female	Under 50	VOLUME DEPLETION	39
Female	Under 50	LYMPHADENOPATHY	38
Female	Under 50	SYMPTOMS OF QUINIDINE-TOXICITY	37
Female	Under 50	COPD	36
Female	Under 50	KIDNEY STONES	36
Female	Under 50	HYPERTHYROIDISM	35
Female	Under 50	ABUSE- DRUG	34

Table 6a. (Continued)

Gender	Age Group	Disease Group	N
Female	Under 50	PERIPHERAL NEUROPATHY	34
Female	Under 50	STRESS DISORDERS	34
Female	Under 50	PREG TERMINATION- CHEMICAL	33
Female	Under 50	SUICIDAL BEHAVIOR	33
Female	Under 50	EPILEPSY	31
Female	Under 50	PLEURAL EFFUSION-D	29
Female	Under 50	ARTHRITIS, OSTEOARTHRITIS	28
Female	Under 50	CHOLELITHIASIS	28
Female	Under 50	GALLSTONES	28
Female	Under 50	CNS DEMYELINATING DIS	26
Female	Under 50	DYSKINESIAS	26
Female	Under 50	GI ULCER	26
Female	Under 50	HEMATEMESIS	25
Female	Under 50	DEEP VEIN THROMBOSIS	24
Female	Under 50	LUPUS	22
Female	Under 50	CONGESTIVE HEART FAILURE	21
Female	Under 50	RENAL DISEASE	21
Female	Under 50	PSYCHOSES	20
Female	Under 50	PULMONARY DISORDERS	19
Female	Under 50	RENAL FAILURE-GENERAL	19
Female	Under 50	BREAST CANCER, FEMALE	18
Female	Under 50	PSORIASIS	18
Female	Under 50	PULMONARY FIBROSIS	18
Female	Under 50	RENAL FAILURE W/O HTN	18
Female	Under 50	ANEURYSM	17
Female	Under 50	BLEEDING RISK DIAGNOSIS	17
Female	Under 50	ANGINA, PECTORIS	16
Female	Under 50	ISCHEMIC HEART DISEASE	16
Female	Under 50	PULMONARY EDEMA	16
Female	Under 50	SUICIDE	16
Female	Under 50	OSTEOPOROSIS	15
Female	Under 50	ANOREXIA	14
Female	Under 50	CROHN'S DISEASE	14
Female	Under 50	LEUKOPENIA	14
Female	Under 50	PRURITUS	14
Female	Under 50	EPISTAXIS	13
Female	Under 50	HEMORRHAGIC DISORDERS	13
Female	Under 50	SEVERE FUNGAL INFECTIONS	13
Female	Under 50	MENOPAUSE	12
Female	Under 50	BOWEL OBSTRUCTION	11
Female	Under 50	RELATED TO FETAL OUTCOMES	11
Female	Under 50	STEATORRHEA	11

Table 6a. (Continued)

Gender	Age Group	Disease Group	N
Female	Under 50	STROKE	11
Female	Under 50	ALBUMINURIA/ NEPHROPATHY	10
Female	Under 50	BRAIN HEMORRHAGE	10
Female	Under 50	THROMBOCYTOPENIA	10
Female	Under 50	THROMBOPHLEBITIS	10
Female	Under 50	URINARY RETENTION	10
Female	Under 50	BULIMIA	9
Female	Under 50	COLON POLYPS	9
Female	Under 50	EXTRAPYRAMIDAL REACTIONS	9
Female	Under 50	HEPATITIS, ALLER CHOLESTATIC	9
Female	Under 50	TELANGLECTASIS	9
Female	Under 50	AGRANULOCYTOSIS	8
Female	Under 50	HEPATIC CIRRHOSIS	8
Female	Under 50	HEPATOMEGALY WITH STEATOSIS	8
Female	Under 50	HYPOTENSION	8
Female	Under 50	MYELOSUPPRESSION	8
Female	Under 50	NEUTROPENIA	8
Female	Under 50	COAGULATION DEFECTS	7
Female	Under 50	ELECTROLYTE DISORDERS	7
Female	Under 50	ILEUS, PARALYTIC	7
Female	Under 50	MYOCARDIAL ISCHEMIA	7
Female	Under 50	NUTRITIONAL/ NEURO DEFICIENCY	7
Female	Under 50	OSTEOSARCOMA	7
Female	Under 50	PULMONARY EMBOLUS	7
Female	Under 50	THROMBOCYTOPENIA, SECONDARY	7
Female	Under 50	UREMIA	7
Female	Under 50	ANGINA, UNSTABLE	6
Female	Under 50	APPENDICITIS	6
Female	Under 50	ARTHROPATHIES, OTHER	6
Female	Under 50	COLITIS	6
Female	Under 50	DELIRIUM	6
Female	Under 50	DEMENTIA	6
Female	Under 50	DRUG INDUCED PSYCH DISORDERS	6
Female	Under 50	GI OBSTRUCTION	6
Female	Under 50	HEMOLYSIS	6
Female	Under 50	INTERSTITIAL PNEUMONITIS	6
Female	Under 50	PANCREATITIS	6
Female	Under 50	PROTEINURIA	6
Female	Under 50	VENTRICULAR ARRHYTHMIA	6
Female	Under 50	ANGIONEUROTIC EDEMA	5
Female	Under 50	COLON LESIONS	5
Female	Under 50	GLAUCOMA	5

Table 6a. (Continued)

Gender	Age Group	Disease Group	N
Female	Under 50	HEMOLYTIC ANEMIA, HERED	5
Female	Under 50	HYPERSECRETORY STATES	5
Female	Under 50	NEUROPATHIES	5
Female	Under 50	ATRIAL FIBRILLATION	4
Female	Under 50	BRADYCARDIA	4
Female	Under 50	CHOLESTATIC JAUNDICE	4
Female	Under 50	ENCEPHALOPATHIC SYNDROME	4
Female	Under 50	EXFOLIATIVE DERMATITIS	4
Female	Under 50	HEMOPTYSIS	4
Female	Under 50	INTRA-ABDOMINAL HEMORRHAGE	4
Female	Under 50	MALIGNANT NEOPLASM, CNS	4
Female	Under 50	NASAL POLYPS	4
Female	Under 50	OPTIC NEURITIS	4
Female	Under 50	PRERENAL AZOTEMIA	4
Female	Under 50	PSEUDOTUMOR CEREBRI	4
Female	Under 50	PULMONARY EMBOLUS, PREVIOUS	4
Female	Under 50	ALCOHOLIC LIVER DISEASE	3
Female	Under 50	ARTHRITIS, PSORIATIC	3
Female	Under 50	CYSTIC FIBROSIS	3
Female	Under 50	HEART BLOCK	3
Female	Under 50	JAUNDICE	3
Female	Under 50	OBSTRUCTIVE UROPATHY	3
Female	Under 50	RENAL CALCIFICATION	3
Female	Under 50	ADDISON'S DISEASE	2
Female	Under 50	ADRENAL INSUFFICIENCY	2
Female	Under 50	ALZHEIMER	2
Female	Under 50	ANEMIA,MEGALOBLASTIC	2
Female	Under 50	BLOOD DYSCRASIAS	2
Female	Under 50	CEREBRAL PALSY	2
Female	Under 50	COLOSTOMY/ ILEOSTOMY	2
Female	Under 50	CRYSTALLURIA	2
Female	Under 50	ERYTHEMA MULTIFORME	2
Female	Under 50	GOUT	2
Female	Under 50	KETOACIDOSIS	2
Female	Under 50	MYASTHENIA GRAVIS	2
Female	Under 50	PSEUDOMEMBRANOUS COLITIS	2
Female	Under 50	RHABDOMYOLYSIS	2
Female	Under 50	SICKLE CELL ANEMIA	2
Female	Under 50	STEVENS JOHNSON SYNDROME	2
Female	Under 50	ALVEOLITIS,FIBROSING	1
Female	Under 50	ANURIA	1
Female	Under 50	AV BLOCK II TO III	1

Table 6a. (Continued)

Gender	Age Group	Disease Group	N
Female	Under 50	BULLOUS RASH	1
Female	Under 50	CEREBRAL ARTERIOSCLEROSIS	1
Female	Under 50	CIRRHOSIS	1
Female	Under 50	FAVISM	1
Female	Under 50	G6PD	1
Female	Under 50	G6PD DEFICIENCY	1
Female	Under 50	GLAUCOMA,NARROW ANGLE	1
Female	Under 50	HALLUCINATIONS	1
Female	Under 50	HEMOLYTIC ANEMIA, ACQ	1
Female	Under 50	HEPATIC FAILURE	1
Female	Under 50	HYPERCALCEMIA	1
Female	Under 50	HYPERSENSITIVITY PNEUMONITIS	1
Female	Under 50	MALIGNANT MELANOMA	1
Female	Under 50	MYOPATHY	1
Female	Under 50	OLIGURIA	1
Female	Under 50	RADIATION THERAPY ICD	1
Female	Under 50	RENAL OSTEODYSTROPHY	1
Female	Under 50	RETROPERITONEAL FIBROSIS	1
Female	Under 50	SUBARACHNOID HEMORRHAGE	1
Female	50+	CARDIOVASCULAR DISEASE	383
Female	50+	HYPERTENSION	356
Female	50+	HYPERSENSITIVITY REACTIONS	315
Female	50+	FRACTURES AND INJURIES	297
Female	50+	DIABETES MELLITUS I AND II	212
Female	50+	RESPIRATORY INFECTIONS	202
Female	50+	LIPID ABNORMALITIES	196
Female	50+	DEPRESSION	144
Female	50+	PSYCHOSES, DRUG INDUCED	138
Female	50+	DIARRHEA, GASTROENTERITIS	118
Female	50+	THYROID DISEASE	111
Female	50+	SYMPTOMS OF GI IRRITATION	92
Female	50+	CNS EXCITATION	79
Female	50+	SYMPTOMS OF DIG-TOXICITY	75
Female	50+	TUBERCULOSIS	66
Female	50+	ABDOMINAL PAIN	65
Female	50+	CANCER	64
Female	50+	GERD	62
Female	50+	ASTHMA	61
Female	50+	HEMATOLOGIC DISORDERS	60
Female	50+	LACTIC ACIDOSIS SYMPTOMS	60
Female	50+	COPD	52
Female	50+	HEPATIC DYSFUNCTION	51

Multiple Medications and Vehicle Crashes: Analysis of Databases

Table 6a. (Continued)

Gender	Age Group	Disease Group	N
Female	50+	ANXIETY DISORDERS	47
Female	50+	OSTEOPOROSIS	43
Female	50+	ARTHRITIS, OSTEOARTHRITIS	42
Female	50+	ISCHEMIC HEART DISEASE	42
Female	50+	MILD FUNGAL INFECTIONS	41
Female	50+	ARRHYTHMIAS	40
Female	50+	HEPATITIS	39
Female	50+	GI HEMORRHAGE	38
Female	50+	COUGH	37
Female	50+	ANKYLOSING SPONDYLITIS	36
Female	50+	BLEEDING	34
Female	50+	COND- REYE SYNDROME RELATED	31
Female	50+	CONGESTIVE HEART FAILURE	30
Female	50+	SYMPTOMS OF ERGOTISM	29
Female	50+	ANEMIAS, OTHER	28
Female	50+	PANCYTOPENIA	28
Female	50+	ANAPHYLACTIC SHOCK	27
Female	50+	BREAST CANCER, FEMALE	27
Female	50+	ANEMIA,DEF.FE,OTH	26
Female	50+	OBESITY	25
Female	50+	EDEMA	24
Female	50+	DIARRHEA	23
Female	50+	GASTRITIS	23
Female	50+	BRONCHOPNEUMONIA	21
Female	50+	HEAD TRAUMA	21
Female	50+	PERIPHERAL NEUROPATHY	21
Female	50+	ATRIAL FIBRILLATION	20
Female	50+	ARTHRITIS, RHEUMATOID	19
Female	50+	HIV	19
Female	50+	MENOPAUSE	19
Female	50+	SYMPTOMS OF QUINIDINE-TOXICITY	19
Female	50+	CHRONIC OTITIS MEDIA	18
Female	50+	DEEP VEIN THROMBOSIS	18
Female	50+	COLON POLYPS	17
Female	50+	HEMATURIA	17
Female	50+	VIRAL ILLNESSES	17
Female	50+	GI ULCER	16
Female	50+	SYNCOPE	16
Female	50+	STROKE	15
Female	50+	ANGINA, PECTORIS	14
Female	50+	RENAL FAILURE-GENERAL	14
Female	50+	ANEURYSM	13

Table 6a. (Continued)

Gender	Age Group	Disease Group	N
Female	50+	BIPOLAR DISORDER	13
Female	50+	HEMATEMESIS	13
Female	50+	RENAL FAILURE W/O HTN	12
Female	50+	CNS DEMYELINATING DIS	11
Female	50+	GLAUCOMA	11
Female	50+	COLON, IRRITABLE	10
Female	50+	DERMATITIS,MACULOPAPULAR	10
Female	50+	MYOCARDIAL ISCHEMIA	10
Female	50+	PLEURAL EFFUSION-D	10
Female	50+	RENAL DISEASE	10
Female	50+	ALCOHOLISM	9
Female	50+	CHOLELITHIASIS	9
Female	50+	DYSKINESIAS	9
Female	50+	GALLSTONES	9
Female	50+	LUPUS	9
Female	50+	NUTRITIONAL/ NEURO DEFICIENCY	9
Female	50+	BLEEDING RISK DIAGNOSIS	8
Female	50+	DEMENTIA	8
Female	50+	EXTRAPYRAMIDAL REACTIONS	8
Female	50+	ARTHROPATHIES, OTHER	7
Female	50+	DEHYDRATION	7
Female	50+	EPILEPSY	7
Female	50+	HEPATIC CIRRHOSIS	7
Female	50+	HYPERTHYROIDISM	7
Female	50+	KIDNEY STONES	7
Female	50+	PULMONARY EMBOLUS	7
Female	50+	STEATORRHEA	7
Female	50+	STRESS DISORDERS	7
Female	50+	VOLUME DEPLETION	7
Female	50+	ACUTE OTITIS MEDIA	6
Female	50+	ALBUMINURIA/ NEPHROPATHY	6
Female	50+	EPISTAXIS	6
Female	50+	GOUT	6
Female	50+	KETOACIDOSIS	6
Female	50+	NEUROPATHIES	6
Female	50+	OSTEOSARCOMA	6
Female	50+	PSYCHOSES	6
Female	50+	PULMONARY DISORDERS	6
Female	50+	PULMONARY FIBROSIS	6
Female	50+	VENTRICULAR ARRHYTHMIA	6
Female	50+	ANGINA, UNSTABLE	5
Female	50+	HYPOTENSION	5

Table 6a. (Continued)

Gender	Age Group	Disease Group	N
Female	50+	INTERSTITIAL PNEUMONITIS	5
Female	50+	PANIC DISORDERS	5
Female	50+	BRAIN HEMORRHAGE	4
Female	50+	CIRRHOSIS	4
Female	50+	CROHN'S DISEASE	4
Female	50+	ELECTROLYTE DISORDERS	4
Female	50+	GI OBSTRUCTION	4
Female	50+	HYPERSECRETORY STATES	4
Female	50+	LEUKOPENIA	4
Female	50+	MYELOSUPPRESSION	4
Female	50+	PSORIASIS	4
Female	50+	PULMONARY EDEMA	4
Female	50+	URINARY RETENTION	4
Female	50+	AGRANULOCYTOSIS	3
Female	50+	BOWEL OBSTRUCTION	3
Female	50+	COAGULATION DEFECTS	3
Female	50+	COLOSTOMY/ ILEOSTOMY	3
Female	50+	DELIRIUM	3
Female	50+	HEART BLOCK	3
Female	50+	HEPATITIS, ALLER CHOLESTATIC	3
Female	50+	HEPATOMEGALY WITH STEATOSIS	3
Female	50+	INTRA-ABDOMINAL HEMORRHAGE	3
Female	50+	NEUTROPENIA	3
Female	50+	PARKINSONISM,PRIMARY	3
Female	50+	PERSONALITY DISORDERS	3
Female	50+	PROTEINURIA	3
Female	50+	PRURITUS	3
Female	50+	RADIATION THERAPY ICD	3
Female	50+	SUICIDAL BEHAVIOR	3
Female	50+	TELANGLECTASIS	3
Female	50+	ANEMIA,MEGALOBLASTIC	2
Female	50+	ANGIONEUROTIC EDEMA	2
Female	50+	APLASTIC ANEMIA	2
Female	50+	BRADYCARDIA	2
Female	50+	COLITIS	2
Female	50+	CRYSTALLURIA	2
Female	50+	HALLUCINATIONS	2
Female	50+	MALIGNANT NEOPLASM, CNS	2
Female	50+	MYELODYSPLASTIC SYNDROME	2
Female	50+	OSTEOMALACIA	2
Female	50+	PULMONARY EMBOLUS, PREVIOUS	2
Female	50+	SEVERE FUNGAL INFECTIONS	2

Table 6a. (Continued)

Gender	Age Group	Disease Group	N
Female	50+	SUBARACHNOID HEMORRHAGE	2
Female	50+	SUICIDE	2
Female	50+	THROMBOPHLEBITIS	2
Female	50+	ADDISON'S DISEASE	1
Female	50+	ADRENAL INSUFFICIENCY	1
Female	50+	ALVEOLITIS,FIBROSING	1
Female	50+	ANOREXIA	1
Female	50+	ARTHRITIS, PSORIATIC	1
Female	50+	AV BLOCK II TO III	1
Female	50+	BLOOD DYSCRASIAS	1
Female	50+	CARDIAC ARREST	1
Female	50+	COLON LESIONS	1
Female	50+	CONTRACEPTION- INJECTION (D)	1
Female	50+	CONTRACEPTIVE MEASURES	1
Female	50+	DRUG INDUCED PSYCH DISORDERS	1
Female	50+	ENCEPHALOPATHIC SYNDROME	1
Female	50+	ERYTHEMA MULTIFORME	1
Female	50+	EXFOLIATIVE DERMATITIS	1
Female	50+	GLAUCOMA,NARROW ANGLE	1
Female	50+	HEMOPTYSIS	1
Female	50+	HEMORRHAGIC DISORDERS	1
Female	50+	HEPATIC FAILURE	1
Female	50+	HYPERCALCEMIA	1
Female	50+	HYPERSENSITIVITY PNEUMONITIS	1
Female	50+	ILEUS, PARALYTIC	1
Female	50+	MALIGNANT MELANOMA	1
Female	50+	NASAL POLYPS	1
Female	50+	OPTIC NEURITIS	1
Female	50+	ORAL CONTRACEPTION	1
Female	50+	PANCREATITIS	1
Female	50+	PREGNANCY	1
Female	50+	PRERENAL AZOTEMIA	1
Female	50+	PSEUDOMEMBRANOUS COLITIS	1
Female	50+	RELATED TO FETAL OUTCOMES	1
Female	50+	RHABDOMYOLYSIS	1
Female	50+	STEVENS JOHNSON SYNDROME	1
Female	50+	THROMBOCYTOPENIA	1
Female	50+	THROMBOCYTOPENIA, SECONDARY	1
Female	50+	UREMIA	1
Male	Under 50	FRACTURES AND INJURIES	1,371
Male	Under 50	HYPERSENSITIVITY REACTIONS	884
Male	Under 50	RESPIRATORY INFECTIONS	828

Table 6a. (Continued)

Gender	Age Group	Disease Group	N
Male	Under 50	SEROTONIN SYNDROME SYMPTOMS	422
Male	Under 50	PSYCHOSES, DRUG INDUCED	320
Male	Under 50	DEPRESSION	305
Male	Under 50	DIARRHEA, GASTROENTERITIS	258
Male	Under 50	CARDIOVASCULAR DISEASE	251
Male	Under 50	HYPERTENSION	225
Male	Under 50	DIABETES MELLITUS I AND II	186
Male	Under 50	CNS EXCITATION	179
Male	Under 50	LIPID ABNORMALITIES	167
Male	Under 50	SYMPTOMS OF GI IRRITATION	150
Male	Under 50	SYMPTOMS OF DIG-TOXICITY	146
Male	Under 50	ABDOMINAL PAIN	141
Male	Under 50	ANXIETY DISORDERS	140
Male	Under 50	LACTIC ACIDOSIS SYMPTOMS	130
Male	Under 50	ASTHMA	129
Male	Under 50	HEAD TRAUMA	119
Male	Under 50	ALCOHOLISM	110
Male	Under 50	COND- REYE SYNDROME RELATED	106
Male	Under 50	COUGH	101
Male	Under 50	TUBERCULOSIS	90
Male	Under 50	GERD	88
Male	Under 50	MILD FUNGAL INFECTIONS	82
Male	Under 50	GI HEMORRHAGE	80
Male	Under 50	CHRONIC OTITIS MEDIA	77
Male	Under 50	HEMATOLOGIC DISORDERS	77
Male	Under 50	HEPATIC DYSFUNCTION	73
Male	Under 50	BLEEDING	68
Male	Under 50	SYMPTOMS OF ERGOTISM	68
Male	Under 50	ARRHYTHMIAS	57
Male	Under 50	VIRAL ILLNESSES	57
Male	Under 50	HEPATITIS	51
Male	Under 50	GASTRITIS	50
Male	Under 50	ANAPHYLACTIC SHOCK	49
Male	Under 50	ACUTE OTITIS MEDIA	44
Male	Under 50	DIARRHEA	44
Male	Under 50	ANEMIAS, OTHER	43
Male	Under 50	BRONCHOPNEUMONIA	42
Male	Under 50	PANCYTOPENIA	39
Male	Under 50	ISCHEMIC HEART DISEASE	35
Male	Under 50	BIPOLAR DISORDER	33
Male	Under 50	CANCER	33
Male	Under 50	COPD	33

Table 6a. (Continued)

Gender	Age Group	Disease Group	N
Male	Under 50	HEMATURIA	33
Male	Under 50	KIDNEY STONES	31
Male	Under 50	SYNCOPE	31
Male	Under 50	ABUSE- DRUG	30
Male	Under 50	SYMPTOMS OF QUINIDINE-TOXICITY	30
Male	Under 50	THYROID DISEASE	30
Male	Under 50	GI ULCER	29
Male	Under 50	CONTRACEPTIVE MEASURES	28
Male	Under 50	PLEURAL EFFUSION-D	28
Male	Under 50	ANEURYSM	25
Male	Under 50	DEEP VEIN THROMBOSIS	25
Male	Under 50	HEMATEMESIS	25
Male	Under 50	ARTHRITIS, OSTEOARTHRITIS	24
Male	Under 50	ANKYLOSING SPONDYLITIS	23
Male	Under 50	DYSKINESIAS	23
Male	Under 50	OBESITY	22
Male	Under 50	PANIC DISORDERS	21
Male	Under 50	EPILEPSY	20
Male	Under 50	PERIPHERAL NEUROPATHY	20
Male	Under 50	BRAIN HEMORRHAGE	19
Male	Under 50	DEHYDRATION	19
Male	Under 50	RENAL DISEASE	19
Male	Under 50	VOLUME DEPLETION	19
Male	Under 50	ANGINA, PECTORIS	16
Male	Under 50	CONGESTIVE HEART FAILURE	16
Male	Under 50	HIV	16
Male	Under 50	PULMONARY DISORDERS	16
Male	Under 50	RENAL FAILURE W/O HTN	16
Male	Under 50	RENAL FAILURE-GENERAL	16
Male	Under 50	STRESS DISORDERS	16
Male	Under 50	EDEMA	15
Male	Under 50	PULMONARY FIBROSIS	15
Male	Under 50	GOUT	14
Male	Under 50	ORAL CONTRACEPTION	13
Male	Under 50	SUICIDE	13
Male	Under 50	BLEEDING RISK DIAGNOSIS	12
Male	Under 50	DERMATITIS,MACULOPAPULAR	12
Male	Under 50	EPISTAXIS	12
Male	Under 50	HEPATITIS, ALLER CHOLESTATIC	12
Male	Under 50	MYOCARDIAL ISCHEMIA	12
Male	Under 50	PSYCHOSES	12
Male	Under 50	ANEMIA,DEF.FE,OTH	11

Table 6a. (Continued)

Gender	Age Group	Disease Group	N
Male	Under 50	ARTHRITIS, RHEUMATOID	11
Male	Under 50	COLON POLYPS	11
Male	Under 50	CONTRACEPTION- INJECTION (D)	11
Male	Under 50	EXTRAPYRAMIDAL REACTIONS	11
Male	Under 50	ANGINA, UNSTABLE	10
Male	Under 50	COLITIS	10
Male	Under 50	COLON, IRRITABLE	10
Male	Under 50	LYMPHADENOPATHY	10
Male	Under 50	PULMONARY EMBOLUS	10
Male	Under 50	STROKE	10
Male	Under 50	ALBUMINURIA/ NEPHROPATHY	9
Male	Under 50	ARTHROPATHIES, OTHER	9
Male	Under 50	ATRIAL FIBRILLATION	9
Male	Under 50	PULMONARY EDEMA	9
Male	Under 50	COAGULATION DEFECTS	8
Male	Under 50	HEPATIC CIRRHOSIS	8
Male	Under 50	HYPOTENSION	8
Male	Under 50	PSORIASIS	8
Male	Under 50	APPENDICITIS	7
Male	Under 50	NUTRITIONAL/ NEURO DEFICIENCY	7
Male	Under 50	PERSONALITY DISORDERS	7
Male	Under 50	SUICIDAL BEHAVIOR	7
Male	Under 50	VENTRICULAR ARRHYTHMIA	7
Male	Under 50	CHOLELITHIASIS	6
Male	Under 50	CROHN'S DISEASE	6
Male	Under 50	GALLSTONES	6
Male	Under 50	GI OBSTRUCTION	6
Male	Under 50	HEMOLYSIS	6
Male	Under 50	HEMOLYTIC ANEMIA, HERED	6
Male	Under 50	INTRA-ABDOMINAL HEMORRHAGE	6
Male	Under 50	STEATORRHEA	6
Male	Under 50	BRADYCARDIA	5
Male	Under 50	CNS DEMYELINATING DIS	5
Male	Under 50	DRUG INDUCED PSYCH DISORDERS	5
Male	Under 50	HEMOPTYSIS	5
Male	Under 50	HEMORRHAGIC DISORDERS	5
Male	Under 50	HEPATOMEGALY WITH STEATOSIS	5
Male	Under 50	NEUROPATHIES	5
Male	Under 50	PANCREATITIS	5
Male	Under 50	SUBARACHNOID HEMORRHAGE	5
Male	Under 50	ALCOHOLIC LIVER DISEASE	4
Male	Under 50	BOWEL OBSTRUCTION	4

Table 6a. (Continued)

Gender	Age Group	Disease Group	N
Male	Under 50	DEMENTIA	4
Male	Under 50	INTERSTITIAL PNEUMONITIS	4
Male	Under 50	MYELOSUPPRESSION	4
Male	Under 50	NASAL POLYPS	4
Male	Under 50	OSTEOSARCOMA	4
Male	Under 50	PROTEINURIA	4
Male	Under 50	SICKLE CELL ANEMIA	4
Male	Under 50	THROMBOPHLEBITIS	4
Male	Under 50	ADRENAL INSUFFICIENCY	3
Male	Under 50	APLASTIC ANEMIA	3
Male	Under 50	CARDIAC ARREST	3
Male	Under 50	CIRRHOSIS	3
Male	Under 50	ENCEPHALOPATHIC SYNDROME	3
Male	Under 50	GLAUCOMA	3
Male	Under 50	HEART BLOCK	3
Male	Under 50	HYPERSECRETORY STATES	3
Male	Under 50	HYPERTHYROIDISM	3
Male	Under 50	ILEUS, PARALYTIC	3
Male	Under 50	LUPUS	3
Male	Under 50	MEASLES	3
Male	Under 50	OSTEOPOROSIS	3
Male	Under 50	PERICARDIAL DISEASE	3
Male	Under 50	PERICARDIAL EFFUSION	3
Male	Under 50	PRURITUS	3
Male	Under 50	RHABDOMYOLYSIS	3
Male	Under 50	THROMBOCYTOPENIA	3
Male	Under 50	UREMIA	3
Male	Under 50	URINARY RETENTION	3
Male	Under 50	ADDISON'S DISEASE	2
Male	Under 50	BLOOD DYSCRASIAS	2
Male	Under 50	CHOLESTATIC JAUNDICE	2
Male	Under 50	COLON LESIONS	2
Male	Under 50	ELECTROLYTE DISORDERS	2
Male	Under 50	JAUNDICE	2
Male	Under 50	KETOACIDOSIS	2
Male	Under 50	LEUKOPENIA	2
Male	Under 50	MALIGNANT MELANOMA	2
Male	Under 50	MYELODYSPLASTIC SYNDROME	2
Male	Under 50	PRERENAL AZOTEMIA	2
Male	Under 50	PULMONARY EMBOLUS, PREVIOUS	2
Male	Under 50	RELATED TO FETAL OUTCOMES	2
Male	Under 50	SEVERE FUNGAL INFECTIONS	2

Multiple Medications and Vehicle Crashes: Analysis of Databases

Table 6a. (Continued)

Gender	Age Group	Disease Group	N
Male	Under 50	TELANGLECTASIS	2
Male	Under 50	THROMBOCYTOPENIA, SECONDARY	2
Male	Under 50	AGRANULOCYTOSIS	1
Male	Under 50	ALVEOLITIS,FIBROSING	1
Male	Under 50	ALZHEIMER	1
Male	Under 50	ANGIONEUROTIC EDEMA	1
Male	Under 50	ANOREXIA	1
Male	Under 50	AV BLOCK II TO III	1
Male	Under 50	BENIGN PROSTATIC HYPERTROPHY	1
Male	Under 50	BLEPHARASPASM	1
Male	Under 50	BOWEL PERFORATION	1
Male	Under 50	BULIMIA	1
Male	Under 50	CEREBRAL PALSY	1
Male	Under 50	COLOSTOMY/ ILEOSTOMY	1
Male	Under 50	CRYSTALLURIA	1
Male	Under 50	CYSTIC FIBROSIS	1
Male	Under 50	DELIRIUM	1
Male	Under 50	EXFOLIATIVE DERMATITIS	1
Male	Under 50	GLAUCOMA,NARROW ANGLE	1
Male	Under 50	HALLUCINATIONS	1
Male	Under 50	MALIGNANT NEOPLASM, CNS	1
Male	Under 50	MEGACOLON	1
Male	Under 50	MYOPATHY	1
Male	Under 50	NEPHROGENIC DIABETES INSIPIDUS	1
Male	Under 50	NEUTROPENIA	1
Male	Under 50	OPTIC NEURITIS	1
Male	Under 50	PARKINSONISM,PRIMARY	1
Male	Under 50	PORPHYRIAS	1
Male	Under 50	PROSTATIC HYPERTROPHY	1
Male	Under 50	RADIATION THERAPY ICD	1
Male	Under 50	RENAL CALCIFICATION	1
Male	Under 50	RETROPERITONEAL FIBROSIS	1
Male	Under 50	THIAMINE DEFICIENCY	1
Male	50+	CARDIOVASCULAR DISEASE	332
Male	50+	HYPERTENSION	293
Male	50+	HYPERSENSITIVITY REACTIONS	245
Male	50+	FRACTURES AND INJURIES	244
Male	50+	DIABETES MELLITUS I AND II	229
Male	50+	LIPID ABNORMALITIES	214
Male	50+	RESPIRATORY INFECTIONS	157
Male	50+	ISCHEMIC HEART DISEASE	114
Male	50+	DIARRHEA, GASTROENTERITIS	96

Table 6a. (Continued)

Gender	Age Group	Disease Group	N
Male	50+	PSYCHOSES, DRUG INDUCED	74
Male	50+	SYMPTOMS OF DIG-TOXICITY	74
Male	50+	SYMPTOMS OF GI IRRITATION	72
Male	50+	DEPRESSION	68
Male	50+	COPD	66
Male	50+	ARRHYTHMIAS	62
Male	50+	HEPATIC DYSFUNCTION	56
Male	50+	HEMATOLOGIC DISORDERS	53
Male	50+	ABDOMINAL PAIN	52
Male	50+	CANCER	50
Male	50+	LACTIC ACIDOSIS SYMPTOMS	49
Male	50+	GERD	45
Male	50+	CONGESTIVE HEART FAILURE	43
Male	50+	BLEEDING	40
Male	50+	CNS EXCITATION	39
Male	50+	SYMPTOMS OF ERGOTISM	39
Male	50+	HEPATITIS	36
Male	50+	SYMPTOMS OF QUINIDINE-TOXICITY	36
Male	50+	COND- REYE SYNDROME RELATED	35
Male	50+	TUBERCULOSIS	35
Male	50+	COUGH	34
Male	50+	ATRIAL FIBRILLATION	33
Male	50+	ANXIETY DISORDERS	31
Male	50+	HEAD TRAUMA	30
Male	50+	ASTHMA	29
Male	50+	GI HEMORRHAGE	29
Male	50+	ANGINA, PECTORIS	28
Male	50+	PANCYTOPENIA	28
Male	50+	BRONCHOPNEUMONIA	27
Male	50+	ANEMIAS, OTHER	25
Male	50+	ALCOHOLISM	24
Male	50+	ARTHRITIS, OSTEOARTHRITIS	24
Male	50+	MILD FUNGAL INFECTIONS	24
Male	50+	ANKYLOSING SPONDYLITIS	23
Male	50+	THYROID DISEASE	23
Male	50+	ANEURYSM	20
Male	50+	COLON POLYPS	20
Male	50+	HEMATURIA	19
Male	50+	STROKE	19
Male	50+	MYOCARDIAL ISCHEMIA	17
Male	50+	SYNCOPE	17
Male	50+	ANAPHYLACTIC SHOCK	16

Table 6a. (Continued)

Gender	Age Group	Disease Group	N
Male	50+	ANEMIA,DEF.FE,OTH	16
Male	50+	EDEMA	16
Male	50+	GLAUCOMA	16
Male	50+	GI ULCER	15
Male	50+	HEMATEMESIS	15
Male	50+	CHRONIC OTITIS MEDIA	14
Male	50+	DIARRHEA	14
Male	50+	RENAL FAILURE-GENERAL	14
Male	50+	ANGINA, UNSTABLE	13
Male	50+	OBESITY	13
Male	50+	RENAL FAILURE W/O HTN	13
Male	50+	DEEP VEIN THROMBOSIS	12
Male	50+	PLEURAL EFFUSION-D	12
Male	50+	PULMONARY EDEMA	12
Male	50+	VIRAL ILLNESSES	12
Male	50+	ACUTE OTITIS MEDIA	11
Male	50+	BLEEDING RISK DIAGNOSIS	11
Male	50+	KIDNEY STONES	11
Male	50+	NUTRITIONAL/ NEURO DEFICIENCY	11
Male	50+	GASTRITIS	10
Male	50+	BENIGN PROSTATIC HYPERTROPHY	9
Male	50+	HEART BLOCK	9
Male	50+	PROSTATIC HYPERTROPHY	9
Male	50+	VENTRICULAR ARRHYTHMIA	9
Male	50+	ALBUMINURIA/ NEPHROPATHY	8
Male	50+	ARTHRITIS, RHEUMATOID	8
Male	50+	CHOLELITHIASIS	8
Male	50+	GALLSTONES	8
Male	50+	PSORIASIS	8
Male	50+	RENAL DISEASE	8
Male	50+	COAGULATION DEFECTS	7
Male	50+	DERMATITIS,MACULOPAPULAR	7
Male	50+	GI OBSTRUCTION	7
Male	50+	HEPATIC CIRRHOSIS	7
Male	50+	HYPOTENSION	7
Male	50+	PERIPHERAL NEUROPATHY	7
Male	50+	PSYCHOSES	7
Male	50+	GOUT	6
Male	50+	STEATORRHEA	6
Male	50+	URINARY RETENTION	6
Male	50+	BOWEL OBSTRUCTION	5
Male	50+	BRAIN HEMORRHAGE	5

Table 6a. (Continued)

Gender	Age Group	Disease Group	N
Male	50+	DYSKINESIAS	5
Male	50+	EXTRAPYRAMIDAL REACTIONS	5
Male	50+	HEMORRHAGIC DISORDERS	5
Male	50+	INTERSTITIAL PNEUMONITIS	5
Male	50+	OSTEOPOROSIS	5
Male	50+	PULMONARY DISORDERS	5
Male	50+	PULMONARY FIBROSIS	5
Male	50+	AV BLOCK II TO III	4
Male	50+	BIPOLAR DISORDER	4
Male	50+	DEHYDRATION	4
Male	50+	DELIRIUM	4
Male	50+	EPILEPSY	4
Male	50+	HEPATITIS, ALLER CHOLESTATIC	4
Male	50+	INTRA-ABDOMINAL HEMORRHAGE	4
Male	50+	KETOACIDOSIS	4
Male	50+	UREMIA	4
Male	50+	VOLUME DEPLETION	4
Male	50+	ADDISON'S DISEASE	3
Male	50+	ADRENAL INSUFFICIENCY	3
Male	50+	ARTHRITIS, PSORIATIC	3
Male	50+	CARDIAC ARREST	3
Male	50+	CIRRHOSIS	3
Male	50+	COLOSTOMY/ ILEOSTOMY	3
Male	50+	CONTRACEPTIVE MEASURES	3
Male	50+	CROHN'S DISEASE	3
Male	50+	DEMENTIA	3
Male	50+	HEMOLYSIS	3
Male	50+	HYPERSECRETORY STATES	3
Male	50+	HYPERTHYROIDISM	3
Male	50+	ILEUS, PARALYTIC	3
Male	50+	LEUKOPENIA	3
Male	50+	MYELODYSPLASTIC SYNDROME	3
Male	50+	NASAL POLYPS	3
Male	50+	PERSONALITY DISORDERS	3
Male	50+	PROTEINURIA	3
Male	50+	ALCOHOLIC LIVER DISEASE	2
Male	50+	ANOREXIA	2
Male	50+	APLASTIC ANEMIA	2
Male	50+	APPENDICITIS	2
Male	50+	BRADYCARDIA	2
Male	50+	COLON, IRRITABLE	2
Male	50+	ELECTROLYTE DISORDERS	2

Table 6a. (Continued)

Gender	Age Group	Disease Group	N
Male	50+	EPISTAXIS	2
Male	50+	GLAUCOMA,NARROW ANGLE	2
Male	50+	HEMOLYTIC ANEMIA, HERED	2
Male	50+	HEPATOMEGALY WITH STEATOSIS	2
Male	50+	MALIGNANT NEOPLASM, CNS	2
Male	50+	MYELOSUPPRESSION	2
Male	50+	NEUROPATHIES	2
Male	50+	PANCREATITIS	2
Male	50+	PANIC DISORDERS	2
Male	50+	PRERENAL AZOTEMIA	2
Male	50+	STRESS DISORDERS	2
Male	50+	TELANGLECTASIS	2
Male	50+	ABUSE- DRUG	1
Male	50+	AGRANULOCYTOSIS	1
Male	50+	ALZHEIMER	1
Male	50+	ANEMIA,MEGALOBLASTIC	1
Male	50+	ANGIONEUROTIC EDEMA	1
Male	50+	ARTHROPATHIES, OTHER	1
Male	50+	BULLOUS RASH	1
Male	50+	CARDIAC VALVE FIBROSIS	1
Male	50+	CEREBRAL PALSY	1
Male	50+	CNS DEMYELINATING DIS	1
Male	50+	COLITIS	1
Male	50+	CRYSTALLURIA	1
Male	50+	ENCEPHALOPATHIC SYNDROME	1
Male	50+	ERYTHEMA MULTIFORME	1
Male	50+	FECAL IMPACTION	1
Male	50+	HEMOLYTIC ANEMIA, ACQ	1
Male	50+	HEMOLYTIC UREMIC SYNDR	1
Male	50+	HEMOPTYSIS	1
Male	50+	HEPATIC FAILURE	1
Male	50+	LYMPHADENOPATHY	1
Male	50+	MALIGNANT MELANOMA	1
Male	50+	MYASTHENIA GRAVIS	1
Male	50+	NEUTROPENIA	1
Male	50+	OBSTRUCTIVE UROPATHY	1
Male	50+	OPTIC NEURITIS	1
Male	50+	ORAL CONTRACEPTION	1
Male	50+	PARKINSONISM,PRIMARY	1
Male	50+	PREGNANCY	1
Male	50+	PULMONARY EMBOLUS	1
Male	50+	RADIATION THERAPY ICD	1

Table 6a. (Continued)

Gender	Age Group	Disease Group	N
Male	50+	RETROPERITONEAL FIBROSIS	1
Male	50+	SICKLE CELL ANEMIA	1
Male	50+	STEVENS JOHNSON SYNDROME	1
Male	50+	SUDDEN DEATH	1
Male	50+	SUICIDAL BEHAVIOR	1
Male	50+	THROMBOCYTOPENIA	1
Male	50+	THROMBOCYTOPENIA, SECONDARY	1
Male	50+	THROMBOPHLEBITIS	1

Table 6b. Number of Control Patients by Age, Gender, and Potential Driver Impairing Disease Groups

Gender	Age Group	Disease Group	N
Female	Under 50	HYPERSENSITIVITY REACTIONS	3,300
Female	Under 50	RESPIRATORY INFECTIONS	2,986
Female	Under 50	FRACTURES AND INJURIES	1,650
Female	Under 50	PREGNANCY	1,513
Female	Under 50	CONTRACEPTIVE MEASURES	1,056
Female	Under 50	DIARRHEA, GASTROENTERITIS	986
Female	Under 50	ORAL CONTRACEPTION	899
Female	Under 50	ABNL PREG TERMINATED OR DELIV	694
Female	Under 50	CNS EXCITATION	596
Female	Under 50	DEPRESSION	578
Female	Under 50	ABDOMINAL PAIN	574
Female	Under 50	PSYCHOSES, DRUG INDUCED	528
Female	Under 50	LACTIC ACIDOSIS SYMPTOMS	513
Female	Under 50	NORMAL PREG TERMINATED	506
Female	Under 50	NORMAL PREGNANCT TERMINATED	506
Female	Under 50	THYROID DISEASE	487
Female	Under 50	HIV	424
Female	Under 50	CARDIOVASCULAR DISEASE	423
Female	Under 50	HYPERTENSION	397
Female	Under 50	ASTHMA	396
Female	Under 50	SYMPTOMS OF DIG-TOXICITY	351
Female	Under 50	LIPID ABNORMALITIES	342
Female	Under 50	CONTRACEPTION- IMPLANTS	330
Female	Under 50	TUBERCULOSIS	319
Female	Under 50	HEMATOLOGIC DISORDERS	316
Female	Under 50	SYMPTOMS OF GI IRRITATION	315
Female	Under 50	DIABETES MELLITUS I AND II	302
Female	Under 50	COUGH	278
Female	Under 50	COND- REYE SYNDROME RELATED	268

Table 6b. (Continued)

Gender	Age Group	Disease Group	N
Female	Under 50	CHRONIC OTITIS MEDIA	251
Female	Under 50	ANXIETY DISORDERS	208
Female	Under 50	PANCYTOPENIA	188
Female	Under 50	OBESITY	175
Female	Under 50	SYMPTOMS OF ERGOTISM	173
Female	Under 50	GERD	171
Female	Under 50	ANAPHYLACTIC SHOCK	166
Female	Under 50	CONTRACEPTION- INJECTION (D)	165
Female	Under 50	MILD FUNGAL INFECTIONS	165
Female	Under 50	ANEMIAS, OTHER	164
Female	Under 50	HEPATIC DYSFUNCTION	158
Female	Under 50	CANCER	146
Female	Under 50	GI HEMORRHAGE	145
Female	Under 50	BLEEDING	128
Female	Under 50	VIRAL ILLNESSES	126
Female	Under 50	HEPATITIS	120
Female	Under 50	ACUTE OTITIS MEDIA	113
Female	Under 50	DIARRHEA	113
Female	Under 50	GASTRITIS	101
Female	Under 50	BRONCHOPNEUMONIA	94
Female	Under 50	HEMATURIA	92
Female	Under 50	ANEMIA,DEF.FE,OTH	85
Female	Under 50	ARTHRITIS, RHEUMATOID	83
Female	Under 50	PREG TERMINATION- CHEMICAL	83
Female	Under 50	ARRHYTHMIAS	78
Female	Under 50	COLON, IRRITABLE	78
Female	Under 50	LYMPHADENOPATHY	78
Female	Under 50	SYNCOPE	70
Female	Under 50	CHOLELITHIASIS	67
Female	Under 50	GALLSTONES	67
Female	Under 50	HYPERTHYROIDISM	63
Female	Under 50	KIDNEY STONES	59
Female	Under 50	DEHYDRATION	54
Female	Under 50	VOLUME DEPLETION	54
Female	Under 50	DERMATITIS,MACULOPAPULAR	50
Female	Under 50	BREAST CANCER, FEMALE	48
Female	Under 50	EDEMA	48
Female	Under 50	PSORIASIS	42
Female	Under 50	ANOREXIA	40
Female	Under 50	ARTHRITIS, OSTEOARTHRITIS	40
Female	Under 50	BIPOLAR DISORDER	40
Female	Under 50	EPILEPSY	40

Table 6b. (Continued)

Gender	Age Group	Disease Group	N
Female	Under 50	ALCOHOLISM	39
Female	Under 50	LUPUS	39
Female	Under 50	CNS DEMYELINATING DIS	38
Female	Under 50	COPD	36
Female	Under 50	PANIC DISORDERS	36
Female	Under 50	PERIPHERAL NEUROPATHY	35
Female	Under 50	GI ULCER	34
Female	Under 50	ANKYLOSING SPONDYLITIS	33
Female	Under 50	DYSKINESIAS	32
Female	Under 50	HEMATEMESIS	32
Female	Under 50	MENOPAUSE	32
Female	Under 50	BLEEDING RISK DIAGNOSIS	31
Female	Under 50	CROHN'S DISEASE	31
Female	Under 50	CRYSTALLURIA	30
Female	Under 50	DEEP VEIN THROMBOSIS	29
Female	Under 50	ALBUMINURIA/ NEPHROPATHY	28
Female	Under 50	OSTEOPOROSIS	28
Female	Under 50	RENAL DISEASE	28
Female	Under 50	SYMPTOMS OF QUINIDINE-TOXICITY	28
Female	Under 50	COLITIS	27
Female	Under 50	COLON POLYPS	27
Female	Under 50	ISCHEMIC HEART DISEASE	26
Female	Under 50	STEATORRHEA	26
Female	Under 50	PRURITUS	25
Female	Under 50	PULMONARY DISORDERS	24
Female	Under 50	PULMONARY FIBROSIS	24
Female	Under 50	RENAL FAILURE-GENERAL	24
Female	Under 50	HEMORRHAGIC DISORDERS	23
Female	Under 50	PLEURAL EFFUSION-D	23
Female	Under 50	EPISTAXIS	22
Female	Under 50	PERSONALITY DISORDERS	22
Female	Under 50	RENAL FAILURE W/O HTN	22
Female	Under 50	PRERENAL AZOTEMIA	21
Female	Under 50	PROTEINURIA	20
Female	Under 50	GI OBSTRUCTION	17
Female	Under 50	LEUKOPENIA	17
Female	Under 50	THROMBOPHLEBITIS	17
Female	Under 50	ABUSE- DRUG	16
Female	Under 50	CONGESTIVE HEART FAILURE	16
Female	Under 50	URINARY RETENTION	16
Female	Under 50	ANGINA, PECTORIS	15
Female	Under 50	EXTRAPYRAMIDAL REACTIONS	15

Table 6b. (Continued)

Gender	Age Group	Disease Group	N
Female	Under 50	MYELOSUPPRESSION	15
Female	Under 50	PSYCHOSES	15
Female	Under 50	STROKE	14
Female	Under 50	SUICIDAL BEHAVIOR	14
Female	Under 50	THROMBOCYTOPENIA	14
Female	Under 50	ANEURYSM	13
Female	Under 50	APPENDICITIS	13
Female	Under 50	HEMOLYSIS	13
Female	Under 50	HEPATITIS, ALLER CHOLESTATIC	13
Female	Under 50	NASAL POLYPS	13
Female	Under 50	PULMONARY EMBOLUS	13
Female	Under 50	TELANGLECTASIS	13
Female	Under 50	ARTHROPATHIES, OTHER	12
Female	Under 50	COLOSTOMY/ ILEOSTOMY	12
Female	Under 50	NUTRITIONAL/ NEURO DEFICIENCY	12
Female	Under 50	SEVERE FUNGAL INFECTIONS	12
Female	Under 50	STRESS DISORDERS	12
Female	Under 50	ANGIONEUROTIC EDEMA	11
Female	Under 50	HEPATIC CIRRHOSIS	11
Female	Under 50	PULMONARY EDEMA	11
Female	Under 50	AGRANULOCYTOSIS	10
Female	Under 50	BOWEL OBSTRUCTION	10
Female	Under 50	BULIMIA	10
Female	Under 50	ENCEPHALOPATHIC SYNDROME	10
Female	Under 50	HEMOLYTIC ANEMIA, HERED	10
Female	Under 50	NEUTROPENIA	10
Female	Under 50	PANCREATITIS	10
Female	Under 50	THROMBOCYTOPENIA, SECONDARY	10
Female	Under 50	COAGULATION DEFECTS	9
Female	Under 50	GLAUCOMA	9
Female	Under 50	HEAD TRAUMA	9
Female	Under 50	HEPATOMEGALY WITH STEATOSIS	9
Female	Under 50	SUICIDE	9
Female	Under 50	VENTRICULAR ARRHYTHMIA	9
Female	Under 50	CHICKEN POX	8
Female	Under 50	MALIGNANT MELANOMA	8
Female	Under 50	RELATED TO FETAL OUTCOMES	8
Female	Under 50	UREMIA	8
Female	Under 50	ANEMIA,MEGALOBLASTIC	7
Female	Under 50	ATRIAL FIBRILLATION	7
Female	Under 50	CEREBRAL PALSY	7
Female	Under 50	CHOLESTATIC JAUNDICE	7

Table 6b. (Continued)

Gender	Age Group	Disease Group	N
Female	Under 50	GOUT	7
Female	Under 50	INTERSTITIAL PNEUMONITIS	7
Female	Under 50	MYOCARDIAL ISCHEMIA	7
Female	Under 50	OPTIC NEURITIS	7
Female	Under 50	ANGINA, UNSTABLE	6
Female	Under 50	EXFOLIATIVE DERMATITIS	6
Female	Under 50	HYPERSECRETORY STATES	6
Female	Under 50	NEUROPATHIES	6
Female	Under 50	SICKLE CELL ANEMIA	6
Female	Under 50	ARTHRITIS, PSORIATIC	5
Female	Under 50	COLON LESIONS	5
Female	Under 50	CYSTIC FIBROSIS	5
Female	Under 50	HEART BLOCK	5
Female	Under 50	JAUNDICE	5
Female	Under 50	MALIGNANT NEOPLASM, CNS	5
Female	Under 50	RENAL CALCIFICATION	5
Female	Under 50	BRAIN HEMORRHAGE	4
Female	Under 50	HEMOPTYSIS	4
Female	Under 50	HYPOTENSION	4
Female	Under 50	INTESTINAL ATONY	4
Female	Under 50	OSTEOSARCOMA	4
Female	Under 50	RADIATION THERAPY ICD	4
Female	Under 50	BRADYCARDIA	3
Female	Under 50	BULLOUS RASH	3
Female	Under 50	CIRRHOSIS	3
Female	Under 50	ELECTROLYTE DISORDERS	3
Female	Under 50	HEMOLYTIC ANEMIA, ACQ	3
Female	Under 50	ILEUS, PARALYTIC	3
Female	Under 50	INTRA-ABDOMINAL HEMORRHAGE	3
Female	Under 50	KETOACIDOSIS	3
Female	Under 50	MYOPATHY	3
Female	Under 50	OBSTRUCTIVE UROPATHY	3
Female	Under 50	PSEUDOTUMOR CEREBRI	3
Female	Under 50	PULMONARY EMBOLUS, PREVIOUS	3
Female	Under 50	RETROPERITONEAL FIBROSIS	3
Female	Under 50	ADDISON'S DISEASE	2
Female	Under 50	ADRENAL INSUFFICIENCY	2
Female	Under 50	ALCOHOLIC LIVER DISEASE	2
Female	Under 50	APLASTIC ANEMIA	2
Female	Under 50	BLEPHARASPASM	2
Female	Under 50	DEMENTIA	2
Female	Under 50	ERYTHEMA MULTIFORME	2

Table 6b. (Continued)

Gender	Age Group	Disease Group	N
Female	Under 50	HALLUCINATIONS	2
Female	Under 50	HEPATIC FAILURE	2
Female	Under 50	MYASTHENIA GRAVIS	2
Female	Under 50	PARKINSONISM,PRIMARY	2
Female	Under 50	PERICARDIAL DISEASE	2
Female	Under 50	PERICARDIAL EFFUSION	2
Female	Under 50	STEVENS JOHNSON SYNDROME	2
Female	Under 50	AV BLOCK II TO III	1
Female	Under 50	BLOOD DYSCRASIAS	1
Female	Under 50	BOWEL PERFORATION	1
Female	Under 50	CEREBRAL ARTERIOSCLEROSIS	1
Female	Under 50	DRUG INDUCED PSYCH DISORDERS	1
Female	Under 50	FECAL IMPACTION	1
Female	Under 50	GLAUCOMA,NARROW ANGLE	1
Female	Under 50	HYPERCALCEMIA	1
Female	Under 50	HYPOPROTHROMINEMIA	1
Female	Under 50	MYELODYSPLASTIC SYNDROME	1
Female	Under 50	SUBARACHNOID HEMORRHAGE	1
Female	50+	CARDIOVASCULAR DISEASE	731
Female	50+	HYPERTENSION	673
Female	50+	HYPERSENSITIVITY REACTIONS	630
Female	50+	LIPID ABNORMALITIES	530
Female	50+	RESPIRATORY INFECTIONS	415
Female	50+	FRACTURES AND INJURIES	369
Female	50+	DIABETES MELLITUS I AND II	294
Female	50+	THYROID DISEASE	229
Female	50+	DIARRHEA, GASTROENTERITIS	204
Female	50+	CANCER	180
Female	50+	SYMPTOMS OF GI IRRITATION	157
Female	50+	SYMPTOMS OF DIG-TOXICITY	140
Female	50+	LACTIC ACIDOSIS SYMPTOMS	136
Female	50+	HEMATOLOGIC DISORDERS	133
Female	50+	PSYCHOSES, DRUG INDUCED	115
Female	50+	ABDOMINAL PAIN	114
Female	50+	TUBERCULOSIS	114
Female	50+	DEPRESSION	113
Female	50+	COUGH	104
Female	50+	HEPATIC DYSFUNCTION	104
Female	50+	OSTEOPOROSIS	104
Female	50+	COPD	102
Female	50+	GERD	100
Female	50+	CNS EXCITATION	99

Table 6b. (Continued)

Gender	Age Group	Disease Group	N
Female	50+	ASTHMA	97
Female	50+	BREAST CANCER, FEMALE	89
Female	50+	HEPATITIS	88
Female	50+	ARTHRITIS, OSTEOARTHRITIS	86
Female	50+	ISCHEMIC HEART DISEASE	85
Female	50+	ARRHYTHMIAS	78
Female	50+	ARTHRITIS, RHEUMATOID	73
Female	50+	GI HEMORRHAGE	71
Female	50+	ANEMIAS, OTHER	66
Female	50+	MENOPAUSE	66
Female	50+	SYMPTOMS OF ERGOTISM	65
Female	50+	MILD FUNGAL INFECTIONS	64
Female	50+	PANCYTOPENIA	64
Female	50+	BLEEDING	60
Female	50+	GLAUCOMA	55
Female	50+	HIV	54
Female	50+	ANEMIA,DEF.FE,OTH	53
Female	50+	CONGESTIVE HEART FAILURE	52
Female	50+	OBESITY	51
Female	50+	COND- REYE SYNDROME RELATED	49
Female	50+	DIARRHEA	47
Female	50+	ANXIETY DISORDERS	46
Female	50+	GASTRITIS	46
Female	50+	ANGINA, PECTORIS	41
Female	50+	ATRIAL FIBRILLATION	40
Female	50+	EDEMA	39
Female	50+	HEMATURIA	36
Female	50+	BRONCHOPNEUMONIA	35
Female	50+	COLON, IRRITABLE	35
Female	50+	COLON POLYPS	34
Female	50+	ANAPHYLACTIC SHOCK	32
Female	50+	ANKYLOSING SPONDYLITIS	31
Female	50+	STROKE	27
Female	50+	GI ULCER	25
Female	50+	SYMPTOMS OF QUINIDINE-TOXICITY	25
Female	50+	MYOCARDIAL ISCHEMIA	23
Female	50+	PERIPHERAL NEUROPATHY	23
Female	50+	PSORIASIS	23
Female	50+	STEATORRHEA	23
Female	50+	ANEURYSM	20
Female	50+	DEEP VEIN THROMBOSIS	20
Female	50+	RENAL FAILURE-GENERAL	20

Table 6b. (Continued)

Gender	Age Group	Disease Group	N
Female	50+	RENAL FAILURE W/O HTN	19
Female	50+	BLEEDING RISK DIAGNOSIS	18
Female	50+	HEMATEMESIS	18
Female	50+	ANGINA, UNSTABLE	17
Female	50+	CHOLELITHIASIS	17
Female	50+	CHRONIC OTITIS MEDIA	17
Female	50+	GALLSTONES	17
Female	50+	DERMATITIS,MACULOPAPULAR	16
Female	50+	DYSKINESIAS	16
Female	50+	SYNCOPE	16
Female	50+	VIRAL ILLNESSES	16
Female	50+	CNS DEMYELINATING DIS	15
Female	50+	DEMENTIA	15
Female	50+	RENAL DISEASE	15
Female	50+	HEART BLOCK	14
Female	50+	ALBUMINURIA/ NEPHROPATHY	13
Female	50+	LUPUS	13
Female	50+	NUTRITIONAL/ NEURO DEFICIENCY	12
Female	50+	ARTHROPATHIES, OTHER	11
Female	50+	DEHYDRATION	11
Female	50+	EXTRAPYRAMIDAL REACTIONS	11
Female	50+	KIDNEY STONES	11
Female	50+	VOLUME DEPLETION	11
Female	50+	HYPERTHYROIDISM	10
Female	50+	LEUKOPENIA	10
Female	50+	LYMPHADENOPATHY	10
Female	50+	MYELOSUPPRESSION	10
Female	50+	ACUTE OTITIS MEDIA	9
Female	50+	AGRANULOCYTOSIS	9
Female	50+	AV BLOCK II TO III	9
Female	50+	BIPOLAR DISORDER	9
Female	50+	COAGULATION DEFECTS	9
Female	50+	NEUROPATHIES	9
Female	50+	NEUTROPENIA	9
Female	50+	PSYCHOSES	9
Female	50+	PULMONARY DISORDERS	9
Female	50+	PULMONARY EDEMA	9
Female	50+	PULMONARY FIBROSIS	9
Female	50+	THROMBOPHLEBITIS	9
Female	50+	COLITIS	8
Female	50+	CROHN'S DISEASE	8
Female	50+	EPILEPSY	8

Table 6b. (Continued)

Gender	Age Group	Disease Group	N
Female	50+	INTERSTITIAL PNEUMONITIS	8
Female	50+	PLEURAL EFFUSION-D	8
Female	50+	TELANGLECTASIS	8
Female	50+	HEMORRHAGIC DISORDERS	7
Female	50+	PANIC DISORDERS	7
Female	50+	PRURITUS	7
Female	50+	ALZHEIMER	6
Female	50+	BOWEL OBSTRUCTION	6
Female	50+	GI OBSTRUCTION	6
Female	50+	GLAUCOMA,NARROW ANGLE	6
Female	50+	HEPATIC CIRRHOSIS	6
Female	50+	HEPATOMEGALY WITH STEATOSIS	6
Female	50+	HYPERSECRETORY STATES	6
Female	50+	OSTEOSARCOMA	6
Female	50+	SEVERE FUNGAL INFECTIONS	6
Female	50+	ALCOHOLISM	5
Female	50+	ANEMIA,MEGALOBLASTIC	5
Female	50+	ARTHRITIS, PSORIATIC	5
Female	50+	BLOOD DYSCRASIAS	5
Female	50+	EPISTAXIS	5
Female	50+	GOUT	5
Female	50+	MYELODYSPLASTIC SYNDROME	5
Female	50+	OPTIC NEURITIS	5
Female	50+	PARKINSONISM,PRIMARY	5
Female	50+	STRESS DISORDERS	5
Female	50+	UREMIA	5
Female	50+	ANOREXIA	4
Female	50+	BRAIN HEMORRHAGE	4
Female	50+	COLOSTOMY/ ILEOSTOMY	4
Female	50+	CRYSTALLURIA	4
Female	50+	ENCEPHALOPATHIC SYNDROME	4
Female	50+	MALIGNANT MELANOMA	4
Female	50+	PERSONALITY DISORDERS	4
Female	50+	PULMONARY EMBOLUS, PREVIOUS	4
Female	50+	THROMBOCYTOPENIA	4
Female	50+	APLASTIC ANEMIA	3
Female	50+	BRADYCARDIA	3
Female	50+	COLON LESIONS	3
Female	50+	DELIRIUM	3
Female	50+	EXFOLIATIVE DERMATITIS	3
Female	50+	HEPATITIS, ALLER CHOLESTATIC	3
Female	50+	HYPERCALCEMIA	3

Table 6b. (Continued)

Gender	Age Group	Disease Group	N
Female	50+	KETOACIDOSIS	3
Female	50+	PANCREATITIS	3
Female	50+	PULMONARY EMBOLUS	3
Female	50+	SUICIDAL BEHAVIOR	3
Female	50+	THROMBOCYTOPENIA, SECONDARY	3
Female	50+	URINARY RETENTION	3
Female	50+	VENTRICULAR ARRHYTHMIA	3
Female	50+	ALVEOLITIS,FIBROSING	2
Female	50+	ANGIONEUROTIC EDEMA	2
Female	50+	CARDIAC VALVE FIBROSIS	2
Female	50+	CEREBRAL PALSY	2
Female	50+	CIRRHOSIS	2
Female	50+	HEMOPTYSIS	2
Female	50+	HYPOPROTHROMINEMIA	2
Female	50+	HYPOTENSION	2
Female	50+	INTRA-ABDOMINAL HEMORRHAGE	2
Female	50+	MALIGNANT NEOPLASM, CNS	2
Female	50+	PROTEINURIA	2
Female	50+	RHABDOMYOLYSIS	2
Female	50+	SUBARACHNOID HEMORRHAGE	2
Female	50+	ABNL PREG TERMINATED OR DELIV	1
Female	50+	ALCOHOLIC LIVER DISEASE	1
Female	50+	APPENDICITIS	1
Female	50+	BLEPHARASPASM	1
Female	50+	BULLOUS RASH	1
Female	50+	CEREBRAL ARTERIOSCLEROSIS	1
Female	50+	CHOLESTATIC JAUNDICE	1
Female	50+	CONTRACEPTIVE MEASURES	1
Female	50+	DRUG INDUCED PSYCH DISORDERS	1
Female	50+	FECAL IMPACTION	1
Female	50+	HALLUCINATIONS	1
Female	50+	HEAD TRAUMA	1
Female	50+	HEPATIC FAILURE	1
Female	50+	ILEUS, PARALYTIC	1
Female	50+	MYOPATHY	1
Female	50+	NASAL POLYPS	1
Female	50+	ORAL CONTRACEPTION	1
Female	50+	RADIATION THERAPY ICD	1
Female	50+	RELATED TO FETAL OUTCOMES	1
Female	50+	RENAL CALCIFICATION	1
Female	50+	SUICIDE	1
Male	Under 50	HYPERSENSITIVITY REACTIONS	1,652

Table 6b. (Continued)

Gender	Age Group	Disease Group	N
Male	Under 50	RESPIRATORY INFECTIONS	1,601
Male	Under 50	FRACTURES AND INJURIES	1,526
Male	Under 50	CARDIOVASCULAR DISEASE	476
Male	Under 50	LIPID ABNORMALITIES	475
Male	Under 50	HYPERTENSION	451
Male	Under 50	DIARRHEA, GASTROENTERITIS	386
Male	Under 50	DIABETES MELLITUS I AND II	274
Male	Under 50	PSYCHOSES, DRUG INDUCED	266
Male	Under 50	DEPRESSION	239
Male	Under 50	SYMPTOMS OF GI IRRITATION	235
Male	Under 50	ASTHMA	215
Male	Under 50	CNS EXCITATION	214
Male	Under 50	LACTIC ACIDOSIS SYMPTOMS	201
Male	Under 50	ABDOMINAL PAIN	196
Male	Under 50	MILD FUNGAL INFECTIONS	178
Male	Under 50	TUBERCULOSIS	178
Male	Under 50	CHRONIC OTITIS MEDIA	177
Male	Under 50	SYMPTOMS OF DIG-TOXICITY	171
Male	Under 50	COUGH	167
Male	Under 50	GERD	150
Male	Under 50	HEPATIC DYSFUNCTION	133
Male	Under 50	COND- REYE SYNDROME RELATED	122
Male	Under 50	ANXIETY DISORDERS	112
Male	Under 50	HEPATITIS	106
Male	Under 50	GI HEMORRHAGE	99
Male	Under 50	CANCER	91
Male	Under 50	ANAPHYLACTIC SHOCK	86
Male	Under 50	BLEEDING	85
Male	Under 50	HEMATOLOGIC DISORDERS	81
Male	Under 50	SYMPTOMS OF ERGOTISM	81
Male	Under 50	VIRAL ILLNESSES	75
Male	Under 50	CONTRACEPTIVE MEASURES	69
Male	Under 50	ACUTE OTITIS MEDIA	66
Male	Under 50	THYROID DISEASE	63
Male	Under 50	BRONCHOPNEUMONIA	62
Male	Under 50	DIARRHEA	61
Male	Under 50	ARRHYTHMIAS	60
Male	Under 50	GASTRITIS	60
Male	Under 50	KIDNEY STONES	57
Male	Under 50	ISCHEMIC HEART DISEASE	53
Male	Under 50	PANCYTOPENIA	52
Male	Under 50	HEMATURIA	50

Table 6b. (Continued)

Gender	Age Group	Disease Group	N
Male	Under 50	PSORIASIS	50
Male	Under 50	OBESITY	45
Male	Under 50	ALCOHOLISM	42
Male	Under 50	HIV	42
Male	Under 50	COPD	37
Male	Under 50	LYMPHADENOPATHY	35
Male	Under 50	ARTHRITIS, RHEUMATOID	34
Male	Under 50	SYNCOPE	34
Male	Under 50	EPILEPSY	33
Male	Under 50	ARTHRITIS, OSTEOARTHRITIS	32
Male	Under 50	ANEMIAS, OTHER	31
Male	Under 50	COLON, IRRITABLE	31
Male	Under 50	RENAL DISEASE	31
Male	Under 50	ORAL CONTRACEPTION	30
Male	Under 50	GOUT	29
Male	Under 50	HEMATEMESIS	29
Male	Under 50	RENAL FAILURE-GENERAL	29
Male	Under 50	SYMPTOMS OF QUINIDINE-TOXICITY	29
Male	Under 50	ANGINA, PECTORIS	27
Male	Under 50	ANKYLOSING SPONDYLITIS	26
Male	Under 50	RENAL FAILURE W/O HTN	26
Male	Under 50	DERMATITIS,MACULOPAPULAR	24
Male	Under 50	GI ULCER	24
Male	Under 50	DEHYDRATION	23
Male	Under 50	VOLUME DEPLETION	23
Male	Under 50	CROHN'S DISEASE	22
Male	Under 50	DYSKINESIAS	22
Male	Under 50	COLON POLYPS	21
Male	Under 50	EPISTAXIS	21
Male	Under 50	PERIPHERAL NEUROPATHY	21
Male	Under 50	ABUSE- DRUG	19
Male	Under 50	CONTRACEPTION- INJECTION (D)	19
Male	Under 50	STEATORRHEA	19
Male	Under 50	ALBUMINURIA/ NEPHROPATHY	18
Male	Under 50	PANIC DISORDERS	18
Male	Under 50	APPENDICITIS	17
Male	Under 50	COLITIS	17
Male	Under 50	EDEMA	17
Male	Under 50	GLAUCOMA	17
Male	Under 50	ATRIAL FIBRILLATION	16
Male	Under 50	BIPOLAR DISORDER	16
Male	Under 50	ARTHRITIS, PSORIATIC	15

Table 6b. (Continued)

Gender	Age Group	Disease Group	N
Male	Under 50	CNS DEMYELINATING DIS	15
Male	Under 50	NUTRITIONAL/ NEURO DEFICIENCY	15
Male	Under 50	CONGESTIVE HEART FAILURE	14
Male	Under 50	DEEP VEIN THROMBOSIS	14
Male	Under 50	HEAD TRAUMA	14
Male	Under 50	BLEEDING RISK DIAGNOSIS	13
Male	Under 50	VENTRICULAR ARRHYTHMIA	13
Male	Under 50	ANEURYSM	12
Male	Under 50	EXTRAPYRAMIDAL REACTIONS	12
Male	Under 50	HEPATITIS, ALLER CHOLESTATIC	12
Male	Under 50	PERSONALITY DISORDERS	12
Male	Under 50	PLEURAL EFFUSION-D	12
Male	Under 50	STROKE	12
Male	Under 50	ARTHROPATHIES, OTHER	11
Male	Under 50	BOWEL OBSTRUCTION	11
Male	Under 50	GI OBSTRUCTION	11
Male	Under 50	HEMORRHAGIC DISORDERS	11
Male	Under 50	PROTEINURIA	11
Male	Under 50	ANEMIA,DEF.FE,OTH	10
Male	Under 50	CHICKEN POX	10
Male	Under 50	HEPATIC CIRRHOSIS	10
Male	Under 50	LEUKOPENIA	10
Male	Under 50	NASAL POLYPS	10
Male	Under 50	PRURITUS	10
Male	Under 50	PULMONARY EDEMA	10
Male	Under 50	STRESS DISORDERS	10
Male	Under 50	THROMBOCYTOPENIA	10
Male	Under 50	URINARY RETENTION	10
Male	Under 50	CEREBRAL PALSY	9
Male	Under 50	CHOLELITHIASIS	9
Male	Under 50	GALLSTONES	9
Male	Under 50	HEART BLOCK	9
Male	Under 50	MYOCARDIAL ISCHEMIA	9
Male	Under 50	THROMBOCYTOPENIA, SECONDARY	9
Male	Under 50	ANGINA, UNSTABLE	8
Male	Under 50	BENIGN PROSTATIC HYPERTROPHY	8
Male	Under 50	HEMOPTYSIS	8
Male	Under 50	HEPATOMEGALY WITH STEATOSIS	8
Male	Under 50	PULMONARY DISORDERS	8
Male	Under 50	SEVERE FUNGAL INFECTIONS	8
Male	Under 50	SUICIDAL BEHAVIOR	8
Male	Under 50	BRAIN HEMORRHAGE	7

Table 6b. (Continued)

Gender	Age Group	Disease Group	N
Male	Under 50	COLOSTOMY/ ILEOSTOMY	7
Male	Under 50	MALIGNANT NEOPLASM, CNS	7
Male	Under 50	NEUROPATHIES	7
Male	Under 50	PERICARDIAL EFFUSION	7
Male	Under 50	PULMONARY FIBROSIS	7
Male	Under 50	ANOREXIA	6
Male	Under 50	COAGULATION DEFECTS	6
Male	Under 50	CYSTIC FIBROSIS	6
Male	Under 50	ENCEPHALOPATHIC SYNDROME	6
Male	Under 50	HYPERSECRETORY STATES	6
Male	Under 50	HYPERTHYROIDISM	6
Male	Under 50	PERICARDIAL DISEASE	6
Male	Under 50	PROSTATIC HYPERTROPHY	6
Male	Under 50	EXFOLIATIVE DERMATITIS	5
Male	Under 50	ILEUS, PARALYTIC	5
Male	Under 50	LUPUS	5
Male	Under 50	MALIGNANT MELANOMA	5
Male	Under 50	MYELOSUPPRESSION	5
Male	Under 50	OSTEOSARCOMA	5
Male	Under 50	PSYCHOSES	5
Male	Under 50	RENAL CALCIFICATION	5
Male	Under 50	AGRANULOCYTOSIS	4
Male	Under 50	HALLUCINATIONS	4
Male	Under 50	NEUTROPENIA	4
Male	Under 50	OBSTRUCTIVE UROPATHY	4
Male	Under 50	OPTIC NEURITIS	4
Male	Under 50	PANCREATITIS	4
Male	Under 50	PRERENAL AZOTEMIA	4
Male	Under 50	RADIATION THERAPY ICD	4
Male	Under 50	SUICIDE	4
Male	Under 50	THROMBOPHLEBITIS	4
Male	Under 50	ANGIONEUROTIC EDEMA	3
Male	Under 50	AV BLOCK II TO III	3
Male	Under 50	CIRRHOSIS	3
Male	Under 50	CRYSTALLURIA	3
Male	Under 50	DRUG INDUCED PSYCH DISORDERS	3
Male	Under 50	KETOACIDOSIS	3
Male	Under 50	MYOCARDITIS	3
Male	Under 50	MYOPATHY	3
Male	Under 50	PARKINSONISM,PRIMARY	3
Male	Under 50	PSEUDOMEMBRANOUS COLITIS	3
Male	Under 50	ALCOHOLIC LIVER DISEASE	2

Table 6b. (Continued)

Gender	Age Group	Disease Group	N
Male	Under 50	APLASTIC ANEMIA	2
Male	Under 50	BRADYCARDIA	2
Male	Under 50	BULLOUS RASH	2
Male	Under 50	CARDIAC VALVE FIBROSIS	2
Male	Under 50	CHOLESTATIC JAUNDICE	2
Male	Under 50	COLON LESIONS	2
Male	Under 50	DEMENTIA	2
Male	Under 50	GLAUCOMA,NARROW ANGLE	2
Male	Under 50	HEMOLYSIS	2
Male	Under 50	HEMOLYTIC ANEMIA, HERED	2
Male	Under 50	INTERSTITIAL PNEUMONITIS	2
Male	Under 50	JAUNDICE	2
Male	Under 50	RELATED TO FETAL OUTCOMES	2
Male	Under 50	RETROPERITONEAL FIBROSIS	2
Male	Under 50	SICKLE CELL ANEMIA	2
Male	Under 50	SUBARACHNOID HEMORRHAGE	2
Male	Under 50	TELANGLECTASIS	2
Male	Under 50	ABNL PREG TERMINATED OR DELIV	1
Male	Under 50	ADDISON'S DISEASE	1
Male	Under 50	ADRENAL INSUFFICIENCY	1
Male	Under 50	ALZHEIMER	1
Male	Under 50	ANEMIA,MEGALOBLASTIC	1
Male	Under 50	BLEPHARASPASM	1
Male	Under 50	BOWEL PERFORATION	1
Male	Under 50	BREAST CANCER, FEMALE	1
Male	Under 50	DELIRIUM	1
Male	Under 50	ERYTHEMA MULTIFORME	1
Male	Under 50	FECAL IMPACTION	1
Male	Under 50	HEPATIC FAILURE	1
Male	Under 50	HYPERSENSITIVITY PNEUMONITIS	1
Male	Under 50	HYPOTENSION	1
Male	Under 50	INTRA-ABDOMINAL HEMORRHAGE	1
Male	Under 50	OSTEOMALACIA	1
Male	Under 50	OSTEOPOROSIS	1
Male	Under 50	PREGNANCY	1
Male	Under 50	PULMONARY EMBOLUS, PREVIOUS	1
Male	Under 50	RENAL OSTEODYSTROPHY	1
Male	Under 50	STEVENS JOHNSON SYNDROME	1
Male	Under 50	UREMIA	1
Male	50+	CARDIOVASCULAR DISEASE	685
Male	50+	HYPERTENSION	621
Male	50+	LIPID ABNORMALITIES	551

Table 6b. (Continued)

Gender	Age Group	Disease Group	N
Male	50+	DIABETES MELLITUS I AND II	390
Male	50+	HYPERSENSITIVITY REACTIONS	350
Male	50+	FRACTURES AND INJURIES	264
Male	50+	RESPIRATORY INFECTIONS	262
Male	50+	CANCER	207
Male	50+	ISCHEMIC HEART DISEASE	205
Male	50+	HEPATIC DYSFUNCTION	136
Male	50+	ARRHYTHMIAS	131
Male	50+	DIARRHEA, GASTROENTERITIS	126
Male	50+	HEPATITIS	112
Male	50+	SYMPTOMS OF GI IRRITATION	110
Male	50+	SYMPTOMS OF DIG-TOXICITY	107
Male	50+	TUBERCULOSIS	107
Male	50+	COPD	104
Male	50+	HEMATOLOGIC DISORDERS	98
Male	50+	BLEEDING	87
Male	50+	ATRIAL FIBRILLATION	79
Male	50+	GI HEMORRHAGE	70
Male	50+	PSYCHOSES, DRUG INDUCED	66
Male	50+	ANGINA, PECTORIS	64
Male	50+	CONGESTIVE HEART FAILURE	64
Male	50+	PANCYTOPENIA	63
Male	50+	ARTHRITIS, OSTEOARTHRITIS	61
Male	50+	ABDOMINAL PAIN	59
Male	50+	ANEMIAS, OTHER	59
Male	50+	GERD	58
Male	50+	DEPRESSION	57
Male	50+	LACTIC ACIDOSIS SYMPTOMS	57
Male	50+	MILD FUNGAL INFECTIONS	55
Male	50+	COUGH	54
Male	50+	GLAUCOMA	52
Male	50+	THYROID DISEASE	50
Male	50+	SYMPTOMS OF QUINIDINE-TOXICITY	49
Male	50+	HEMATURIA	46
Male	50+	ASTHMA	43
Male	50+	COLON POLYPS	43
Male	50+	CNS EXCITATION	42
Male	50+	SYMPTOMS OF ERGOTISM	41
Male	50+	GI ULCER	40
Male	50+	COND- REYE SYNDROME RELATED	38
Male	50+	HEMATEMESIS	37
Male	50+	STROKE	37

Table 6b. (Continued)

Gender	Age Group	Disease Group	N
Male	50+	BENIGN PROSTATIC HYPERTROPHY	36
Male	50+	ANEMIA,DEF.FE,OTH	35
Male	50+	BRONCHOPNEUMONIA	34
Male	50+	ANXIETY DISORDERS	32
Male	50+	PROSTATIC HYPERTROPHY	32
Male	50+	OBESITY	31
Male	50+	PERIPHERAL NEUROPATHY	31
Male	50+	RENAL FAILURE W/O HTN	31
Male	50+	GASTRITIS	30
Male	50+	RENAL FAILURE-GENERAL	30
Male	50+	ANEURYSM	29
Male	50+	EDEMA	29
Male	50+	MYOCARDIAL ISCHEMIA	28
Male	50+	CHRONIC OTITIS MEDIA	26
Male	50+	KIDNEY STONES	25
Male	50+	NUTRITIONAL/ NEURO DEFICIENCY	24
Male	50+	ANKYLOSING SPONDYLITIS	22
Male	50+	ARTHRITIS, RHEUMATOID	22
Male	50+	GOUT	22
Male	50+	PSORIASIS	22
Male	50+	ALBUMINURIA/ NEPHROPATHY	21
Male	50+	RENAL DISEASE	21
Male	50+	STEATORRHEA	21
Male	50+	VENTRICULAR ARRHYTHMIA	21
Male	50+	SYNCOPE	20
Male	50+	DIARRHEA	19
Male	50+	DEEP VEIN THROMBOSIS	18
Male	50+	ALCOHOLISM	16
Male	50+	ANAPHYLACTIC SHOCK	16
Male	50+	BLEEDING RISK DIAGNOSIS	16
Male	50+	VIRAL ILLNESSES	15
Male	50+	ACUTE OTITIS MEDIA	14
Male	50+	HEART BLOCK	14
Male	50+	HEPATIC CIRRHOSIS	13
Male	50+	ANGINA, UNSTABLE	12
Male	50+	BOWEL OBSTRUCTION	12
Male	50+	COLON, IRRITABLE	12
Male	50+	AV BLOCK II TO III	11
Male	50+	DEHYDRATION	11
Male	50+	HEMORRHAGIC DISORDERS	11
Male	50+	URINARY RETENTION	11
Male	50+	VOLUME DEPLETION	11

Table 6b. (Continued)

Gender	Age Group	Disease Group	N
Male	50+	CIRRHOSIS	10
Male	50+	NEUROPATHIES	10
Male	50+	PULMONARY DISORDERS	10
Male	50+	PULMONARY FIBROSIS	10
Male	50+	BIPOLAR DISORDER	9
Male	50+	BRADYCARDIA	9
Male	50+	COAGULATION DEFECTS	9
Male	50+	COLOSTOMY/ ILEOSTOMY	9
Male	50+	DERMATITIS,MACULOPAPULAR	9
Male	50+	INTERSTITIAL PNEUMONITIS	9
Male	50+	LYMPHADENOPATHY	9
Male	50+	PARKINSONISM,PRIMARY	9
Male	50+	DEMENTIA	8
Male	50+	GI OBSTRUCTION	8
Male	50+	HIV	8
Male	50+	PULMONARY EDEMA	8
Male	50+	CNS DEMYELINATING DIS	7
Male	50+	HYPOTENSION	7
Male	50+	ILEUS, PARALYTIC	7
Male	50+	NASAL POLYPS	7
Male	50+	OSTEOPOROSIS	7
Male	50+	PLEURAL EFFUSION-D	7
Male	50+	UREMIA	7
Male	50+	CROHN'S DISEASE	6
Male	50+	EPILEPSY	6
Male	50+	HEPATITIS, ALLER CHOLESTATIC	6
Male	50+	HYPERSECRETORY STATES	6
Male	50+	MYELOSUPPRESSION	6
Male	50+	THROMBOCYTOPENIA	6
Male	50+	THROMBOPHLEBITIS	6
Male	50+	CHOLELITHIASIS	5
Male	50+	GALLSTONES	5
Male	50+	OPTIC NEURITIS	5
Male	50+	OSTEOSARCOMA	5
Male	50+	THROMBOCYTOPENIA, SECONDARY	5
Male	50+	ALCOHOLIC LIVER DISEASE	4
Male	50+	ALZHEIMER	4
Male	50+	ANOREXIA	4
Male	50+	APLASTIC ANEMIA	4
Male	50+	ARTHROPATHIES, OTHER	4
Male	50+	BRAIN HEMORRHAGE	4
Male	50+	COLITIS	4

Table 6b. (Continued)

Gender	Age Group	Disease Group	N
Male	50+	DYSKINESIAS	4
Male	50+	HEAD TRAUMA	4
Male	50+	LEUKOPENIA	4
Male	50+	MYELODYSPLASTIC SYNDROME	4
Male	50+	PANIC DISORDERS	4
Male	50+	PRERENAL AZOTEMIA	4
Male	50+	PRURITUS	4
Male	50+	PULMONARY EMBOLUS	4
Male	50+	RADIATION THERAPY ICD	4
Male	50+	ANEMIA,MEGALOBLASTIC	3
Male	50+	COLON LESIONS	3
Male	50+	ENCEPHALOPATHIC SYNDROME	3
Male	50+	EPISTAXIS	3
Male	50+	EXFOLIATIVE DERMATITIS	3
Male	50+	HEMOPTYSIS	3
Male	50+	MALIGNANT MELANOMA	3
Male	50+	PROTEINURIA	3
Male	50+	PSYCHOSES	3
Male	50+	SEVERE FUNGAL INFECTIONS	3
Male	50+	AGRANULOCYTOSIS	2
Male	50+	APPENDICITIS	2
Male	50+	ARTHRITIS, PSORIATIC	2
Male	50+	HEPATOMEGALY WITH STEATOSIS	2
Male	50+	HYPERCALCEMIA	2
Male	50+	HYPERTHYROIDISM	2
Male	50+	KETOACIDOSIS	2
Male	50+	MALIGNANT NEOPLASM, CNS	2
Male	50+	MYASTHENIA GRAVIS	2
Male	50+	NEUTROPENIA	2
Male	50+	PANCREATITIS	2
Male	50+	ALVEOLITIS,FIBROSING	1
Male	50+	BOWEL PERFORATION	1
Male	50+	CARDIAC ARREST	1
Male	50+	EXTRAPYRAMIDAL REACTIONS	1
Male	50+	GLAUCOMA,NARROW ANGLE	1
Male	50+	HALLUCINATIONS	1
Male	50+	HEMOLYSIS	1
Male	50+	HEMOLYTIC ANEMIA, HERED	1
Male	50+	MEASLES	1
Male	50+	MYOPATHY	1
Male	50+	OBSTRUCTIVE UROPATHY	1
Male	50+	OSTEOMALACIA	1

Table 6b. (Continued)

Gender	Age Group	Disease Group	N
Male	50+	PERICARDIAL EFFUSION	1
Male	50+	PULMONARY EMBOLUS, PREVIOUS	1
Male	50+	RENAL CALCIFICATION	1
Male	50+	RHABDOMYOLYSIS	1
Male	50+	SUBARACHNOID HEMORRHAGE	1
Male	50+	TELANGLECTASIS	1

Table 7a. Number of Patients by Age, Gender, and Number of Driver Impairing Disease Groups Case Group

Age Group	Number of Potential Impairing Disease Groups	Gender					
		Female		Male		Both	
		N	PCTN	N	PCTN	N	PCTN
Under 50	0	8,603	56	8,944	70	17,547	62
	1	2,433	16	1,602	13	4,035	14
	2	1,574	10	892	7	2,466	9
	3	1,052	7	508	4	1,560	6
	4	625	4	266	2	891	3
	5	366	2	169	1	535	2
	6	270	2	105	1	375	1
	7	182	1	76	1	258	1
	8	125	1	59	0	184	1
	9	84	1	33	0	117	0
	10	56	0	21	0	77	0
	11	28	0	17	0	45	0
	12	33	0	9	0	42	0
	13	11	0	6	0	17	0
	14	13	0	10	0	23	0
	15	1	0	4	0	5	0
	16	4	0	2	0	6	0
	17	7	0	3	0	10	0
	18	4	0			4	0
	19	2	0			2	0
	20	1	0			1	0
	21	2	0			2	0
	22			1	0	1	0
	24	1	0			1	0

Table 7a. (Continued)

		Gender				Both	
		Female		Male			
		N	PCTN	N	PCTN	N	PCTN
Age Group Under 50	Number of Potential Impairing Disease Groups						
	26	1	0	1	0	2	0
	27	1	0			1	0
	All	15,479	100	12,728	100	28,207	100
50+	Number of Potential Impairing Disease Groups						
	0	1,321	46	1,338	52	2,659	49
	1	351	12	260	10	611	11
	2	312	11	248	10	560	10
	3	228	8	206	8	434	8
	4	167	6	112	4	279	5
	5	140	5	107	4	247	5
	6	90	3	75	3	165	3
	7	66	2	58	2	124	2
	8	45	2	40	2	85	2
	9	32	1	23	1	55	1
	10	21	1	16	1	37	1
	11	24	1	18	1	42	1
	12	9	0	15	1	24	0
	13	10	0	6	0	16	0
	14	7	0	9	0	16	0
	15	4	0	7	0	11	0
	16	8	0	5	0	13	0
	17	2	0	1	0	3	0

Multiple Medications and Vehicle Crashes: Analysis of Databases

Table 7a. (Continued)

| | | Gender | | | | Both | |
| | | Female | | Male | | | |
		N	PCTN	N	PCTN	N	PCTN
Age Group 50+	Number of Potential Impairing Disease Groups						
	18	3	0	3	0	6	0
	19	1	0	1	0	2	0
	20	1	0	2	0	3	0
	21			2	0	2	0
	22			1	0	1	0
	24			3	0	3	0
	All	2,842	100	2,556	100	5,398	100
All Age	Number of Potential Impairing Disease Groups						
	0	9,924	54	10,282	67	20,206	60
	1	2,784	15	1,862	12	4,646	14
	2	1,886	10	1,140	7	3,026	9
	3	1,280	7	714	5	1,994	6
	4	792	4	378	2	1,170	3
	5	506	3	276	2	782	2
	6	360	2	180	1	540	2
	7	248	1	134	1	382	1
	8	170	1	99	1	269	1
	9	116	1	56	0	172	1
	10	77	0	37	0	114	0
	11	52	0	35	0	87	0
	12	42	0	24	0	66	0
	13	21	0	12	0	33	0

Table 7a. (Continued)

| | | Gender | | | | | |
| | | Female | | Male | | Both | |
		N	PCTN	N	PCTN	N	PCTN
All Age	Number of Potential Impairing Disease Groups						
	14	20	0	19	0	39	0
	15	5	0	11	0	16	0
	16	12	0	7	0	19	0
	17	9	0	4	0	13	0
	18	7	0	3	0	10	0
	19	3	0	1	0	4	0
	20	2	0	2	0	4	0
	21	2	0	2	0	4	0
	22			2	0	2	0
	24	1	0	3	0	4	0
	26	1	0	1	0	2	0
	27	1	0			1	0
	All	18,321	100	15,284	100	33,605	100

Table 7b. Number of Patients by Age, Gender, and Number of Driver Impairing Disease Groups Control Group

| | | Gender | | | | | |
| | | Female | | Male | | Both | |
		N	PCTN	N	PCTN	N	PCTN
Age Group Under 50	Number of Potential Impairing Disease Groups						
	0	34,038	73	31,710	83	65,748	78
	1	4,821	10	2,798	7	7,619	9
	2	3,275	7	1,836	5	5,111	6
	3	2,018	4	862	2	2,880	3
	4	991	2	357	1	1,348	2
	5	500	1	276	1	776	1
	6	307	1	137	0	444	1
	7	201	0	87	0	288	0
	8	88	0	53	0	141	0
	9	70	0	23	0	93	0
	10	53	0	22	0	75	0
	11	22	0	8	0	30	0
	12	21	0	4	0	25	0

Multiple Medications and Vehicle Crashes: Analysis of Databases

Table 7b. (Continued)

| | | Gender | | | | | |
| | | Female | | Male | | Both | |
		N	PCTN	N	PCTN	N	PCTN
	13	8	0	5	0	13	0
	14	8	0	2	0	10	0
	15	3	0	3	0	6	0
	16	5	0			5	0
	17	4	0			4	0
	18	1	0			1	0
	20			1	0	1	0
	21	1	0			1	0
	22	2	0			2	0
	All	46,437	100	38,184	100	84,621	100
Age Group 50+	Number of Potential Impairing Disease Groups						
	0	5,325	62	5,069	66	10,394	64
	1	829	10	621	8	1,450	9
	2	768	9	629	8	1,397	9
	3	553	6	454	6	1,007	6
	4	286	3	216	3	502	3
	5	261	3	235	3	496	3
	6	168	2	131	2	299	2
	7	115	1	107	1	222	1
	8	72	1	63	1	135	1
	9	51	1	32	0	83	1
	10	34	0	35	0	69	0
	11	20	0	17	0	37	0
	12	12	0	16	0	28	0
	13	10	0	6	0	16	0
	14	3	0	7	0	10	0
	15	4	0	10	0	14	0
	16	5	0	3	0	8	0
	17	3	0	4	0	7	0
	18	1	0	5	0	6	0
	19	2	0	3	0	5	0
	20	2	0	1	0	3	0
	21	1	0	1	0	2	0
	22			2	0	2	0
	23			1	0	1	0

Table 7b. (Continued)

| | | Gender | | | | | |
| | | Female | | Male | | Both | |
		N	PCTN	N	PCTN	N	PCTN
Age Group 50+	Number of Potential Impairing Disease Groups						
	34	1	0			1	0
	All	8,526	100	7,668	100	16,194	100
All Age	Number of Potential Impairing Disease Groups						
	0	39,363	72	36,779	80	76,142	76
	1	5,650	10	3,419	7	9,069	9
	2	4,043	7	2,465	5	6,508	6
	3	2,571	5	1,316	3	3,887	4
	4	1,277	2	573	1	1,850	2
	5	761	1	511	1	1,272	1
	6	475	1	268	1	743	1
	7	316	1	194	0	510	1
	8	160	0	116	0	276	0
	9	121	0	55	0	176	0
	10	87	0	57	0	144	0
	11	42	0	25	0	67	0
	12	33	0	20	0	53	0
	13	18	0	11	0	29	0
	14	11	0	9	0	20	0
	15	7	0	13	0	20	0
	16	10	0	3	0	13	0
	17	7	0	4	0	11	0
	18	2	0	5	0	7	0
All Age	Number of Potential Impairing Disease Groups						
	19	2	0	3	0	5	0
	20	2	0	2	0	4	0
	21	2	0	1	0	3	0
	22	2	0	2	0	4	0
	23			1	0	1	0
	34	1	0			1	0
	All	54,963	100	45,852	100	100815	100

Multiple Medications and Vehicle Crashes: Analysis of Databases

Table 8a. Number of Patients by Age, Gender, and Number of Disease-Drug Conflicts
Case Group

| | | Gender | | | | | |
| | | Female | | Male | | Both | |
		N	PCTN	N	PCTN	N	PCTN
Age Group Under 50	Number of Disease-Drug Conflicts						
	0	15,172	98	12,543	99	27,715	98
	1	192	1	115	1	307	1
	2	46	0	40	0	86	0
	3	32	0	12	0	44	0
	4	13	0	4	0	17	0
	5	5	0	3	0	8	0
	6	4	0	6	0	10	0
	7	1	0	2	0	3	0
	8	6	0	1	0	7	0
	9	2	0			2	0
	10			1	0	1	0
	12	1	0	1	0	2	0
	13	1	0			1	0
	17	1	0			1	0
	18	1	0			1	0
	20	1	0			1	0
	27	1	0			1	0
	All	15,479	100	12,728	100	28,207	100
50+	Number of Disease-Drug Conflicts						
	0	2,603	92	2,364	92	4,967	92
	1	143	5	102	4	245	5
	2	48	2	40	2	88	2
	3	13	0	13	1	26	0

Table 8a. (Continued)

		Gender				Both	
		Female		Male			
		N	PCTN	N	PCTN	N	PCTN
Age Group 50+	Number of Disease-Drug Conflicts						
	4	11	0	16	1	27	1
	5	5	0	6	0	11	0
	6	4	0	5	0	9	0
	7	7	0	3	0	10	0
	8	2	0	2	0	4	0
	9	1	0	3	0	4	0
	10	1	0	1	0	2	0
	11	1	0			1	0
	13	1	0			1	0
	18	1	0			1	0
	19	1	0			1	0
	21			1	0	1	0
	All	2,842	100	2,556	100	5,398	100
All Age	Number of Disease-Drug Conflicts						
	0	17,775	97	14,907	98	32,682	97
	1	335	2	217	1	552	2
	2	94	1	80	1	174	1
	3	45	0	25	0	70	0
	4	24	0	20	0	44	0
	5	10	0	9	0	19	0
	6	8	0	11	0	19	0
	7	8	0	5	0	13	0
	8	8	0	3	0	11	0

Multiple Medications and Vehicle Crashes: Analysis of Databases

Table 8a. (Continued)

		Female		Male		Both	
		N	PCTN	N	PCTN	N	PCTN
All Age	Number of Disease-Drug Conflicts						
	9	3	0	3	0	6	0
	10	1	0	2	0	3	0
	11	1	0			1	0
	12	1	0	1	0	2	0
	13	2	0			2	0
	17	1	0			1	0
	18	2	0			2	0
	19	1	0			1	0
	20	1	0			1	0
	21			1	0	1	0
	27	1	0			1	0
	All	18,321	100	15,284	100	33,605	100

Table 8b. Number of Patients by Age, Gender, and Number of Disease-Drug Conflicts Control Group

		Female		Male		Both	
		N	PCTN	N	PCTN	N	PCTN
Age Group	Number of Disease-Drug Conflicts						
Under 50	0	46,150	99	37,982	99	84,132	99
	1	193	0	137	0	330	0
	2	52	0	31	0	83	0
	3	19	0	14	0	33	0
	4	9	0	8	0	17	0
	5	3	0	3	0	6	0
	6	3	0	3	0	6	0
	7	3	0			3	0
	8	3	0	2	0	5	0
	10			2	0	2	0
	11			2	0	2	0
	25	1	0			1	0
	26	1	0			1	0
	All	46,437	100	38,184	100	84,621	100

Table 8b. (Continued)

		Gender					
		Female		Male		Both	
		N	PCTN	N	PCTN	N	PCTN
50+	Number of Disease-Drug Conflicts						
	0	8,178	96	7,312	95	15,490	96
	1	209	2	205	3	414	3
	2	67	1	67	1	134	1
	3	29	0	30	0	59	0
	4	13	0	19	0	32	0
	5	10	0	7	0	17	0
	6	6	0	11	0	17	0
	7	3	0	2	0	5	0

		Gender					
		Female		Male		Both	
		N	PCTN	N	PCTN	N	PCTN
Age Group 50+	Number of Disease-Drug Conflicts						
	8	3	0	5	0	8	0
	9	1	0	4	0	5	0
	10	1	0	1	0	2	0
	11	2	0	2	0	4	0
	12			1	0	1	0
	17	2	0			2	0
	21	1	0	1	0	2	0
	24	1	0			1	0
	26			1	0	1	0
	All	8,526	100	7,668	100	16,194	100

Multiple Medications and Vehicle Crashes: Analysis of Databases

Table 8b. (Continued)

| | | Gender | | | | | |
| | | Female | | Male | | Both | |
		N	PCTN	N	PCTN	N	PCTN
All Age	Number of Disease-Drug Conflicts						
	0	54,328	99	45,294	99	99,622	99
	1	402	1	342	1	744	1
	2	119	0	98	0	217	0
	3	48	0	44	0	92	0
	4	22	0	27	0	49	0
	5	13	0	10	0	23	0
	6	9	0	14	0	23	0
	7	6	0	2	0	8	0
	8	6	0	7	0	13	0
	9	1	0	4	0	5	0
	10	1	0	3	0	4	0
	11	2	0	4	0	6	0
All Age	Number of Disease-Drug Conflicts						
	12			1	0	1	0
	17	2	0			2	0
	21	1	0	1	0	2	0
	24	1	0			1	0
	25	1	0			1	0
	26	1	0	1	0	2	0
	All	54,963	100	45,852	100	100815	100

Appendix VIII. Table 1A. Odds Ratios for Driver Impairing Drugs

HIC3	DRUG_NAME	OR	L_OR	U_OR	P-VALUE	A	B	C	D
H2D	BARBITURATES	7.50	2.35	23.91	0.00	10	4499	4	13523
H2W	TRICYCLIC ANTIDEPRESSANT/PHENOTHIAZINE COMBINATNS	4.50	0.75	26.93	0.10	3	4506	2	13525
H2X	TRICYCLIC ANTIDEPRESSANT/BENZODIAZEPINE COMBINATNS	4.00	0.90	17.87	0.07	4	4505	3	13524
B3A	MUCOLYTICS	3.00	0.19	47.96	0.44	1	4508	1	13526
H7P	ANTIPSYCHOTICS,DOPAMINE ANTAGONISTS, THIOXANTHENES	3.00	0.42	21.30	0.27	2	4507	2	13525
N1D	PLATELET REDUCING AGENTS	3.00	0.19	47.96	0.44	1	4508	1	13526
R1R	URICOSURIC AGENTS	3.00	0.42	21.30	0.27	2	4507	2	13525
Z2F	MAST CELL STABILIZERS	3.00	1.05	8.55	0.04	7	4502	7	13520
J5G	BETA-ADRENERGICS AND GLUCOCORTICOIDS COMBINATION	2.40	0.95	6.08	0.06	8	4501	10	13517
H6C	ANTITUSSIVES,NON-NARCOTIC	2.23	1.30	3.82	0.00	23	4486	31	13496
H3A	ANALGESICS,NARCOTICS	2.22	1.98	2.49	0.00	557	3952	806	12721
H7T	ANTIPSYCHOTICS,ATYPICAL,DOPAMINE,& SEROTONIN ANTAG	2.20	1.37	3.52	0.00	30	4479	41	13486
H6H	SKELETAL MUSCLE RELAXANTS	2.09	1.71	2.55	0.00	167	4342	247	13280
M9K	HEPARIN AND RELATED PREPARATIONS	2.00	0.33	11.97	0.45	2	4507	3	13524
H2F	ANTI-ANXIETY DRUGS	2.00	1.72	2.31	0.00	315	4194	490	13037
H4B	ANTICONVULSANTS	1.97	1.64	2.38	0.00	189	4320	295	13232
H7E	SEROTONIN-2 ANTAGONIST/REUPTAKE INHIBITORS (SARIS)	1.90	1.49	2.44	0.00	105	4404	167	13360
H7B	ALPHA-2 RECEPTOR ANTAGONIST ANTIDEPRESSANTS	1.88	0.85	4.13	0.12	10	4499	16	13511
J2A	BELLADONNA ALKALOIDS	1.85	1.08	3.19	0.03	21	4488	34	13493
S2J	ANTI-INFLAMMATORY TUMOR NECROSIS FACTOR INHIBITOR	1.80	0.43	7.53	0.42	3	4506	5	13522
C4G	INSULINS	1.80	1.45	2.22	0.00	140	4369	237	13290
A4B	HYPOTENSIVES,SYMPATHOLYTIC	1.79	1.17	2.74	0.01	34	4475	57	13470
H7C	SEROTONIN-NOREPINEPHRINE REUPTAKE-INHIB (SNRIS)	1.78	1.19	2.66	0.00	38	4471	64	13463
Q6S	EYE SULFONAMIDES	1.76	0.81	3.85	0.15	10	4499	17	13510
M9P	PLATELET AGGREGATION INHIBITORS	1.69	1.17	2.43	0.01	46	4463	83	13444
Q6R	EYE ANTIHISTAMINES	1.67	0.89	3.13	0.11	15	4494	27	13500
H6J	ANTIEMETIC/ANTIVERTIGO AGENTS	1.63	1.17	2.28	0.00	54	4455	100	13427
H6A	ANTIPARKINSONISM DRUGS,OTHER	1.62	0.99	2.66	0.05	25	4484	47	13480

HIC3	DRUG_NAME	OR	L_OR	U_OR	P-VALUE	A	B	C	D
B3K	COUGH AND/OR COLD PREPARATIONS	1.62	1.19	2.20	0.00	63	4446	118	13409
H2S	SEROTONIN SPECIFIC REUPTAKE INHIBITOR (SSRIS)	1.59	1.40	1.81	0.00	380	4129	741	12786
B3J	EXPECTORANTS	1.58	1.28	1.94	0.00	142	4367	275	13252
S2B	NSAIDS, CYCLOOXYGENASE INHIBITOR - TYPE	1.58	1.41	1.76	0.00	534	3975	1066	12461
Z2A	ANTIHISTAMINES	1.55	1.36	1.78	0.00	349	4160	693	12834
D4K	GASTRIC ACID SECRETION REDUCERS	1.55	1.38	1.73	0.00	491	4018	995	12532
H3D	ANALGESIC/ANTIPYRETICS, SALICYLATES	1.51	0.98	2.33	0.06	31	4478	62	13465
C4K	HYPOGLYCEMICS, INSULIN-RELEASE STIMULANT TYPE	1.50	1.28	1.76	0.00	238	4271	486	13041
C4M	HYPOGLYCEMICS, ALPHA-GLUCOSIDASE INHIB TYPE (N-S)	1.50	0.51	4.39	0.46	5	4504	10	13517
P3L	ANTITHYROID PREPARATIONS	1.50	0.45	4.98	0.51	4	4505	8	13519
C4L	HYPOGLYCEMICS, BIGUANIDE TYPE (NON-SULFONYLUREAS)	1.49	1.23	1.80	0.00	169	4340	345	13182
H2E	SEDATIVE-HYPNOTICS,NON-BARBITURATE	1.48	1.16	1.88	0.00	100	4409	206	13321
A2A	ANTIARRHYTHMICS	1.46	0.83	2.56	0.19	18	4491	37	13490
H2U	TRICYCLIC ANTIDEPRESSANTS & REL. NON-SEL. RU-INHIB	1.41	1.15	1.73	0.00	139	4370	300	13227
H2V	ANTI-NARCOLEPSY/ANTI-HYPERKINESIS, STIMULANT-TYPE	1.41	0.72	2.75	0.32	13	4496	28	13499
C7A	HYPERURICEMIA TX - PURINE INHIBITORS	1.36	0.95	1.94	0.09	45	4464	100	13427
J5D	BETA-ADRENERGIC AGENTS	1.35	1.12	1.64	0.00	157	4352	352	13175
C4N	HYPOGLYCEMICS, INSULIN-RESPONSE ENHANCER (N-S)	1.35	1.01	1.80	0.04	68	4441	152	13375
R1M	LOOP DIURETICS	1.35	1.10	1.65	0.00	136	4373	306	13221
S2A	COLCHICINE	1.34	0.70	2.59	0.37	13	4496	29	13498
W4A	ANTIMALARIAL DRUGS	1.34	0.90	2.00	0.15	36	4473	81	13446
R1L	POTASSIUM SPARING DIURETICS IN COMBINATION	1.33	1.10	1.61	0.00	161	4348	366	13161
A7B	VASODILATORS,CORONARY	1.31	1.04	1.66	0.02	103	4406	237	13290
M9L	ORAL ANTICOAGULANTS,COUMARIN TYPE	1.31	1.01	1.70	0.04	84	4425	193	13334
P3A	THYROID HORMONES	1.29	1.12	1.48	0.00	307	4202	730	12797
A1A	DIGITALIS GLYCOSIDES	1.29	0.96	1.72	0.09	67	4442	157	13370
J8A	ANOREXIC AGENTS	1.29	0.33	4.97	0.72	3	4506	7	13520
H3F	ANTIMIGRAINE PREPARATIONS	1.26	0.92	1.73	0.14	57	4452	136	13391
H3E	ANALGESIC/ANTIPYRETICS,NON-SALICYLATE	1.26	0.82	1.95	0.30	29	4480	69	13458

Appendix VIII. Table 1A. (Continued)

HIC3	DRUG_NAME	OR	L_OR	U_OR	P-VALUE	A	B	C	D
A9A	CALCIUM CHANNEL BLOCKING AGENTS	1.25	1.10	1.41	0.00	401	4108	985	12542
H2M	ANTI-MANIA DRUGS	1.24	0.63	2.43	0.53	12	4497	29	13498
A4D	HYPOTENSIVES, ACE INHIBITORS	1.23	1.11	1.37	0.00	534	3975	1330	12197
D4B	ANTACIDS	1.20	0.23	6.23	0.83	2	4507	5	13522
J2D	ANTICHOLINERGICS/ANTISPASMODICS	1.20	0.61	2.34	0.59	12	4497	30	13497
R1H	POTASSIUM SPARING DIURETICS	1.20	0.69	2.07	0.51	18	4491	45	13482
H7D	NOREPINEPHRINE AND DOPAMINE REUPTAKE INHIB (NDRIS)	1.19	0.87	1.62	0.27	57	4452	144	13383
J7B	ALPHA-ADRENERGIC BLOCKING AGENTS	1.19	0.95	1.49	0.13	112	4397	284	13243
J9B	ANTISPASMODIC AGENTS	1.15	0.41	3.24	0.79	5	4504	13	13514
A4A	HYPOTENSIVES,VASODILATORS	1.13	0.44	2.88	0.81	6	4503	16	13511
Q6W	OPHTHALMIC ANTIBIOTICS	1.05	0.68	1.63	0.82	27	4482	77	13450
H2G	ANTI-PSYCHOTICS,PHENOTHIAZINES	1.05	0.44	2.48	0.91	7	4502	20	13507
M4E	LIPOTROPICS	1.00	0.91	1.11	0.94	588	3921	1758	11769
J7A	ALPHA/BETA-ADRENERGIC BLOCKING AGENTS	1.00	0.56	1.79	1.00	15	4494	45	13482
Q6I	EYE ANTIBIOTIC-CORTICOID COMBINATIONS	1.00	0.58	1.73	1.00	17	4492	51	13476
A4F	HYPOTENSIVES,ANGIOTENSIN RECEPTOR ANTAGONIST	0.99	0.80	1.22	0.94	118	4391	357	13170
Z4B	LEUKOTRIENE RECEPTOR ANTAGONISTS	0.99	0.64	1.52	0.96	28	4481	85	13442
R1F	THIAZIDE AND RELATED DIURETICS	0.97	0.79	1.18	0.74	126	4383	391	13136
J1B	CHOLINESTERASE INHIBITORS	0.96	0.46	2.04	0.92	9	4500	28	13499
H6B	ANTIPARKINSONISM DRUGS,ANTICHOLINERGIC	0.94	0.34	2.56	0.90	5	4504	16	13511
D4E	ANTI-ULCER PREPARATIONS	0.91	0.39	2.13	0.83	7	4502	23	13504
A4K	ACE INHIBITOR/CALCIUM CHANNEL BLOCKER COMBINATION	0.91	0.55	1.50	0.71	20	4489	66	13461
J7C	BETA-ADRENERGIC BLOCKING AGENTS	0.90	0.79	1.02	0.09	349	4160	1154	12373
Q6G	MIOTICS/OTHER INTRAOC. PRESSURE REDUCERS	0.83	0.62	1.12	0.22	56	4453	202	13325
J2B	ANTICHOLINERGICS,QUATERNARY AMMONIUM	0.80	0.27	2.41	0.69	4	4505	15	13512
D4F	ANTI-ULCER-H.PYLORI AGENTS	0.75	0.08	6.71	0.80	1	4508	4	13523
H7O	ANTIPSYCHOTICS,DOPAMINE ANTAGONISTS,BUTYROPHENONES	0.75	0.16	3.53	0.72	2	4507	8	13519
A4Y	HYPOTENSIVES,MISCELLANEOUS	0.74	0.49	1.12	0.15	29	4480	117	13410
Q6P	EYE ANTIINFLAMMATORY AGENTS	0.74	0.41	1.32	0.31	14	4495	57	13470

Appendix VIII. Table 1A. (Continued)

HIC3	DRUG_NAME	OR	L_OR	U_OR	P-VALUE	A	B	C	D
Q6J	MYDRIATICS	0.60	0.07	5.14	0.64	1	4508	5	13522
R1S	URINARY PH MODIFIERS	0.60	0.07	5.14	0.64	1	4508	5	13522
R1E	CARBONIC ANHYDRASE INHIBITORS	0.38	0.05	3.00	0.36	1	4508	8	13519

Appendix VIII. Table 1B. Significant Odds Ratios for Driver Impairing Drugs

HIC3	DRUG_NAME	OR	L_OR	U_OR	P-VALUE	A	B	C	D
H2D	BARBITURATES	7.50	2.35	23.91	0.00	10	4499	4	13523
Z2F	MAST CELL STABILIZERS	3.00	1.05	8.55	0.04	7	4502	7	13520
H6C	ANTITUSSIVES,NON-NARCOTIC	2.23	1.30	3.82	0.00	23	4486	31	13496
H3A	ANALGESICS,NARCOTICS	2.22	1.98	2.49	0.00	557	3952	806	12721
H7T	ANTIPSYCHOTICS,ATYPICAL,DOPAMINE,& SEROTONIN ANTAG	2.20	1.37	3.52	0.00	30	4479	41	13486
H6H	SKELETAL MUSCLE RELAXANTS	2.09	1.71	2.55	0.00	167	4342	247	13280
H2F	ANTI-ANXIETY DRUGS	2.00	1.72	2.31	0.00	315	4194	490	13037
H4B	ANTICONVULSANTS	1.97	1.64	2.38	0.00	189	4320	295	13232
H7E	SEROTONIN-2 ANTAGONIST/REUPTAKE INHIBITORS (SARIS)	1.90	1.49	2.44	0.00	105	4404	167	13360
J2A	BELLADONNA ALKALOIDS	1.85	1.08	3.19	0.03	21	4488	34	13493
C4G	INSULINS	1.80	1.45	2.22	0.00	140	4369	237	13290
A4B	HYPOTENSIVES,SYMPATHOLYTIC	1.79	1.17	2.74	0.01	34	4475	57	13470
H7C	SEROTONIN-NOREPINEPHRINE REUPTAKE-INHIB (SNRIS)	1.78	1.19	2.66	0.00	38	4471	64	13463
M9P	PLATELET AGGREGATION INHIBITORS	1.69	1.17	2.43	0.01	46	4463	83	13444
H6J	ANTIEMETIC/ANTIVERTIGO AGENTS	1.63	1.17	2.28	0.00	54	4455	100	13427
H6A	ANTIPARKINSONISM DRUGS,OTHER	1.62	0.99	2.66	0.05	25	4484	47	13480
B3K	COUGH AND/OR COLD PREPARATIONS	1.62	1.19	2.20	0.00	63	4446	118	13409
H2S	SEROTONIN SPECIFIC REUPTAKE INHIBITOR (SSRIS)	1.59	1.40	1.81	0.00	380	4129	741	12786
B3J	EXPECTORANTS	1.58	1.28	1.94	0.00	142	4367	275	13252
S2B	NSAIDS, CYCLOOXYGENASE INHIBITOR - TYPE	1.58	1.41	1.76	0.00	534	3975	1066	12461
Z2A	ANTIHISTAMINES	1.55	1.36	1.78	0.00	349	4160	693	12834

Appendix VIII. Table 1B. (Continued)

HIC3	DRUG_NAME	OR	L_OR	U_OR	P-VALUE	A	B	C	D
D4K	GASTRIC ACID SECRETION REDUCERS	1.55	1.38	1.73	0.00	491	4018	995	12532
C4K	HYPOGLYCEMICS, INSULIN-RELEASE STIMULANT TYPE	1.50	1.28	1.76	0.00	238	4271	486	13041
C4L	HYPOGLYCEMICS, BIGUANIDE TYPE (NON-SULFONYLUREAS)	1.49	1.23	1.80	0.00	169	4340	345	13182
H2E	SEDATIVE-HYPNOTICS,NON-BARBITURATE	1.48	1.16	1.88	0.00	100	4409	206	13321
H2U	TRICYCLIC ANTIDEPRESSANTS & REL. NON-SEL. RU-INHIB	1.41	1.15	1.73	0.00	139	4370	300	13227
J5D	BETA-ADRENERGIC AGENTS	1.35	1.12	1.64	0.00	157	4352	352	13175
C4N	HYPOGLYCEMICS, INSULIN-RESPONSE ENHANCER (N-S)	1.35	1.01	1.80	0.04	68	4441	152	13375
R1M	LOOP DIURETICS	1.35	1.10	1.65	0.00	136	4373	306	13221
R1L	POTASSIUM SPARING DIURETICS IN COMBINATION	1.33	1.10	1.61	0.00	161	4348	366	13161
A7B	VASODILATORS,CORONARY	1.31	1.04	1.66	0.02	103	4406	237	13290
M9L	ORAL ANTICOAGULANTS,COUMARIN TYPE	1.31	1.01	1.70	0.04	84	4425	193	13334
P3A	THYROID HORMONES	1.29	1.12	1.48	0.00	307	4202	730	12797
A9A	CALCIUM CHANNEL BLOCKING AGENTS	1.25	1.10	1.41	0.00	401	4108	985	12542
A4D	HYPOTENSIVES, ACE INHIBITORS	1.23	1.11	1.37	0.00	534	3975	1330	12197

Appendix VIII. Table 2A. Odds Ratios for Driver Impairing Diseases

ICD GROUP	ICD GROUP NAME	OR	L_OR	U_OR	P-VALUE	A	B	C	D
424	HEAD TRAUMA	36.00	11.09	116.90	0.00	36	4473	3	13524
369	LACTIC ACIDOSIS	15.00	1.75	128.40	0.01	5	4504	1	13526
1894	SUICIDAL BEHAVIOR	12.00	1.34	107.37	0.03	4	4505	1	13526
1702	DELIRIUM	10.50	2.18	50.55	0.00	7	4502	2	13525
286	CARDIAC ARREST	9.00	0.94	86.53	0.06	3	4506	1	13526
336	HEMOLYSIS	9.00	0.94	86.53	0.06	3	4506	1	13526
1563	PERSONALITY DISORDERS	9.00	1.82	44.59	0.01	6	4503	2	13525
3178	DROWSINESS	9.00	2.90	27.91	0.00	12	4497	4	13523
265	HEMOLYTIC ANEMIA, HERED	6.00	0.54	66.17	0.14	2	4507	1	13526
330	HALLUCINATIONS	6.00	0.54	66.17	0.14	2	4507	1	13526

Appendix VIII. Table 2A. (Continued)

ICD GROUP	ICD GROUP NAME	OR	L_OR	U_OR	P-VALUE	A	B	C	D
340	HEPATIC FAILURE	6.00	0.54	66.17	0.14	2	4507	1	13526
393	OSTEOMALACIA	6.00	0.54	66.17	0.14	2	4507	1	13526
1363	INTRA-ABDOMINAL HEMORRHAGE	6.00	1.10	32.76	0.04	4	4505	2	13525
262	ALCOHOLISM	5.44	2.95	10.01	0.00	29	4480	16	13511
945	KETOACIDOSIS	5.40	1.81	16.11	0.00	9	4500	5	13522
1564	STRESS DISORDERS	5.40	1.81	16.11	0.00	9	4500	5	13522
3084	VISUAL DISTURBANCES	4.71	1.83	12.16	0.00	11	4498	7	13520
361	ANGIONEUROTIC EDEMA	4.50	0.75	26.93	0.10	3	4506	2	13525
2469	OCULAR HERPES SIMPLEX	4.50	0.75	26.93	0.10	3	4506	2	13525
314	DEPRESSION	3.99	3.19	4.99	0.00	185	4324	145	13382
2662	PSYCHOSES, DRUG INDUCED	3.72	2.99	4.63	0.00	184	4325	155	13372
1710	PLEURAL EFFUSION-D	3.69	1.78	7.68	0.00	16	4493	13	13514
397	EXTRAPYRAMIDAL REACTIONS	3.60	1.56	8.33	0.00	12	4497	10	13517
408	PULMONARY EMBOLUS	3.50	1.18	10.41	0.02	7	4502	6	13521
2002	SURGERY	3.46	1.65	7.27	0.00	15	4494	13	13514
2658	ANKYLOSING SPONDYLITIS	3.33	2.23	4.96	0.00	51	4458	46	13481
1561	PSYCHOSES	3.27	1.44	7.42	0.00	12	4497	11	13516
1963	HEPATIC CIRRHOSIS	3.25	1.48	7.12	0.00	13	4496	12	13515
3177	LACK OF COORDINATION	3.19	1.61	6.31	0.00	17	4492	16	13511
2820	INSOMNIA	3.16	1.69	5.92	0.00	20	4489	19	13508
325	ALVEOLITIS,FIBROSING	3.00	0.19	47.96	0.44	1	4508	1	13526
390	OBSTRUCTIVE UROPATHY	3.00	0.19	47.96	0.44	1	4508	1	13526
1421	RELATED TO FETAL OUTCOMES	3.00	0.19	47.96	0.44	1	4508	1	13526
1567	DRUG INDUCED PSYCH DISORDERS	3.00	0.19	47.96	0.44	1	4508	1	13526
1986	ALCOHOLIC LIVER DISEASE	3.00	0.42	21.30	0.27	2	4507	2	13525
2190	APPENDICITIS	3.00	0.42	21.30	0.27	2	4507	2	13525
421	MALIGNANT NEOPLASM, CNS	3.00	0.75	12.00	0.12	4	4505	4	13523

ICD GROUP	ICD GROUP NAME	OR	L_OR	U_OR	P-VALUE	A	B	C	D
1081	PROTEINURIA	3.00	0.75	12.00	0.12	4	4505	4	13523
1203	BRAIN HEMORRHAGE	3.00	0.97	9.30	0.06	6	4503	6	13521
351	HYPOTENSION	3.00	1.13	7.99	0.03	8	4501	8	13519
949	SYNCOPE	3.00	1.76	5.11	0.00	27	4482	27	13500
1562	ANXIETY DISORDERS	2.87	2.03	4.04	0.00	64	4445	67	13460
315	BIPOLAR DISORDER	2.81	1.39	5.69	0.00	15	4494	16	13511
360	ANAPHYLACTIC SHOCK	2.78	1.77	4.34	0.00	37	4472	40	13487
339	HEPATIC DYSFUNCTION	2.73	1.75	4.26	0.00	38	4471	43	13484
348	HYPERTHYROIDISM	2.73	1.16	6.42	0.02	10	4499	11	13516
306	CIRRHOSIS	2.63	0.95	7.24	0.06	7	4502	8	13519
407	PULMONARY EDEMA	2.63	1.28	5.38	0.01	14	4495	16	13511
2187	GI OBSTRUCTION	2.57	0.86	7.65	0.09	6	4503	7	13520
1409	CNS EXCITATION	2.55	1.94	3.35	0.00	97	4412	116	13411
3545	BLURRED VSION	2.50	0.76	8.19	0.13	5	4504	6	13521
311	DEEP VEIN THROMBOSIS	2.42	1.43	4.10	0.00	25	4484	31	13496
3203	BACK PAIN	2.42	2.03	2.88	0.00	234	4275	297	13230
1300	RADIATION THERAPY ICD	2.40	0.64	8.94	0.19	4	4505	5	13522
1406	HEPATOMEGALY WITH STEATOSIS	2.40	0.64	8.94	0.19	4	4505	5	13522
2642	ACUTE OTITIS MEDIA	2.40	1.24	4.63	0.01	16	4493	20	13507
2541	URINARY RETENTION	2.36	0.97	5.78	0.06	9	4500	12	13515
2624	FRACTURES AND INJURIES	2.34	2.04	2.69	0.00	382	4127	522	13005
1972	SYMPTOMS OF QUINIDINE-TOXICITY	2.31	1.58	3.37	0.00	48	4461	63	13464
1205	EPISTAXIS	2.25	0.78	6.48	0.13	6	4503	8	13519
2461	PANIC DISORDERS	2.25	0.78	6.48	0.13	6	4503	8	13519
2062	GERD	2.23	1.71	2.91	0.00	96	4413	130	13397
304	CHOLELITHIASIS	2.21	1.11	4.41	0.02	14	4495	19	13508
327	GALLSTONES	2.21	1.11	4.41	0.02	14	4495	19	13508

Appendix VIII. Table 2A. (Continued)

ICD GROUP	ICD GROUP NAME	OR	L_OR	U_OR	P-VALUE	A	B	C	D
1709	LUPUS	2.18	0.88	5.42	0.09	8	4501	11	13516
269	ANGINA, UNSTABLE	2.18	1.15	4.15	0.02	16	4493	22	13505
317	DYSKINESIAS	2.17	1.06	4.42	0.03	13	4496	18	13509
283	BRONCHOPNEUMONIA	2.17	1.44	3.27	0.00	39	4470	54	13473
1703	COND- REYE SYNDROME RELATED	2.15	1.50	3.09	0.00	51	4458	71	13456
3205	MUSCLE SPASMS	2.15	1.33	3.50	0.00	28	4481	39	13488
380	MYELODYSPLASTIC SYNDROME	2.14	0.68	6.75	0.19	5	4504	7	13520
2203	EDEMA	2.13	1.40	3.25	0.00	37	4472	52	13475
2644	CHRONIC OTITIS MEDIA	2.13	1.30	3.47	0.00	28	4481	40	13487
102	CONGESTIVE HEART FAILURE	2.10	1.53	2.89	0.00	65	4444	94	13433
274	ASTHMA	2.08	1.55	2.80	0.00	75	4434	109	13418
320	EPILEPSY	2.08	0.89	4.86	0.09	9	4500	13	13514
422	DIABETES MELLITUS I AND II	2.07	1.81	2.37	0.00	372	4137	568	12959
1942	TEST	2.07	1.81	2.37	0.00	372	4137	568	12959
2581	SYMPTOMS OF ERGOTISM	2.07	1.49	2.88	0.00	60	4449	87	13440
2153	ABDOMINAL PAIN	2.04	1.57	2.65	0.00	95	4414	142	13385
2443	SYMPTOMS OF GI IRRITATION	2.01	1.63	2.49	0.00	144	4365	218	13309
310	CRYSTALLURIA	2.00	0.33	11.97	0.45	2	4507	3	13524
1994	COAGULATION DEFECTS	2.00	0.90	4.45	0.09	10	4499	15	13512
1880	ANEURYSM	1.97	1.20	3.25	0.01	26	4483	40	13487
1282	DIARRHEA, GASTROENTERITIS	1.97	1.62	2.39	0.00	175	4334	273	13254
309	COPD	1.89	1.47	2.43	0.00	101	4408	163	13364
263	HEPATITIS, ALLER CHOLESTATIC	1.88	0.61	5.73	0.27	5	4504	8	13519
398	HEPATITIS,PELIOSIS	1.88	0.61	5.73	0.27	5	4504	8	13519
200	BLEEDING RISK DIAGNOSIS	1.86	1.03	3.35	0.04	18	4491	29	13498
373	DERMATITIS,MACULOPAPULAR	1.86	0.93	3.71	0.08	13	4496	21	13506
2971	SLEEP APNEA	1.83	1.26	2.67	0.00	44	4465	72	13455

Appendix VIII. Table 2A. (Continued)

ICD GROUP	ICD GROUP NAME	OR	L_OR	U_OR	P-VALUE	A	B	C	D
1381	ISCHEMIC HEART DISEASE	1.83	1.48	2.27	0.00	142	4367	240	13287
101	MILD FUNGAL INFECTIONS	1.83	1.31	2.54	0.00	57	4452	94	13433
919	SYMPTOMS OF DIG-TOXICITY	1.82	1.46	2.28	0.00	126	4383	211	13316
1084	DIARRHEA	1.75	1.13	2.70	0.01	32	4477	55	13472
378	MYOCARDIAL ISCHEMIA	1.74	1.07	2.86	0.03	25	4484	43	13484
1683	HYPERSENSITIVITY REACTIONS	1.71	1.47	2.00	0.00	264	4245	472	13055
400	PERIPHERAL NEUROPATHY	1.70	1.05	2.74	0.03	26	4483	46	13481
287	CARDIOVASCULAR DISEASE	1.69	1.52	1.88	0.00	620	3889	1174	12353
561	RENAL FAILURE-GENERAL	1.69	1.02	2.80	0.04	24	4485	43	13484
2648	STROKE	1.69	1.07	2.67	0.03	29	4480	52	13475
1700	VIRAL ILLNESSES	1.69	0.97	2.93	0.06	20	4489	36	13491
2673	POLYMYALGIA RHEUMATICA	1.67	0.56	4.97	0.36	5	4504	9	13518
542	GI HEMORRHAGE	1.66	1.28	2.16	0.00	90	4419	163	13364
347	HYPERTENSION	1.65	1.48	1.84	0.00	557	3952	1075	12452
2185	COLOSTOMY/ ILEOSTOMY	1.64	0.61	4.42	0.33	6	4503	11	13516
2603	ARTHROPATHIES, OTHER	1.64	0.61	4.42	0.33	6	4503	11	13516
2652	OSTEOSARCOMA	1.64	0.61	4.42	0.33	6	4503	11	13516
1102	VENTRICULAR ARRHYTHMIA	1.64	0.81	3.31	0.17	12	4497	22	13505
1343	LACTIC ACIDOSIS SYMPTOMS	1.63	1.26	2.11	0.00	88	4421	162	13365
356	INTERSTITIAL PNEUMONITIS	1.62	0.64	4.05	0.31	7	4502	13	13514
365	INTERSTITIAL PNEUMONITIS	1.62	0.64	4.05	0.31	7	4502	13	13514
370	LEUKOPENIA	1.62	0.64	4.05	0.31	7	4502	13	13514
861	RENAL DISEASE	1.61	0.86	3.01	0.14	15	4494	28	13499
3168	DIZZINESS	1.60	1.09	2.35	0.02	41	4468	78	13449
307	CNS DEMYELINATING DIS	1.57	0.76	3.26	0.22	11	4498	21	13506
2515	RESPIRATORY INFECTIONS	1.56	1.35	1.82	0.00	270	4239	527	13000
1340	COUGH	1.56	1.15	2.11	0.00	64	4445	124	13403

Appendix VIII. Table 2A. (Continued)

ICD GROUP	ICD GROUP NAME	OR	L_OR	U_OR	P-VALUE	A	B	C	D
2602	ARTHRITIS, OSTEOARTHRITIS	1.54	1.12	2.11	0.01	59	4450	117	13410
1999	BLEEDING	1.51	1.11	2.05	0.01	62	4447	123	13404
301	CEREBRAL PALSY	1.50	0.14	16.54	0.74	1	4508	2	13525
363	RHABDOMYOLYSIS	1.50	0.14	16.54	0.74	1	4508	2	13525
1159	CARDIAC VALVE FIBROSIS	1.50	0.14	16.54	0.74	1	4508	2	13525
402	PRERENAL AZOTEMIA	1.50	0.27	8.19	0.64	2	4507	4	13523
1204	HEMOPTYSIS	1.50	0.27	8.19	0.64	2	4507	4	13523
353	ILEUS, PARALYTIC	1.50	0.38	6.00	0.57	3	4506	6	13521
1996	NASAL POLYPS	1.50	0.38	6.00	0.57	3	4506	6	13521
2654	CROHN'S DISEASE	1.50	0.56	4.00	0.42	6	4503	12	13515
406	PULMONARY FIBROSIS	1.50	0.61	3.72	0.38	7	4502	14	13513
1321	PULMONARY DISORDERS	1.50	0.61	3.72	0.38	7	4502	14	13513
1671	NUTRITIONAL/ NEURO DEFICIENCY	1.50	0.82	2.73	0.19	16	4493	32	13495
1202	HEMATEMESIS	1.50	0.91	2.47	0.11	23	4486	46	13481
273	ARRHYTHMIAS	1.50	1.16	1.94	0.00	89	4420	180	13347
1445	RENAL FAILURE W/O HTN	1.47	0.82	2.64	0.20	17	4492	35	13492
333	HEMATOLOGIC DISORDERS	1.44	1.13	1.85	0.00	95	4414	199	13328
266	ANEMIA,DEF.FE,OTH	1.43	0.95	2.15	0.08	35	4474	74	13453
268	ANGINA, PECTORIS	1.42	0.96	2.09	0.08	38	4471	81	13446
313	DEMENTIA	1.41	0.61	3.28	0.42	9	4500	20	13507
1407	OBESITY	1.40	0.93	2.10	0.11	34	4475	73	13454
1082	HEMATURIA	1.39	0.91	2.12	0.12	32	4477	69	13458
331	HEART BLOCK	1.38	0.70	2.74	0.35	12	4497	26	13501
868	THYROID DISEASE	1.37	1.09	1.73	0.01	108	4401	237	13290
341	HEPATITIS	1.36	0.65	2.88	0.42	10	4499	22	13505
275	ATRIAL FIBRILLATION	1.36	0.96	1.93	0.08	47	4462	104	13423
2000	COLON POLYPS	1.36	0.87	2.13	0.18	28	4481	62	13465

Appendix VIII. Table 2A. (Continued)

ICD GROUP	ICD GROUP NAME	OR	L_OR	U_OR	P-VALUE	A	B	C	D
312	DEHYDRATION	1.35	0.61	2.96	0.45	9	4500	20	13507
1460	VOLUME DEPLETION	1.35	0.61	2.96	0.45	9	4500	20	13507
2015	OSTEOPOROSIS	1.33	0.92	1.94	0.13	41	4468	93	13434
367	KIDNEY STONES	1.32	0.72	2.43	0.37	15	4494	34	13493
329	GOUT	1.30	0.62	2.74	0.48	10	4499	23	13504
352	HYPOTHYROIDISM	1.30	1.02	1.66	0.04	93	4416	215	13312
272	APLASTIC ANEMIA	1.29	0.33	4.97	0.72	3	4506	7	13520
1997	TELANGLECTASIS	1.29	0.33	4.97	0.72	3	4506	7	13520
2657	ARTHRITIS, PSORIATIC	1.29	0.33	4.97	0.72	3	4506	7	13520
2663	GASTRITIS	1.27	0.81	1.98	0.30	27	4482	64	13463
381	PANCYTOPENIA	1.23	0.87	1.74	0.23	46	4463	112	13415
281	BRADYCARDIA	1.20	0.38	3.83	0.76	4	4505	10	13517
328	GI ULCER	1.20	0.73	1.97	0.47	22	4487	55	13472
2513	NEUROPATHIES	1.17	0.49	2.79	0.73	7	4502	18	13509
2563	HYPERLIPIDEMIA-2	1.13	0.99	1.29	0.07	332	4177	890	12637
270	ANOREXIA	1.13	0.30	4.24	0.86	3	4506	8	13519
1083	PRURITUS	1.13	0.30	4.24	0.86	3	4506	8	13519
371	LIPID ABNORMALITIES	1.12	0.99	1.28	0.08	343	4166	925	12602
267	ANEMIAS, OTHER	1.12	0.78	1.61	0.54	41	4468	110	13417
261	AGRANULOCYTOSIS	1.09	0.35	3.43	0.88	4	4505	11	13516
279	BOWEL OBSTRUCTION	1.09	0.35	3.43	0.88	4	4505	11	13516
388	NEUTROPENIA	1.09	0.35	3.43	0.88	4	4505	11	13516
2066	HYPERSECRETORY STATES	1.09	0.35	3.43	0.88	4	4505	11	13516
1101	SUBARACHNOID HEMORRHAGE	1.00	0.10	9.61	1.00	1	4508	3	13524
2667	POLYMYOSITIS	1.00	0.10	9.61	1.00	1	4508	3	13524
385	GLAUCOMA,NARROW ANGLE	1.00	0.20	4.95	1.00	2	4507	6	13521
395	PARKINSONISM,PRIMARY	1.00	0.32	3.10	1.00	4	4505	12	13515

ICD GROUP	ICD GROUP NAME	OR	L_OR	U_OR	P-VALUE	A	B	C	D
2601	ARTHRITIS, RHEUMATOID	1.00	0.63	1.59	1.00	24	4485	72	13455
860	MYELOSUPPRESSION	0.94	0.34	2.56	0.90	5	4504	16	13511
2069	STEATORRHEA	0.92	0.48	1.76	0.81	12	4497	39	13488
323	COLITIS	0.90	0.25	3.27	0.87	3	4506	10	13517
1756	MENOPAUSE	0.89	0.52	1.54	0.69	17	4492	57	13470
338	HEMORRHAGIC DISORDERS	0.88	0.33	2.39	0.81	5	4504	17	13510
374	MALIGNANT MELANOMA	0.86	0.18	4.13	0.85	2	4507	7	13520
376	ANEMIA,MEGALOBLASTIC	0.86	0.18	4.13	0.85	2	4507	7	13520
2083	GLAUCOMA	0.84	0.53	1.32	0.44	24	4485	86	13441
276	AV BLOCK II TO III	0.83	0.31	2.24	0.72	5	4504	18	13509
282	BREAST CANCER, FEMALE	0.83	0.51	1.34	0.45	21	4488	76	13451
2070	ALBUMINURIA/ NEPHROPATHY	0.83	0.38	1.81	0.64	8	4501	29	13498
2511	CANCER	0.83	0.65	1.04	0.11	91	4418	330	13197
2202	UREMIA	0.82	0.23	2.93	0.76	3	4506	11	13516
409	PULMONARY EMBOLUS, PREVIOUS	0.75	0.08	6.71	0.80	1	4508	4	13523
2150	HYPERCALCEMIA	0.75	0.08	6.71	0.80	1	4508	4	13523
103	SEVERE FUNGAL INFECTIONS	0.75	0.16	3.53	0.72	2	4507	8	13519
342	HIV	0.75	0.16	3.53	0.72	2	4507	8	13519
867	THROMBOPHLEBITIS	0.75	0.21	2.66	0.66	3	4506	12	13515
2084	PROSTATIC HYPERTROPHY	0.75	0.33	1.72	0.50	7	4502	28	13499
2013	COLON, IRRITABLE	0.69	0.34	1.43	0.32	9	4500	39	13488
2528	BENIGN PROSTATIC HYPERTROPHY	0.67	0.29	1.54	0.34	7	4502	31	13496
405	PSORIASIS	0.63	0.31	1.29	0.20	9	4500	43	13484
278	BLOOD DYSCRASIAS	0.60	0.07	5.14	0.64	1	4508	5	13522
394	PANCREATITIS	0.60	0.07	5.14	0.64	1	4508	5	13522
319	ENCEPHALOPATHIC SYNDROME	0.43	0.05	3.48	0.43	1	4508	7	13520
2646	ALZHEIMER	0.43	0.05	3.48	0.43	1	4508	7	13520

ICD GROUP	ICD GROUP NAME	OR	L_OR	U_OR	P-VALUE	A	B	C	D
865	THROMBOCYTOPENIA, SECONDARY	0.38	0.05	3.00	0.36	1	4508	8	13519
392	OPTIC NEURITIS	0.33	0.04	2.63	0.30	1	4508	9	13518
866	THROMBOCYTOPENIA	0.30	0.04	2.34	0.25	1	4508	10	13517
372	LYMPHADENOPATHY	0.14	0.02	1.01	0.05	1	4508	22	13505

Appendix VIII. Table 2B. Significant Odds Ratios for Driver Impairing Diseases

ICD GROUP	ICD GROUP NAME	OR	L_OR	U_OR	P-VALUE	A	B	C	D	
424	HEAD TRAUMA	36.00	11.09	116.90	0.000	36	4473	3	13524	
369	LACTIC ACIDOSIS	15.00	1.75	128.40	0.013	5	4504	1	13526	ACIDOSIS
1894	SUICIDAL BEHAVIOR/NEUROTIC DISORDER UNSPEC.	12.00	1.34	107.37	0.026	4	4505	1	13526	neurotic disorder unspec
1702	DELIRIUM	10.50	2.18	50.55	0.003	7	4502	2	13525	DELIRIUM TREMENS, DELIRIUM ACUTE, SUBACUTE
3178	DROWSINESS	9.00	2.90	27.91	0.000	12	4497	4	13523	CONSCIOUSNESS ALTER OTH
1563	PERSONALITY DISORDERS	9.00	1.82	44.59	0.007	6	4503	2	13525	neurotic disorder, PERSONALITY DISORDERS
1363	INTRA-ABDOMINAL HEMORRHAGE	6.00	1.10	32.76	0.039	4	4505	2	13525	
262	ALCOHOLISM	5.44	2.95	10.01	0.000	29	4480	16	13511	
945	KETOACIDOSIS	5.40	1.81	16.11	0.002	9	4500	5	13522	DIABETIC KETOACIDOSIS
1564	STRESS DISORDERS	5.40	1.81	16.11	0.002	9	4500	5	13522	STRESS DISORDERS
3084	VISUAL DISTURBANCES	4.71	1.83	12.16	0.001	11	4498	7	13520	VISUAL DISTURBANCES NOS

Appendix VIII. Table 2B. (Continued)

ICD GROUP	ICD GROUP NAME	OR	L_OR	U_OR	P-VALUE	A	B	C	D	
314	DEPRESSION	3.99	3.19	4.99	0.000	185	4324	145	13382	
2662	PSYCHOSES, DRUG INDUCED	3.72	2.99	4.63	0.000	184	4325	155	13372	drug induced sx, schizophrenia, mania, depression, confusion, anxiety, paranoia
1710	PLEURAL EFFUSION-D	3.69	1.78	7.68	0.000	16	4493	13	13514	
397	EXTRAPYRAMIDAL REACTIONS	3.60	1.56	8.33	0.003	12	4497	10	13517	TREMOR, EXTRAPYRAMIDAL SX
408	PULMONARY EMBOLUS	3.50	1.18	10.41	0.024	7	4502	6	13521	
2002	SURGERY	3.46	1.65	7.27	0.001	15	4494	13	13514	
2658	ANKYLOSING SPONDYLITIS	3.33	2.23	4.96	0.000	51	4458	46	13481	
1561	PSYCHOSES	3.27	1.44	7.42	0.005	12	4497	11	13516	
1963	HEPATIC CIRRHOSIS	3.25	1.48	7.12	0.003	13	4496	12	13515	
3177	LACK OF COORDINATION	3.19	1.61	6.31	0.001	17	4492	16	13511	
2820	INSOMNIA	3.16	1.69	5.92	0.000	20	4489	19	13508	
949	SYNCOPE	3.00	1.76	5.11	0.000	27	4482	27	13500	
351	HYPOTENSION	3.00	1.13	7.99	0.028	8	4501	8	13519	
1562	ANXIETY DISORDERS	2.87	2.03	4.04	0.000	64	4445	67	13460	anxiety, panic, phobias
315	BIPOLAR DISORDER	2.81	1.39	5.69	0.004	15	4494	16	13511	
360	ANAPHYLACTIC SHOCK	2.78	1.77	4.34	0.000	37	4472	40	13487	urticaria, wheezing, anaphylactic shock, adverse eff of med, allergy unspec
339	HEPATIC DYSFUNCTION	2.73	1.75	4.26	0.000	38	4471	43	13484	
348	HYPERTHYROIDISM	2.73	1.16	6.42	0.022	10	4499	11	13516	
407	PULMONARY EDEMA	2.63	1.28	5.38	0.008	14	4495	16	13511	
1409	CNS EXCITATION	2.55	1.94	3.35	0.000	97	4412	116	13411	nervousness, headache, confusion

Appendix VIII. Table 2B. (Continued)

ICD GROUP	ICD GROUP NAME	OR	L_OR	U_OR	P-VALUE	A	B	C	D	
311	DEEP VEIN THROMBOSIS	2.42	1.43	4.10	0.001	25	4484	31	13496	
3203	BACK PAIN	2.42	2.03	2.88	0.000	234	4275	297	13230	sciatica, lumbago, backache
2642	ACUTE OTITIS MEDIA	2.40	1.24	4.63	0.009	16	4493	20	13507	
2624	FRACTURES AND INJURIES	2.34	2.04	2.69	0.000	382	4127	522	13005	
1972	SYMPTOMS OF QUINIDINE-TOXICITY	2.31	1.58	3.37	0.000	48	4461	63	13464	hypotension, bradycardia, v tach, av block, acute lung edema
2062	GERD	2.23	1.71	2.91	0.000	96	4413	130	13397	reflux esophagitis
304	CHOLELITHIASIS	2.21	1.11	4.41	0.024	14	4495	19	13508	
327	GALLSTONES	2.21	1.11	4.41	0.024	14	4495	19	13508	
269	ANGINA, UNSTABLE	2.18	1.15	4.15	0.018	16	4493	22	13505	
283	BRONCHOPNEUMONIA	2.17	1.44	3.27	0.000	39	4470	54	13473	pneumonias
317	DYSKINESIAS	2.17	1.06	4.42	0.034	13	4496	18	13509	
1703	COND- REYE SYNDROME RELATED	2.15	1.50	3.09	0.000	51	4458	71	13456	
3205	MUSCLE SPASMS	2.15	1.33	3.50	0.002	28	4481	39	13488	spasm of muscle
2203	EDEMA	2.13	1.40	3.25	0.000	37	4472	52	13475	
2644	CHRONIC OTITIS MEDIA	2.13	1.30	3.47	0.002	28	4481	40	13487	
102	CONGESTIVE HEART FAILURE	2.10	1.53	2.89	0.000	65	4444	94	13433	
274	ASTHMA	2.08	1.55	2.80	0.000	75	4434	109	13418	
422	DIABETES MELLITUS I AND II	2.07	1.81	2.37	0.000	372	4137	568	12959	
1942	TEST	2.07	1.81	2.37	0.000	372	4137	568	12959	
2581	SYMPTOMS OF ERGOTISM	2.07	1.49	2.88	0.000	60	4449	87	13440	
2153	ABDOMINAL PAIN	2.04	1.57	2.65	0.000	95	4414	142	13385	abdominal pain unspec
2443	SYMPTOMS OF GI IRRITATION	2.01	1.63	2.49	0.000	144	4365	218	13309	esophagitis, gastritis
1880	ANEURYSM	1.97	1.20	3.25	0.008	26	4483	40	13487	cva, subarachnoid hemorrhage

ICD GROUP	ICD GROUP NAME	OR	L_OR	U_OR	P-VALUE	A	B	C	D	
1282	DIARRHEA, GASTROENTERITIS	1.97	1.62	2.39	0.000	175	4334	273	13254	abdominal pain, enteritis, ulcerative colitis
309	COPD	1.89	1.47	2.43	0.000	101	4408	163	13364	
200	BLEEDING RISK DIAGNOSIS	1.86	1.03	3.35	0.038	18	4491	29	13498	
2971	SLEEP APNEA	1.83	1.26	2.67	0.002	44	4465	72	13455	
1381	ISCHEMIC HEART DISEASE	1.83	1.48	2.27	0.000	142	4367	240	13287	coronary atherosclerosis
101	MILD FUNGAL INFECTIONS	1.83	1.31	2.54	0.000	57	4452	94	13433	
919	SYMPTOMS OF DIG-TOXICITY	1.82	1.46	2.28	0.000	126	4383	211	13316	nausea, vomiting, visual disturbances, arrhythmias, hypokalemia, hypomagnesemia
1084	DIARRHEA	1.75	1.13	2.70	0.012	32	4477	55	13472	
378	MYOCARDIAL ISCHEMIA	1.74	1.07	2.86	0.027	25	4484	43	13484	
1683	HYPERSENSITIVITY REACTIONS	1.71	1.47	2.00	0.000	264	4245	472	13055	allergy, wheezing, shock, hypotension
400	PERIPHERAL NEUROPATHY	1.70	1.05	2.74	0.031	26	4483	46	13481	
287	CARDIOVASCULAR DISEASE	1.69	1.52	1.88	0.000	620	3889	1174	12353	htn, chf, cardiomyopathy
561	RENAL FAILURE-GENERAL	1.69	1.02	2.80	0.041	24	4485	43	13484	diabetic & hypertensive renal dis, acute renal failure
2648	STROKE	1.69	1.07	2.67	0.025	29	4480	52	13475	cva, cerebral thrombosis
542	GI HEMORRHAGE	1.66	1.28	2.16	0.000	90	4419	163	13364	gi ulcer w/hemorrhage
347	HYPERTENSION	1.65	1.48	1.84	0.000	557	3952	1075	12452	
1343	LACTIC ACIDOSIS SYMPTOMS	1.63	1.26	2.11	0.000	88	4421	162	13365	
3168	DIZZINESS	1.60	1.09	2.35	0.017	41	4468	78	13449	

Appendix VIII. Table 2B. (Continued)

ICD GROUP	ICD GROUP NAME	OR	L_OR	U_OR	P-VALUE	A	B	C	D	
2515	RESPIRATORY INFECTIONS	1.56	1.35	1.82	0.000	270	4239	527	13000	sinusitis, bronchitis
1340	COUGH	1.56	1.15	2.11	0.004	64	4445	124	13403	
2602	ARTHRITIS, OSTEOARTHRITIS	1.54	1.12	2.11	0.008	59	4450	117	13410	
1999	BLEEDING	1.51	1.11	2.05	0.008	62	4447	123	13404	
273	ARRHYTHMIAS	1.50	1.16	1.94	0.002	89	4420	180	13347	
333	HEMATOLOGIC DISORDERS	1.44	1.13	1.85	0.004	95	4414	199	13328	anemias, sickle cell, thrombocytopenia, blood disease unspec.
868	THYROID DISEASE	1.37	1.09	1.73	0.007	108	4401	237	13290	
352	HYPOTHYROIDISM	1.30	1.02	1.66	0.035	93	4416	215	13312	
372	LYMPHADENOPATHY	0.14	0.02	1.01	0.051	1	4508	22	13505	

Appendix VIII. Table 3A. Odds Ratios for Drug Interactions

DRUG_DRUG	DRUG 1	DRUG 2	OR	L_OR	U_OR	P-VALUE	A	B	C	D
H4B W3B	ANTICONVULSANTS	ANTIFUNGAL AGENTS	21.00	2.58	170.69	0.00	7	4502	1	13526
H7C W1Q	SEROTONIN-NOREPINEPHRINE REUPTAKE-INHIB (SNRIS)	QUINOLONES	21.00	2.58	170.69	0.00	7	4502	1	13526
H6H H7T	SKELETAL MUSCLE RELAXANTS	ANTIPSYCHOTICS,ATYPICAL,DOP AMINE,& SEROTONIN ANTAG	18.00	2.17	149.52	0.01	6	4503	1	13526
C4K W2A	HYPOGLYCEMICS, INSULIN-RELEASE STIMULANT TYPE	ABSORBABLE SULFONAMIDES	15.00	1.75	128.40	0.01	5	4504	1	13526
H2S H7B	SEROTONIN SPECIFIC REUPTAKE INHIBITOR (SSRIS)	ALPHA-2 RECEPTOR ANTAGONIST ANTIDEPRESSANTS	15.00	1.75	128.40	0.01	5	4504	1	13526
H4B J2A	ANTICONVULSANTS	BELLADONNA ALKALOIDS	12.00	1.34	107.37	0.03	4	4505	1	13526
H2U H7T	TRICYCLIC ANTIDEPRESSANTS & REL. NON-SEL. RU-INHIB	ANTIPSYCHOTICS,ATYPICAL,DOP AMINE,& SEROTONIN ANTAG	10.50	2.18	50.55	0.00	7	4502	2	13525
C4M D4K	HYPOGLYCEMICS, ALPHA-GLUCOSIDASE INHIB TYPE (N-S)	GASTRIC ACID SECRETION REDUCERS	9.00	0.94	86.53	0.06	3	4506	1	13526
H2F W1K	ANTI-ANXIETY DRUGS	LINCOSAMIDES	7.50	1.46	38.66	0.02	5	4504	2	13525

DRUG_DRUG	DRUG 1	DRUG 2	OR	L_OR	U_OR	P-VALUE	A	B	C	D
H2S H7C	SEROTONIN SPECIFIC REUPTAKE INHIBITOR (SSRIS)	SEROTONIN-NOREPINEPHRINE REUPTAKE-INHIB (SNRIS)	7.50	1.46	38.66	0.02	5	4504	2	13525
A2A W1Q	ANTIARRHYTHMICS	QUINOLONES	6.00	0.54	66.17	0.14	2	4507	1	13526
B3J H2V	EXPECTORANTS	ANTI-NARCOLEPSY/ANTI-HYPERKINESIS, STIMULANT-TYPE	6.00	0.54	66.17	0.14	2	4507	1	13526
C4G H3E	INSULINS	ANALGESIC/ANTIPYRETICS,NON-SALICYLATE	6.00	0.54	66.17	0.14	2	4507	1	13526
C4G H7C	INSULINS	SEROTONIN-NOREPINEPHRINE REUPTAKE-INHIB (SNRIS)	6.00	1.10	32.76	0.04	4	4505	2	13525
C4L W1K	HYPOGLYCEMICS, BIGUANIDE TYPE (NON-SULFONYLUREAS)	LINCOSAMIDES	6.00	0.54	66.17	0.14	2	4507	1	13526
C4N H7C	HYPOGLYCEMICS, INSULIN-RESPONSE ENHANCER (N-S)	SEROTONIN-NOREPINEPHRINE REUPTAKE-INHIB (SNRIS)	6.00	0.54	66.17	0.14	2	4507	1	13526
H2D H3A	BARBITURATES	ANALGESICS,NARCOTICS	6.00	0.54	66.17	0.14	2	4507	1	13526
H2D H4B	BARBITURATES	ANTICONVULSANTS	6.00	1.50	23.99	0.01	6	4503	3	13524
H2F H7B	ANTI-ANXIETY DRUGS	ALPHA-2 RECEPTOR ANTAGONIST ANTIDEPRESSANTS	6.00	0.54	66.17	0.14	2	4507	1	13526
H2V W1D	ANTI-NARCOLEPSY/ANTI-HYPERKINESIS, STIMULANT-TYPE	MACROLIDES	6.00	0.54	66.17	0.14	2	4507	1	13526
H2V W1Q	ANTI-NARCOLEPSY/ANTI-HYPERKINESIS, STIMULANT-TYPE	QUINOLONES	6.00	0.54	66.17	0.14	2	4507	1	13526
H3D M9L	ANALGESIC/ANTIPYRETICS, SALICYLATES	ORAL ANTICOAGULANTS, COUMARIN TYPE	6.00	0.54	66.17	0.14	2	4507	1	13526
H4B W3A	ANTICONVULSANTS	ANTIFUNGAL ANTIBIOTICS	6.00	0.54	66.17	0.14	2	4507	1	13526
H6J H7T	ANTIEMETIC/ANTIVERTIGO AGENTS	ANTIPSYCHOTICS,ATYPICAL,DOPAMINE,& SEROTONIN ANTAG	6.00	0.54	66.17	0.14	2	4507	1	13526
H7C W3B	SEROTONIN-NOREPINEPHRINE REUPTAKE-INHIB (SNRIS)	ANTIFUNGAL AGENTS	6.00	0.54	66.17	0.14	2	4507	1	13526
M9L W1K	ORAL ANTICOAGULANTS, COUMARIN TYPE	LINCOSAMIDES	6.00	0.54	66.17	0.14	2	4507	1	13526
A1A W1D	DIGITALIS GLYCOSIDES	MACROLIDES	4.50	0.75	26.93	0.10	3	4506	2	13525
B3J H7T	EXPECTORANTS	ANTIPSYCHOTICS,ATYPICAL,DOPAMINE,& SEROTONIN ANTAG	4.50	0.75	26.93	0.10	3	4506	2	13525

DRUG_DRUG	DRUG 1	DRUG 2	OR	L_OR	U_OR	P-VALUE	A	B	C	D
C4K H2U	HYPOGLYCEMICS, INSULIN-RELEASE STIMULANT TYPE	TRICYCLIC ANTIDEPRESSANTS & REL. NON-SEL. RU-INHIB	4.50	2.02	10.02	0.00	15	4494	10	13517
C7A W1D	HYPERURICEMIA TX - PURINE INHIBITORS	MACROLIDES	4.50	0.75	26.93	0.10	3	4506	2	13525
H2E J2A	SEDATIVE-HYPNOTICS,NON-BARBITURATE	BELLADONNA ALKALOIDS	4.50	0.75	26.93	0.10	3	4506	2	13525
H2G H2S	ANTI-PSYCHOTICS,PHENOTHIAZINES	SEROTONIN SPECIFIC REUPTAKE INHIBITOR (SSRIS)	4.50	0.75	26.93	0.10	3	4506	2	13525
H7C W5A	SEROTONIN-NOREPINEPHRINE REUPTAKE-INHIB (SNRIS)	ANTIVIRALS, GENERAL	4.50	0.75	26.93	0.10	3	4506	2	13525
H7T W1D	ANTIPSYCHOTICS,ATYPICAL,DOP AMINE,& SEROTONIN ANTAG	MACROLIDES	4.50	0.75	26.93	0.10	3	4506	2	13525
J5D W2F	BETA-ADRENERGIC AGENTS	NITROFURAN DERIVATIVES	4.50	0.75	26.93	0.10	3	4506	2	13525
Q6R R1M	EYE ANTIHISTAMINES	LOOP DIURETICS	4.50	0.75	26.93	0.10	3	4506	2	13525
H7T Z2A	ANTIPSYCHOTICS,ATYPICAL,DOP AMINE,& SEROTONIN ANTAG	ANTIHISTAMINES	4.20	1.33	13.23	0.01	7	4502	5	13522
M9L S2B	ORAL ANTICOAGULANTS, COUMARIN TYPE	NSAIDS, CYCLOOXYGENASE INHIBITOR - TYPE	4.15	2.04	8.48	0.00	18	4491	13	13514
H6H W1D	SKELETAL MUSCLE RELAXANTS	MACROLIDES	4.07	2.04	8.12	0.00	19	4490	14	13513
H2S W1Q	SEROTONIN SPECIFIC REUPTAKE INHIBITOR (SSRIS)	QUINOLONES	4.00	2.17	7.37	0.00	24	4485	18	13509
H2U W3B	TRICYCLIC ANTIDEPRESSANTS & REL. NON-SEL. RU-INHIB	ANTIFUNGAL AGENTS	4.00	0.90	17.87	0.07	4	4505	3	13524
R1F Z4B	THIAZIDE AND RELATED DIURETICS	LEUKOTRIENE RECEPTOR ANTAGONISTS	4.00	0.90	17.87	0.07	4	4505	3	13524
H2E H4B	SEDATIVE-HYPNOTICS,NON-BARBITURATE	ANTICONVULSANTS	3.92	1.91	8.08	0.00	17	4492	13	13514
B3J W5A	EXPECTORANTS	ANTIVIRALS, GENERAL	3.75	1.01	13.97	0.05	5	4504	4	13523
H3A H7T	ANALGESICS,NARCOTICS	ANTIPSYCHOTICS,ATYPICAL,DOP AMINE,& SEROTONIN ANTAG	3.75	1.48	9.50	0.01	10	4499	8	13519
H7T J7C	ANTIPSYCHOTICS,ATYPICAL,DOP AMINE,& SEROTONIN ANTAG	BETA-ADRENERGIC BLOCKING AGENTS	3.75	1.01	13.97	0.05	5	4504	4	13523

DRUG_DRUG	DRUG 1	DRUG 2	OR	L_OR	U_OR	P-VALUE	A	B	C	D
H4B H7C	ANTICONVULSANTS	SEROTONIN-NOREPINEPHRINE REUPTAKE-INHIB (SNRIS)	3.67	1.52	8.85	0.00	11	4498	9	13518
H2S H3A	SEROTONIN SPECIFIC REUPTAKE INHIBITOR (SSRIS)	ANALGESICS,NARCOTICS	3.64	2.72	4.85	0.00	104	4405	88	13439
J5D Z2F	BETA-ADRENERGIC AGENTS	MAST CELL STABILIZERS	3.60	1.10	11.80	0.03	6	4503	5	13522
M4E W1K	LIPOTROPICS	LINCOSAMIDES	3.60	1.10	11.80	0.03	6	4503	5	13522
M9L W1W	ORAL ANTICOAGULANTS, COUMARIN TYPE	CEPHALOSPORINS - 1ST GENERATION	3.60	1.10	11.80	0.03	6	4503	5	13522
H2F H7C	ANTI-ANXIETY DRUGS	SEROTONIN-NOREPINEPHRINE REUPTAKE-INHIB (SNRIS)	3.55	1.59	7.91	0.00	13	4496	11	13516
H2F W3B	ANTI-ANXIETY DRUGS	ANTIFUNGAL AGENTS	3.43	1.24	9.45	0.02	8	4501	7	13520
H2F H2U	ANTI-ANXIETY DRUGS	TRICYCLIC ANTIDEPRESSANTS & REL. NON-SEL. RU-INHIB	3.40	2.08	5.56	0.00	34	4475	30	13497
H2S H7T	SEROTONIN SPECIFIC REUPTAKE INHIBITOR (SSRIS)	ANTIPSYCHOTICS,ATYPICAL,DOP AMINE,& SEROTONIN ANTAG	3.40	1.70	6.81	0.00	17	4492	15	13512
A1A A2A	DIGITALIS GLYCOSIDES	ANTIARRHYTHMICS	3.38	1.30	8.75	0.01	9	4500	8	13519
C4N H2S	HYPOGLYCEMICS, INSULIN-RESPONSE ENHANCER (N-S)	SEROTONIN SPECIFIC REUPTAKE INHIBITOR (SSRIS)	3.30	1.40	7.77	0.01	11	4498	10	13517
H6H W1Q	SKELETAL MUSCLE RELAXANTS	QUINOLONES	3.27	1.44	7.42	0.00	12	4497	11	13516
A1A W1C	DIGITALIS GLYCOSIDES	TETRACYCLINES	3.00	0.19	47.96	0.44	1	4508	1	13526
A1A W3B	DIGITALIS GLYCOSIDES	ANTIFUNGAL AGENTS	3.00	0.19	47.96	0.44	1	4508	1	13526
A4K A9A	ACE INHIBITOR/CALCIUM CHANNEL BLOCKER COMBINATION	CALCIUM CHANNEL BLOCKING AGENTS	3.00	0.19	47.96	0.44	1	4508	1	13526
A4K J7A	ACE INHIBITOR/CALCIUM CHANNEL BLOCKER COMBINATION	ALPHA/BETA-ADRENERGIC BLOCKING AGENTS	3.00	0.19	47.96	0.44	1	4508	1	13526
A9A W3A	CALCIUM CHANNEL BLOCKING AGENTS	ANTIFUNGAL ANTIBIOTICS	3.00	0.19	47.96	0.44	1	4508	1	13526
C4G W2F	INSULINS	NITROFURAN DERIVATIVES	3.00	0.42	21.30	0.27	2	4507	2	13525
C4G W5A	INSULINS	ANTIVIRALS, GENERAL	3.00	0.19	47.96	0.44	1	4508	1	13526
C4K H2W	HYPOGLYCEMICS, INSULIN-RELEASE STIMULANT TYPE	TRICYCLIC ANTI-DEPRESSANT/ PHENOTHIAZINE COMBINATNS	3.00	0.19	47.96	0.44	1	4508	1	13526

Appendix VIII. Table 3A. (Continued)

DRUG_DRUG	DRUG 1	DRUG 2	OR	L_OR	U_OR	P-VALUE	A	B	C	D
C4K H3D	HYPOGLYCEMICS, INSULIN-RELEASE STIMULANT TYPE	ANALGESIC/ANTIPYRETICS, SALICYLATES	3.00	0.42	21.30	0.27	2	4507	2	13525
C4K H3E	HYPOGLYCEMICS, INSULIN-RELEASE STIMULANT TYPE	ANALGESIC/ANTIPYRETICS,NON-SALICYLATE	3.00	0.42	21.30	0.27	2	4507	2	13525
C4K W3B	HYPOGLYCEMICS, INSULIN-RELEASE STIMULANT TYPE	ANTIFUNGAL AGENTS	3.00	0.97	9.30	0.06	6	4503	6	13521
C4L H3D	HYPOGLYCEMICS, BIGUANIDE TYPE (NON-SULFONYLUREAS)	ANALGESIC/ANTIPYRETICS, SALICYLATES	3.00	0.19	47.96	0.44	1	4508	1	13526
C4N J7A	HYPOGLYCEMICS, INSULIN-RESPONSE ENHANCER (N-S)	ALPHA/BETA-ADRENERGIC BLOCKING AGENTS	3.00	0.61	14.86	0.18	3	4506	3	13524
C4N M9L	HYPOGLYCEMICS, INSULIN-RESPONSE ENHANCER (N-S)	ORAL ANTICOAGULANTS, COUMARIN TYPE	3.00	0.61	14.86	0.18	3	4506	3	13524
C7A W5A	HYPERURICEMIA TX - PURINE INHIBITORS	ANTIVIRALS, GENERAL	3.00	0.19	47.96	0.44	1	4508	1	13526
H2F W3A	ANTI-ANXIETY DRUGS	ANTIFUNGAL ANTIBIOTICS	3.00	0.19	47.96	0.44	1	4508	1	13526
H2F Z2E	ANTI-ANXIETY DRUGS	IMMUNOSUPPRESSIVES	3.00	0.19	47.96	0.44	1	4508	1	13526
H2G H2U	ANTI-PSYCHOTICS,PHENOTHIAZINES	TRICYCLIC ANTIDEPRESSANTS & REL. NON-SEL. RU-INHIB	3.00	0.42	21.30	0.27	2	4507	2	13525
H2G W1D	ANTI-PSYCHOTICS,PHENOTHIAZINES	MACROLIDES	3.00	0.42	21.30	0.27	2	4507	2	13525
H2S H2X	SEROTONIN SPECIFIC REUPTAKE INHIBITOR (SSRIS)	TRICYCLIC ANTIDEPRESSANT/ BENZODIAZEPI NE COMBINATNS	3.00	0.19	47.96	0.44	1	4508	1	13526
H2S W1K	SEROTONIN SPECIFIC REUPTAKE INHIBITOR (SSRIS)	LINCOSAMIDES	3.00	0.61	14.86	0.18	3	4506	3	13524
H2U H2V	TRICYCLIC ANTIDEPRESSANTS & REL. NON-SEL. RU-INHIB	ANTI-NARCOLEPSY/ANTI-HYPERKINESIS, STIMULANT-TYPE	3.00	0.42	21.30	0.27	2	4507	2	13525
H2U H7P	TRICYCLIC ANTIDEPRESSANTS & REL. NON-SEL. RU-INHIB	ANTIPSYCHOTICS,DOPAMINE ANTAGONISTS, THIOXANTHENES	3.00	0.19	47.96	0.44	1	4508	1	13526
H2U W1D	TRICYCLIC ANTIDEPRESSANTS & REL. NON-SEL. RU-INHIB	MACROLIDES	3.00	1.39	6.47	0.01	13	4496	13	13514
H2U W3A	TRICYCLIC ANTIDEPRESSANTS & REL. NON-SEL. RU-INHIB	ANTIFUNGAL ANTIBIOTICS	3.00	0.19	47.96	0.44	1	4508	1	13526
H2U W5A	TRICYCLIC ANTIDEPRESSANTS & REL. NON-SEL. RU-INHIB	ANTIVIRALS, GENERAL	3.00	0.42	21.30	0.27	2	4507	2	13525

Appendix VIII. Table 3A. (Continued)

DRUG_DRUG	DRUG 1	DRUG 2	OR	L_OR	U_OR	P-VALUE	A	B	C	D
H3A H7O	ANALGESICS,NARCOTICS	ANTIPSYCHOTICS,DOPAMINE ANTAGONISTS,BUTYROPHENONES	3.00	0.19	47.96	0.44	1	4508	1	13526
H3D M9P	ANALGESIC/ANTIPYRETICS, SALICYLATES	PLATELET AGGREGATION INHIBITORS	3.00	0.19	47.96	0.44	1	4508	1	13526
H3F H7C	ANTIMIGRAINE PREPARATIONS	SEROTONIN-NOREPINEPHRINE REUPTAKE-INHIB (SNRIS)	3.00	0.42	21.30	0.27	2	4507	2	13525
H6H H7B	SKELETAL MUSCLE RELAXANTS	ALPHA-2 RECEPTOR ANTAGONIST ANTIDEPRESSANTS	3.00	0.19	47.96	0.44	1	4508	1	13526
H6H H7C	SKELETAL MUSCLE RELAXANTS	SEROTONIN-NOREPINEPHRINE REUPTAKE-INHIB (SNRIS)	3.00	0.75	12.00	0.12	4	4505	4	13523
H6H W2F	SKELETAL MUSCLE RELAXANTS	NITROFURAN DERIVATIVES	3.00	0.61	14.86	0.18	3	4506	3	13524
H6J H7C	ANTIEMETIC/ANTIVERTIGO AGENTS	SEROTONIN-NOREPINEPHRINE REUPTAKE-INHIB (SNRIS)	3.00	0.42	21.30	0.27	2	4507	2	13525
H7B H7T	ALPHA-2 RECEPTOR ANTAGONIST ANTIDEPRESSANTS	ANTIPSYCHOTICS,ATYPICAL,DOP AMINE,& SEROTONIN ANTAG	3.00	0.42	21.30	0.27	2	4507	2	13525
H7C W1D	SEROTONIN-NOREPINEPHRINE REUPTAKE-INHIB (SNRIS)	MACROLIDES	3.00	0.75	12.00	0.12	4	4505	4	13523
H7D J7A	NOREPINEPHRINE AND DOPAMINE REUPTAKE INHIB (NDRIS)	ALPHA/BETA-ADRENERGIC BLOCKING AGENTS	3.00	0.19	47.96	0.44	1	4508	1	13526
H7T W1Q	ANTIPSYCHOTICS,ATYPICAL,DOP AMINE,& SEROTONIN ANTAG	QUINOLONES	3.00	0.19	47.96	0.44	1	4508	1	13526
H7T W4A	ANTIPSYCHOTICS,ATYPICAL,DOP AMINE,& SEROTONIN ANTAG	ANTIMALARIAL DRUGS	3.00	0.19	47.96	0.44	1	4508	1	13526
H7T W5A	ANTIPSYCHOTICS,ATYPICAL,DOP AMINE,& SEROTONIN ANTAG	ANTIVIRALS, GENERAL	3.00	0.19	47.96	0.44	1	4508	1	13526
J2A M9L	BELLADONNA ALKALOIDS	ORAL ANTICOAGULANTS, COUMARIN TYPE	3.00	0.19	47.96	0.44	1	4508	1	13526
J2A W2F	BELLADONNA ALKALOIDS	NITROFURAN DERIVATIVES	3.00	0.19	47.96	0.44	1	4508	1	13526
J5G J7C	BETA-ADRENERGICS AND GLUCOCORTICOIDS COMBINATION	BETA-ADRENERGIC BLOCKING AGENTS	3.00	0.19	47.96	0.44	1	4508	1	13526
M9K W1W	HEPARIN AND RELATED PREPARATIONS	CEPHALOSPORINS - 1ST GENERATION	3.00	0.19	47.96	0.44	1	4508	1	13526

DRUG_DRUG	DRUG 1	DRUG 2	OR	L_OR	U_OR	P-VALUE	A	B	C	D
M9L M9P	ORAL ANTICOAGULANTS, COUMARIN TYPE	PLATELET AGGREGATION INHIBITORS	3.00	1.05	8.55	0.04	7	4502	7	13520
M9L Z2E	ORAL ANTICOAGULANTS, COUMARIN TYPE	IMMUNOSUPPRESSIVES	3.00	0.19	47.96	0.44	1	4508	1	13526
Q6R W1Q	EYE ANTIHISTAMINES	QUINOLONES	3.00	0.19	47.96	0.44	1	4508	1	13526
R1M Z2F	LOOP DIURETICS	MAST CELL STABILIZERS	3.00	0.19	47.96	0.44	1	4508	1	13526
S2A W1Q	COLCHICINE	QUINOLONES	3.00	0.19	47.96	0.44	1	4508	1	13526
W5A W5J	ANTIVIRALS, GENERAL	ANTIVIRALS, HIV-SPECIFIC, NUCLEOSIDE ANALOG, RTI	3.00	0.19	47.96	0.44	1	4508	1	13526
W5A W5K	ANTIVIRALS, GENERAL	ANTIVIRALS, HIV-SPECIFIC, NON-NUCLEOSIDE, RTI	3.00	0.19	47.96	0.44	1	4508	1	13526
W5J W5K	ANTIVIRALS, HIV-SPECIFIC, NUCLEOSIDE ANALOG, RTI	ANTIVIRALS, HIV-SPECIFIC, NON-NUCLEOSIDE, RTI	3.00	0.19	47.96	0.44	1	4508	1	13526
Z2F Z4B	MAST CELL STABILIZERS	LEUKOTRIENE RECEPTOR ANTAGONISTS	3.00	0.61	14.86	0.18	3	4506	3	13524
B3J H2S	EXPECTORANTS	SEROTONIN SPECIFIC REUPTAKE INHIBITOR (SSRIS)	2.96	1.70	5.17	0.00	25	4484	26	13501
H4B M9L	ANTICONVULSANTS	ORAL ANTICOAGULANTS, COUMARIN TYPE	2.93	1.39	6.19	0.00	14	4495	15	13512
H4B W1D	ANTICONVULSANTS	MACROLIDES	2.80	1.35	5.80	0.01	14	4495	15	13512
H2E H3A	SEDATIVE-HYPNOTICS,NON-BARBITURATE	ANALGESICS,NARCOTICS	2.79	1.85	4.20	0.00	45	4464	49	13478
H2F H2S	ANTI-ANXIETY DRUGS	SEROTONIN SPECIFIC REUPTAKE INHIBITOR (SSRIS)	2.71	2.02	3.64	0.00	85	4424	94	13433
C4L H2S	HYPOGLYCEMICS, BIGUANIDE TYPE (NON-SULFONYLUREAS)	SEROTONIN SPECIFIC REUPTAKE INHIBITOR (SSRIS)	2.68	1.40	5.16	0.00	17	4492	19	13508
A1A R1F	DIGITALIS GLYCOSIDES	THIAZIDE AND RELATED DIURETICS	2.67	1.03	6.91	0.04	8	4501	9	13518
A9A H7E	CALCIUM CHANNEL BLOCKING AGENTS	SEROTONIN-2 ANTAGONIST/REUPTAKE INHIBITORS (SARIS)	2.63	1.28	5.38	0.01	14	4495	16	13511
A2A A9A	ANTIARRHYTHMICS	CALCIUM CHANNEL BLOCKING AGENTS	2.57	0.86	7.65	0.09	6	4503	7	13520

DRUG_DRUG	DRUG 1	DRUG 2	OR	L_OR	U_OR	P-VALUE	A	B	C	D
C4G W1D	INSULINS	MACROLIDES	2.57	0.86	7.65	0.09	6	4503	7	13520
H2S M9L	SEROTONIN SPECIFIC REUPTAKE INHIBITOR (SSRIS)	ORAL ANTICOAGULANTS, COUMARIN TYPE	2.57	1.19	5.56	0.02	12	4497	14	13513
A9A H7C	CALCIUM CHANNEL BLOCKING AGENTS	SEROTONIN-NOREPINEPHRINE REUPTAKE-INHIB (SNRIS)	2.50	0.76	8.19	0.13	5	4504	6	13521
H2S W2F	SEROTONIN SPECIFIC REUPTAKE INHIBITOR (SSRIS)	NITROFURAN DERIVATIVES	2.50	0.76	8.19	0.13	5	4504	6	13521
H2S W5A	SEROTONIN SPECIFIC REUPTAKE INHIBITOR (SSRIS)	ANTIVIRALS, GENERAL	2.50	0.76	8.19		5	4504	6	13521
H2U W1Q	TRICYCLIC ANTIDEPRESSANTS & REL. NON-SEL. RU-INHIB	QUINOLONES	2.45	1.02	5.92	0.05	9	4500	11	13516
C4K H2S	HYPOGLYCEMICS, INSULIN-RELEASE STIMULANT TYPE	SEROTONIN SPECIFIC REUPTAKE INHIBITOR (SSRIS)	2.44	1.39	4.29	0.00	22	4487	27	13500
H2F W1D	ANTI-ANXIETY DRUGS	MACROLIDES	2.42	1.36	4.31	0.00	21	4488	26	13501
H2F J5D	ANTI-ANXIETY DRUGS	BETA-ADRENERGIC AGENTS	2.36	1.41	3.95	0.00	26	4483	33	13494
H2S H3F	SEROTONIN SPECIFIC REUPTAKE INHIBITOR (SSRIS)	ANTIMIGRAINE PREPARATIONS	2.35	1.27	4.35	0.01	18	4491	23	13504
H2U H3A	TRICYCLIC ANTIDEPRESSANTS & REL. NON-SEL. RU-INHIB	ANALGESICS,NARCOTICS	2.34	1.62	3.39	0.00	50	4459	64	13463
A1A H2F	DIGITALIS GLYCOSIDES	ANTI-ANXIETY DRUGS	2.33	0.87	6.27	0.09	7	4502	9	13518
A4K J7C	ACE INHIBITOR/CALCIUM CHANNEL BLOCKER COMBINATION	BETA-ADRENERGIC BLOCKING AGENTS	2.33	0.87	6.27	0.09	7	4502	9	13518
H6C Z2A	ANTITUSSIVES,NON-NARCOTIC	ANTIHISTAMINES	2.33	0.87	6.27	0.09	7	4502	9	13518
P5A W1D	GLUCOCORTICOIDS	MACROLIDES	2.31	1.51	3.55	0.00	37	4472	48	13479
C4L H2U	HYPOGLYCEMICS, BIGUANIDE TYPE (NON-SULFONYLUREAS)	TRICYCLIC ANTIDEPRESSANTS & REL. NON-SEL. RU-INHIB	2.29	1.11	4.72	0.02	13	4496	17	13510
A2A D4K	ANTIARRHYTHMICS	GASTRIC ACID SECRETION REDUCERS	2.25	0.50	10.05	0.29	3	4506	4	13523
C4G M9P	INSULINS	PLATELET AGGREGATION INHIBITORS	2.25	0.78	6.48	0.13	6	4503	8	13519
H7C H7T	SEROTONIN-NOREPINEPHRINE REUPTAKE-INHIB (SNRIS)	ANTIPSYCHOTICS,ATYPICAL,DOPAMINE,& SEROTONIN ANTAG	2.25	0.50	10.05	0.29	3	4506	4	13523
H7C M4E	SEROTONIN-NOREPINEPHRINE REUPTAKE-INHIB (SNRIS)	LIPOTROPICS	2.25	0.78	6.48	0.13	6	4503	8	13519

DRUG_DRUG	DRUG 1	DRUG 2	OR	L_OR	U_OR	P-VALUE	A	B	C	D
M9L W1D	ORAL ANTICOAGULANTS, COUMARIN TYPE	MACROLIDES	2.25	0.50	10.05	0.29	3	4506	4	13523
C4G D4K	INSULINS	GASTRIC ACID SECRETION REDUCERS	2.21	1.32	3.70	0.00	25	4484	34	13493
H2F W1Q	ANTI-ANXIETY DRUGS	QUINOLONES	2.20	1.27	3.81	0.00	22	4487	30	13497
H7C J7C	SEROTONIN-NOREPINEPHRINE REUPTAKE-INHIB (SNRIS)	BETA-ADRENERGIC BLOCKING AGENTS	2.14	0.68	6.75	0.19	5	4504	7	13520
C7A D4K	HYPERURICEMIA TX - PURINE INHIBITORS	GASTRIC ACID SECRETION REDUCERS	2.12	1.01	4.46	0.05	12	4497	17	13510
C4K W1D	HYPOGLYCEMICS, INSULIN-RELEASE STIMULANT TYPE	MACROLIDES	2.05	1.06	3.94	0.03	15	4494	22	13505
B3J H7C	EXPECTORANTS	SEROTONIN-NOREPINEPHRINE REUPTAKE-INHIB (SNRIS)	2.00	0.33	11.97	0.45	2	4507	3	13524
C4L W2A	HYPOGLYCEMICS, BIGUANIDE TYPE (NON-SULFONYLUREAS)	ABSORBABLE SULFONAMIDES	2.00	0.33	11.97	0.45	2	4507	3	13524
C4L W2F	HYPOGLYCEMICS, BIGUANIDE TYPE (NON-SULFONYLUREAS)	NITROFURAN DERIVATIVES	2.00	0.33	11.97	0.45	2	4507	3	13524
C7A W1Q	HYPERURICEMIA TX - PURINE INHIBITORS	QUINOLONES	2.00	0.33	11.97	0.45	2	4507	3	13524
H2E W3B	SEDATIVE-HYPNOTICS,NON-BARBITURATE	ANTIFUNGAL AGENTS	2.00	0.56	7.09	0.28	4	4505	6	13521
H2F W2F	ANTI-ANXIETY DRUGS	NITROFURAN DERIVATIVES	2.00	0.33	11.97	0.45	2	4507	3	13524
H2S W3B	SEROTONIN SPECIFIC REUPTAKE INHIBITOR (SSRIS)	ANTIFUNGAL AGENTS	2.00	0.71	5.62	0.19	6	4503	9	13518
H4B H7B	ANTICONVULSANTS	ALPHA-2 RECEPTOR ANTAGONIST ANTIDEPRESSANTS	2.00	0.33	11.97	0.45	2	4507	3	13524
P5A W1K	GLUCOCORTICOIDS	LINCOSAMIDES	2.00	0.33	11.97	0.45	2	4507	3	13524
H2U M9L	TRICYCLIC ANTIDEPRESSANTS & REL. NON-SEL. RU-INHIB	ORAL ANTICOAGULANTS, COUMARIN TYPE	1.88	0.61	5.73	0.27	5	4504	8	13519
M9L W1Q	ORAL ANTICOAGULANTS, COUMARIN TYPE	QUINOLONES	1.88	0.61	5.73	0.27	5	4504	8	13519
C4K C4M	HYPOGLYCEMICS, INSULIN-RELEASE STIMULANT TYPE	HYPOGLYCEMICS, ALPHA-GLUCOSIDASE INHIB TYPE (N-S)	1.80	0.43	7.53	0.42	3	4506	5	13522

DRUG_DRUG	DRUG 1	DRUG 2	OR	L_OR	U_OR	P-VALUE	A	B	C	D
C4M M4E	HYPOGLYCEMICS, ALPHA-GLUCOSIDASE INHIB TYPE (N-S)	LIPOTROPICS	1.80	0.43	7.53	0.42	3	4506	5	13522
H2S H6B	SEROTONIN SPECIFIC REUPTAKE INHIBITOR (SSRIS)	ANTIPARKINSONISM DRUGS,ANTICHOLINERGIC	1.80	0.43	7.53	0.42	3	4506	5	13522
H2U H7C	TRICYCLIC ANTIDEPRESSANTS & REL. NON-SEL. RU-INHIB	SEROTONIN-NOREPINEPHRINE REUPTAKE-INHIB (SNRIS)	1.80	0.43	7.53	0.42	3	4506	5	13522
M9P S2B	PLATELET AGGREGATION INHIBITORS	NSAIDS, CYCLOOXYGENASE INHIBITOR - TYPE	1.80	0.65	4.95	0.26	6	4503	10	13517
A9A D4K	CALCIUM CHANNEL BLOCKING AGENTS	GASTRIC ACID SECRETION REDUCERS	1.77	1.35	2.33	0.00	85	4424	145	13382
C4K D4K	HYPOGLYCEMICS, INSULIN-RELEASE STIMULANT TYPE	GASTRIC ACID SECRETION REDUCERS	1.75	1.13	2.73	0.01	31	4478	53	13474
H2S M4E	SEROTONIN SPECIFIC REUPTAKE INHIBITOR (SSRIS)	LIPOTROPICS	1.75	1.33	2.32	0.00	79	4430	136	13391
M9P P3A	PLATELET AGGREGATION INHIBITORS	THYROID HORMONES	1.75	0.69	4.45	0.24	7	4502	12	13515
B3J Z2A	EXPECTORANTS	ANTIHISTAMINES	1.74	1.06	2.86	0.03	25	4484	43	13484
H4B M9P	ANTICONVULSANTS	PLATELET AGGREGATION INHIBITORS	1.71	0.50	5.86	0.39	4	4505	7	13520
C4G H2S	INSULINS	SEROTONIN SPECIFIC REUPTAKE INHIBITOR (SSRIS)	1.69	0.75	3.82	0.21	9	4500	16	13511
C4L W1D	HYPOGLYCEMICS, BIGUANIDE TYPE (NON-SULFONYLUREAS)	MACROLIDES	1.69	0.75	3.82	0.21	9	4500	16	13511
A1A J7A	DIGITALIS GLYCOSIDES	ALPHA/BETA-ADRENERGIC BLOCKING AGENTS	1.67	0.56	4.97	0.36	5	4504	9	13518
A9A W1D	CALCIUM CHANNEL BLOCKING AGENTS	MACROLIDES	1.67	0.96	2.88	0.07	20	4489	36	13491
C4G W1Q	INSULINS	QUINOLONES	1.67	0.77	3.61	0.20	10	4499	18	13509
C4L M9P	HYPOGLYCEMICS, BIGUANIDE TYPE (NON-SULFONYLUREAS)	PLATELET AGGREGATION INHIBITORS	1.67	0.56	4.97	0.36	5	4504	9	13518
C4G J7C	INSULINS	BETA-ADRENERGIC BLOCKING AGENTS	1.62	0.95	2.75	0.08	21	4488	39	13488
H7E J7C	SEROTONIN-2 ANTAGONIST/ REUPTAKE INHIBITORS (SARIS)	BETA-ADRENERGIC BLOCKING AGENTS	1.62	0.64	4.05	0.31	7	4502	13	13514

DRUG_DRUG	DRUG 1	DRUG 2	OR	L_OR	U_OR	P-VALUE	A	B	C	D
H2S W1D	SEROTONIN SPECIFIC REUPTAKE INHIBITOR (SSRIS)	MACROLIDES	1.61	0.96	2.70	0.07	22	4487	41	13486
M4E W3B	LIPOTROPICS	ANTIFUNGAL AGENTS	1.59	0.71	3.56	0.26	9	4500	17	13510
M4E W1Q	LIPOTROPICS	QUINOLONES	1.55	1.02	2.34	0.04	34	4475	66	13461
A9A J7B	CALCIUM CHANNEL BLOCKING AGENTS	ALPHA-ADRENERGIC BLOCKING AGENTS	1.53	0.96	2.43	0.07	27	4482	53	13474
J5D W1D	BETA-ADRENERGIC AGENTS	MACROLIDES	1.53	0.98	2.37	0.06	30	4479	59	13468
H2S H2U	SEROTONIN SPECIFIC REUPTAKE INHIBITOR (SSRIS)	TRICYCLIC ANTIDEPRESSANTS & REL. NON-SEL. RU-INHIB	1.51	0.91	2.50	0.11	23	4486	46	13481
A1A R1L	DIGITALIS GLYCOSIDES	POTASSIUM SPARING DIURETICS IN COMBINATION	1.50	0.38	6.00	0.57	3	4506	6	13521
A9A J1B	CALCIUM CHANNEL BLOCKING AGENTS	CHOLINESTERASE INHIBITORS	1.50	0.14	16.54	0.74	1	4508	2	13525
B3J H2U	EXPECTORANTS	TRICYCLIC ANTIDEPRESSANTS & REL. NON-SEL. RU-INHIB	1.50	0.51	4.39	0.46	5	4504	10	13517
C4G H2U	INSULINS	TRICYCLIC ANTIDEPRESSANTS & REL. NON-SEL. RU-INHIB	1.50	0.67	3.34	0.32	9	4500	18	13509
C4G W2A	INSULINS	ABSORBABLE SULFONAMIDES	1.50	0.51	4.39	0.46	5	4504	10	13517
C4K W1K	HYPOGLYCEMICS, INSULIN-RELEASE STIMULANT TYPE	LINCOSAMIDES	1.50	0.14	16.54	0.74	1	4508	2	13525
C4K W2F	HYPOGLYCEMICS, INSULIN-RELEASE STIMULANT TYPE	NITROFURAN DERIVATIVES	1.50	0.14	16.54	0.74	1	4508	2	13525
C4L H7C	HYPOGLYCEMICS, BIGUANIDE TYPE (NON-SULFONYLUREAS)	SEROTONIN-NOREPINEPHRINE REUPTAKE-INHIB (SNRIS)	1.50	0.27	8.19	0.64	2	4507	4	13523
C4L M9L	HYPOGLYCEMICS, BIGUANIDE TYPE (NON-SULFONYLUREAS)	ORAL ANTICOAGULANTS, COUMARIN TYPE	1.50	0.56	4.00	0.42	6	4503	12	13515
C4N M9P	HYPOGLYCEMICS, INSULIN-RESPONSE ENHANCER (N-S)	PLATELET AGGREGATION INHIBITORS	1.50	0.38	6.00	0.57	3	4506	6	13521
C4N W2F	HYPOGLYCEMICS, INSULIN-RESPONSE ENHANCER (N-S)	NITROFURAN DERIVATIVES	1.50	0.14	16.54	0.74	1	4508	2	13525
H2E W3A	SEDATIVE-HYPNOTICS,NON-BARBITURATE	ANTIFUNGAL ANTIBIOTICS	1.50	0.14	16.54	0.74	1	4508	2	13525

DRUG_DRUG	DRUG 1	DRUG 2	OR	L_OR	U_OR	P-VALUE	A	B	C	D
H2F Z4B	ANTI-ANXIETY DRUGS	LEUKOTRIENE RECEPTOR ANTAGONISTS	1.50	0.51	4.39	0.46	5	4504	10	13517
H2S H6A	SEROTONIN SPECIFIC REUPTAKE INHIBITOR (SSRIS)	ANTIPARKINSONISM DRUGS,OTHER	1.50	0.27	8.19	0.64	2	4507	4	13523
H4B W1K	ANTICONVULSANTS	LINCOSAMIDES	1.50	0.14	16.54	0.74	1	4508	2	13525
H4B W2F	ANTICONVULSANTS	NITROFURAN DERIVATIVES	1.50	0.27	8.19	0.64	2	4507	4	13523
H4B Z2E	ANTICONVULSANTS	IMMUNOSUPPRESSIVES	1.50	0.14	16.54	0.74	1	4508	2	13525
H6H M9P	SKELETAL MUSCLE RELAXANTS	PLATELET AGGREGATION INHIBITORS	1.50	0.27	8.19	0.64	2	4507	4	13523
H6H W1K	SKELETAL MUSCLE RELAXANTS	LINCOSAMIDES	1.50	0.14	16.54	0.74	1	4508	2	13525
H7C M9L	SEROTONIN-NOREPINEPHRINE REUPTAKE-INHIB (SNRIS)	ORAL ANTICOAGULANTS, COUMARIN TYPE	1.50	0.14	16.54	0.74	1	4508	2	13525
H7D J7C	NOREPINEPHRINE AND DOPAMINE REUPTAKE INHIB (NDRIS)	BETA-ADRENERGIC BLOCKING AGENTS	1.50	0.56	4.00	0.42	6	4503	12	13515
J2A W1D	BELLADONNA ALKALOIDS	MACROLIDES	1.50	0.27	8.19	0.64	2	4507	4	13523
J2A W3B	BELLADONNA ALKALOIDS	ANTIFUNGAL AGENTS	1.50	0.14	16.54	0.74	1	4508	2	13525
J5D J5G	BETA-ADRENERGIC AGENTS	BETA-ADRENERGICS AND GLUCO-CORTICOIDS COMBINATION	1.50	0.38	6.00	0.57	3	4506	6	13521
J5D W1K	BETA-ADRENERGIC AGENTS	LINCOSAMIDES	1.50	0.27	8.19	0.64	2	4507	4	13523
J5G Z4B	BETA-ADRENERGICS AND GLUCOCORTICOIDS COMBINATION	LEUKOTRIENE RECEPTOR ANTAGONISTS	1.50	0.14	16.54	0.74	1	4508	2	13525
J7A J7C	ALPHA/BETA-ADRENERGIC BLOCKING AGENTS	BETA-ADRENERGIC BLOCKING AGENTS	1.50	0.14	16.54	0.74	1	4508	2	13525
M4E W2F	LIPOTROPICS	NITROFURAN DERIVATIVES	1.50	0.51	4.39	0.46	5	4504	10	13517
M9K M9L	HEPARIN AND RELATED PREPARATIONS	ORAL ANTICOAGULANTS, COUMARIN TYPE	1.50	0.14	16.54	0.74	1	4508	2	13525
M9L W1X	ORAL ANTICOAGULANTS, COUMARIN TYPE	CEPHALOSPORINS - 2ND GENERATION	1.50	0.14	16.54	0.74	1	4508	2	13525
M9P W1Q	PLATELET AGGREGATION INHIBITORS	QUINOLONES	1.50	0.38	6.00	0.57	3	4506	6	13521

DRUG_DRUG	DRUG 1	DRUG 2	OR	L_OR	U_OR	P-VALUE	A	B	C	D
Q6R R1L	EYE ANTIHISTAMINES	POTASSIUM SPARING DIURETICS IN COMBINATION	1.50	0.14	16.54	0.74	1	4508	2	13525
Q6R W1D	EYE ANTIHISTAMINES	MACROLIDES	1.50	0.14	16.54	0.74	1	4508	2	13525
R1L Z4B	POTASSIUM SPARING DIURETICS IN COMBINATION	LEUKOTRIENE RECEPTOR ANTAGONISTS	1.50	0.27	8.19	0.64	2	4507	4	13523
R1M Z4B	LOOP DIURETICS	LEUKOTRIENE RECEPTOR ANTAGONISTS	1.50	0.27	8.19	0.64	2	4507	4	13523
S2A W1D	COLCHICINE	MACROLIDES	1.50	0.14	16.54	0.74	1	4508	2	13525
C4L D4K	HYPOGLYCEMICS, BIGUANIDE TYPE (NON-SULFONYLUREAS)	GASTRIC ACID SECRETION REDUCERS	1.47	0.87	2.47	0.15	21	4488	43	13484
C4G C4K	INSULINS	HYPOGLYCEMICS, INSULIN-RELEASE STIMULANT TYPE	1.45	0.78	2.69	0.24	15	4494	31	13496
H6H J7C	SKELETAL MUSCLE RELAXANTS	BETA-ADRENERGIC BLOCKING AGENTS	1.45	0.77	2.74	0.26	14	4495	29	13498
C4K C4L	HYPOGLYCEMICS, INSULIN-RELEASE STIMULANT TYPE	HYPOGLYCEMICS, BIGUANIDE TYPE (NON-SULFONYLUREAS)	1.44	1.13	1.85	0.00	94	4415	196	13331
H3F J7C	ANTIMIGRAINE PREPARATIONS	BETA-ADRENERGIC BLOCKING AGENTS	1.44	0.72	2.87	0.30	12	4497	25	13502
C4K C4N	HYPOGLYCEMICS, INSULIN-RELEASE STIMULANT TYPE	HYPOGLYCEMICS, INSULIN-RESPONSE ENHANCER (N-S)	1.44	0.95	2.16	0.08	34	4475	71	13456
M4E W1D	LIPOTROPICS	MACROLIDES	1.42	0.91	2.23	0.12	28	4481	59	13468
R1H R1M	POTASSIUM SPARING DIURETICS	LOOP DIURETICS	1.38	0.67	2.81	0.38	11	4498	24	13503
C4G W3B	INSULINS	ANTIFUNGAL AGENTS	1.36	0.47	3.92	0.57	5	4504	11	13516
C4L W1Q	HYPOGLYCEMICS, BIGUANIDE TYPE (NON-SULFONYLUREAS)	QUINOLONES	1.33	0.58	3.07	0.50	8	4501	18	13509
H6H M9L	SKELETAL MUSCLE RELAXANTS	ORAL ANTICOAGULANTS, COUMARIN TYPE	1.33	0.41	4.33	0.63	4	4505	9	13518
M4E Z2E	LIPOTROPICS	IMMUNOSUPPRESSIVES	1.33	0.41	4.33	0.63	4	4505	9	13518
P5A Z2E	GLUCOCORTICOIDS	IMMUNOSUPPRESSIVES	1.33	0.41	4.33	0.63	4	4505	9	13518
C4G M4E	INSULINS	LIPOTROPICS	1.32	0.91	1.91	0.14	40	4469	91	13436
A4D A9A	HYPOTENSIVES, ACE INHIBITORS	CALCIUM CHANNEL BLOCKING AGENTS	1.31	1.03	1.66	0.03	100	4409	230	13297
A1A R1M	DIGITALIS GLYCOSIDES	LOOP DIURETICS	1.29	0.81	2.07	0.28	25	4484	58	13469

DRUG_DRUG	DRUG 1	DRUG 2	OR	L_OR	U_OR	P-VALUE	A	B	C	D
J7C W4A	BETA-ADRENERGIC BLOCKING AGENTS	ANTIMALARIAL DRUGS	1.29	0.33	4.97	0.72	3	4506	7	13520
C4L C4N	HYPOGLYCEMICS, BIGUANIDE TYPE (NON-SULFONYLUREAS)	HYPOGLYCEMICS, INSULIN-RESPONSE ENHANCER (N-S)	1.28	0.81	2.04	0.29	26	4483	61	13466
C4K M9L	HYPOGLYCEMICS, INSULIN-RELEASE STIMULANT TYPE	ORAL ANTICOAGULANTS, COUMARIN TYPE	1.28	0.55	2.98	0.57	8	4501	19	13508
C4G C4N	INSULINS	HYPOGLYCEMICS, INSULIN-RESPONSE ENHANCER (N-S)	1.27	0.74	2.17	0.39	19	4490	45	13482
H2U M4E	TRICYCLIC ANTIDEPRESSANTS & REL. NON-SEL. RU-INHIB	LIPOTROPICS	1.24	0.80	1.92	0.35	28	4481	68	13459
C4N J7C	HYPOGLYCEMICS, INSULIN-RESPONSE ENHANCER (N-S)	BETA-ADRENERGIC BLOCKING AGENTS	1.22	0.64	2.32	0.55	13	4496	32	13495
C4K W1Q	HYPOGLYCEMICS, INSULIN-RELEASE STIMULANT TYPE	QUINOLONES	1.21	0.52	2.80	0.66	8	4501	20	13507
A1A A9A	DIGITALIS GLYCOSIDES	CALCIUM CHANNEL BLOCKING AGENTS	1.20	0.67	2.14	0.54	16	4493	40	13487
A9A H7D	CALCIUM CHANNEL BLOCKING AGENTS	NOREPINEPHRINE AND DOPAMINE REUPTAKE INHIB (NDRIS)	1.20	0.47	3.09	0.71	6	4503	15	13512
A9A W1K	CALCIUM CHANNEL BLOCKING AGENTS	LINCOSAMIDES	1.20	0.23	6.19	0.83	2	4507	5	13522
A9A W3B	CALCIUM CHANNEL BLOCKING AGENTS	ANTIFUNGAL AGENTS	1.20	0.38	3.83	0.76	4	4505	10	13517
C4N W3B	HYPOGLYCEMICS, INSULIN-RESPONSE ENHANCER (N-S)	ANTIFUNGAL AGENTS	1.20	0.23	6.19	0.83	2	4507	5	13522
C4L M4E	HYPOGLYCEMICS, BIGUANIDE TYPE (NON-SULFONYLUREAS)	LIPOTROPICS	1.19	0.87	1.63	0.28	56	4453	142	13385
A4D R1L	HYPOTENSIVES, ACE INHIBITORS	POTASSIUM SPARING DIURETICS IN COMBINATION	1.13	0.68	1.89	0.64	20	4489	53	13474
C4K M9P	HYPOGLYCEMICS, INSULIN-RELEASE STIMULANT TYPE	PLATELET AGGREGATION INHIBITORS	1.13	0.30	4.24	0.86	3	4506	8	13519
A4D R1M	HYPOTENSIVES, ACE INHIBITORS	LOOP DIURETICS	1.12	0.79	1.58	0.53	44	4465	118	13409
A9A J7C	CALCIUM CHANNEL BLOCKING AGENTS	BETA-ADRENERGIC BLOCKING AGENTS	1.12	0.84	1.49	0.45	65	4444	175	13352

Appendix VIII. Table 3A. (Continued)

DRUG_DRUG	DRUG 1	DRUG 2	OR	L_OR	U_OR	P-VALUE	A	B	C	D
J5D J7C	BETA-ADRENERGIC AGENTS	BETA-ADRENERGIC BLOCKING AGENTS	1.11	0.54	2.30	0.78	10	4499	27	13500
C4G C4L	INSULINS	HYPOGLYCEMICS, BIGUANIDE TYPE (NON-SULFONYLUREAS)	1.10	0.64	1.89	0.72	18	4491	49	13478
H2S H2V	SEROTONIN SPECIFIC REUPTAKE INHIBITOR (SSRIS)	ANTI-NARCOLEPSY/ANTI-HYPERKINESIS, STIMULANT-TYPE	1.09	0.35	3.43	0.88	4	4505	11	13516
A4D R1F	HYPOTENSIVES, ACE INHIBITORS	THIAZIDE AND RELATED DIURETICS	1.07	0.76	1.50	0.69	46	4463	129	13398
C4N D4K	HYPOGLYCEMICS, INSULIN-RESPONSE ENHANCER (N-S)	GASTRIC ACID SECRETION REDUCERS	1.04	0.47	2.33	0.92	8	4501	23	13504
C4N M4E	HYPOGLYCEMICS, INSULIN-RESPONSE ENHANCER (N-S)	LIPOTROPICS	1.01	0.65	1.57	0.96	27	4482	80	13447
A1A R1H	DIGITALIS GLYCOSIDES	POTASSIUM SPARING DIURETICS	1.00	0.27	3.69	1.00	3	4506	9	13518
A4K D4K	ACE INHIBITOR/CALCIUM CHANNEL BLOCKER COMBINATION	GASTRIC ACID SECRETION REDUCERS	1.00	0.20	4.95	1.00	2	4507	6	13521
A4K J7B	ACE INHIBITOR/CALCIUM CHANNEL BLOCKER COMBINATION	ALPHA-ADRENERGIC BLOCKING AGENTS	1.00	0.20	4.95	1.00	2	4507	6	13521
A4K R1F	ACE INHIBITOR/CALCIUM CHANNEL BLOCKER COMBINATION	THIAZIDE AND RELATED DIURETICS	1.00	0.20	4.95	1.00	2	4507	6	13521
A4K R1L	ACE INHIBITOR/CALCIUM CHANNEL BLOCKER COMBINATION	POTASSIUM SPARING DIURETICS IN COMBINATION	1.00	0.10	9.61	1.00	1	4508	3	13524
A4K R1M	ACE INHIBITOR/CALCIUM CHANNEL BLOCKER COMBINATION	LOOP DIURETICS	1.00	0.10	9.61	1.00	1	4508	3	13524
A9A D4E	CALCIUM CHANNEL BLOCKING AGENTS	ANTI-ULCER PREPARATIONS	1.00	0.10	9.61	1.00	1	4508	3	13524
A9A Z2E	CALCIUM CHANNEL BLOCKING AGENTS	IMMUNOSUPPRESSIVES	1.00	0.27	3.69	1.00	3	4506	9	13518
C4G J7A	INSULINS	ALPHA/BETA-ADRENERGIC BLOCKING AGENTS	1.00	0.10	9.61	1.00	1	4508	3	13524

DRUG_DRUG	DRUG 1	DRUG 2	OR	L_OR	U_OR	P-VALUE	A	B	C	D
C4K H7C	HYPOGLYCEMICS, INSULIN-RELEASE STIMULANT TYPE	SEROTONIN-NOREPINEPHRINE REUPTAKE-INHIB (SNRIS)	1.00	0.10	9.61	1.00	1	4508	3	13524
C4L C4M	HYPOGLYCEMICS, BIGUANIDE TYPE (NON-SULFONYLUREAS)	HYPOGLYCEMICS, ALPHA-GLUCOSIDASE INHIB TYPE (N-S)	1.00	0.27	3.69	1.00	3	4506	9	13518
C4L W3B	HYPOGLYCEMICS, BIGUANIDE TYPE (NON-SULFONYLUREAS)	ANTIFUNGAL AGENTS	1.00	0.20	4.95	1.00	2	4507	6	13521
C4L W5A	HYPOGLYCEMICS, BIGUANIDE TYPE (NON-SULFONYLUREAS)	ANTIVIRALS, GENERAL	1.00	0.10	9.61	1.00	1	4508	3	13524
C4N H3D	HYPOGLYCEMICS, INSULIN-RESPONSE ENHANCER (N-S)	ANALGESIC/ANTIPYRETICS, SALICYLATES	1.00	0.10	9.61	1.00	1	4508	3	13524
H2U H3F	TRICYCLIC ANTIDEPRESSANTS & REL. NON-SEL. RU-INHIB	ANTIMIGRAINE PREPARATIONS	1.00	0.43	2.35	1.00	7	4502	21	13506
H2U H6A	TRICYCLIC ANTIDEPRESSANTS & REL. NON-SEL. RU-INHIB	ANTIPARKINSONISM DRUGS,OTHER	1.00	0.10	9.61	1.00	1	4508	3	13524
H3E M9P	ANALGESIC/ANTIPYRETICS,NON-SALICYLATE	PLATELET AGGREGATION INHIBITORS	1.00	0.10	9.61	1.00	1	4508	3	13524
H7T J5D	ANTIPSYCHOTICS,ATYPICAL,DOPAMINE,& SEROTONIN ANTAG	BETA-ADRENERGIC AGENTS	1.00	0.10	9.61	1.00	1	4508	3	13524
J5D Z4B	BETA-ADRENERGIC AGENTS	LEUKOTRIENE RECEPTOR ANTAGONISTS	1.00	0.56	1.77	1.00	16	4493	48	13479
P5A W2F	GLUCOCORTICOIDS	NITROFURAN DERIVATIVES	1.00	0.10	9.61	1.00	1	4508	3	13524
Q6P W1Q	EYE ANTIINFLAMMATORY AGENTS	QUINOLONES	1.00	0.10	9.61	1.00	1	4508	3	13524
R1F R1L	THIAZIDE AND RELATED DIURETICS	POTASSIUM SPARING DIURETICS IN COMBINATION	1.00	0.10	9.61	1.00	1	4508	3	13524
W5C W5J	ANTIVIRALS, HIV-SPECIFIC, PROTEASE INHIBITORS	ANTIVIRALS, HIV-SPECIFIC, NUCLEOSIDE ANALOG, RTI	1.00	0.10	9.61	1.00	1	4508	3	13524
C4K M4E	HYPOGLYCEMICS, INSULIN-RELEASE STIMULANT TYPE	LIPOTROPICS	0.96	0.71	1.29	0.79	58	4451	181	13346
C4L J7C	HYPOGLYCEMICS, BIGUANIDE TYPE (NON-SULFONYLUREAS)	BETA-ADRENERGIC BLOCKING AGENTS	0.95	0.57	1.59	0.85	19	4490	60	13467
H2F W5A	ANTI-ANXIETY DRUGS	ANTIVIRALS, GENERAL	0.90	0.25	3.27	0.87	3	4506	10	13517
C4K J7C	HYPOGLYCEMICS, INSULIN-RELEASE STIMULANT TYPE	BETA-ADRENERGIC BLOCKING AGENTS	0.88	0.58	1.35	0.56	28	4481	95	13432

Appendix VIII. Table 3A. (Continued)

DRUG_DRUG	DRUG 1	DRUG 2	OR	L_OR	U_OR	P-VALUE	A	B	C	D
A1A A4F	DIGITALIS GLYCOSIDES	HYPOTENSIVES,ANGIOTENSIN RECEPTOR ANTAGONIST	0.88	0.33	2.39	0.81	5	4504	17	13510
A1A J7C	DIGITALIS GLYCOSIDES	BETA-ADRENERGIC BLOCKING AGENTS	0.86	0.50	1.48	0.60	17	4492	59	13468
A4D R1H	HYPOTENSIVES, ACE INHIBITORS	POTASSIUM SPARING DIURETICS	0.86	0.28	2.60	0.79	4	4505	14	13513
C4N H2U	HYPOGLYCEMICS, INSULIN-RESPONSE ENHANCER (N-S)	TRICYCLIC ANTIDEPRESSANTS & REL. NON-SEL. RU-INHIB	0.86	0.18	4.13	0.85	2	4507	7	13520
R1F R1M	THIAZIDE AND RELATED DIURETICS	LOOP DIURETICS	0.80	0.27	2.41	0.69	4	4505	15	13512
J7B J7C	ALPHA-ADRENERGIC BLOCKING AGENTS	BETA-ADRENERGIC BLOCKING AGENTS	0.79	0.44	1.43	0.44	14	4495	53	13474
M9L P3A	ORAL ANTICOAGULANTS, COUMARIN TYPE	THYROID HORMONES	0.79	0.29	2.11	0.64	5	4504	19	13508
C4M C4N	HYPOGLYCEMICS, ALPHA-GLUCOSIDASE INHIB TYPE (N-S)	HYPOGLYCEMICS, INSULIN-RESPONSE ENHANCER (N-S)	0.75	0.08	6.71	0.80	1	4508	4	13523
H2S M9P	SEROTONIN SPECIFIC REUPTAKE INHIBITOR (SSRIS)	PLATELET AGGREGATION INHIBITORS	0.75	0.16	3.53	0.72	2	4507	8	13519
P5A W3A	GLUCOCORTICOIDS	ANTIFUNGAL ANTIBIOTICS	0.75	0.08	6.71	0.80	1	4508	4	13523
C4K W5A	HYPOGLYCEMICS, INSULIN-RELEASE STIMULANT TYPE	ANTIVIRALS, GENERAL	0.60	0.07	5.14	0.64	1	4508	5	13522
J1B J7C	CHOLINESTERASE INHIBITORS	BETA-ADRENERGIC BLOCKING AGENTS	0.60	0.07	5.14	0.64	1	4508	5	13522
M4E W5A	LIPOTROPICS	ANTIVIRALS, GENERAL	0.60	0.17	2.07	0.42	3	4506	15	13512
M9L W2A	ORAL ANTICOAGULANTS, COUMARIN TYPE	ABSORBABLE SULFONAMIDES	0.60	0.07	5.14	0.64	1	4508	5	13522
P5A W3B	GLUCOCORTICOIDS	ANTIFUNGAL AGENTS	0.56	0.16	1.93	0.36	3	4506	16	13511
C4G M9L	INSULINS	ORAL ANTICOAGULANTS, COUMARIN TYPE	0.55	0.12	2.46	0.43	2	4507	11	13516
C4K J7A	HYPOGLYCEMICS, INSULIN-RELEASE STIMULANT TYPE	ALPHA/BETA-ADRENERGIC BLOCKING AGENTS	0.50	0.06	4.15	0.52	1	4508	6	13521
R1L R1M	POTASSIUM SPARING DIURETICS IN COMBINATION	LOOP DIURETICS	0.50	0.06	4.15	0.52	1	4508	6	13521
C4N W1Q	HYPOGLYCEMICS, INSULIN-RESPONSE ENHANCER (N-S)	QUINOLONES	0.43	0.05	3.48	0.43	1	4508	7	13520

DRUG_DRUG	DRUG 1	DRUG 2	OR	L_OR	U_OR	P-VALUE	A	B	C	D
H2U M9P	TRICYCLIC ANTIDEPRESSANTS & REL. NON-SEL. RU-INHIB	PLATELET AGGREGATION INHIBITORS	0.43	0.05	3.48	0.43	1	4508	7	13520
C4N W1D	HYPOGLYCEMICS, INSULIN-RESPONSE ENHANCER (N-S)	MACROLIDES	0.38	0.05	3.00	0.36	1	4508	8	13519
A9A J7A	CALCIUM CHANNEL BLOCKING AGENTS	ALPHA/BETA-ADRENERGIC BLOCKING AGENTS	0.30	0.04	2.34	0.25	1	4508	10	13517
A2A M4E	ANTIARRHYTHMICS	LIPOTROPICS	0.27	0.04	2.11	0.21	1	4508	11	13516

Appendix VIII. Table 3B. Significant Odds Ratios for Drug Interactions

	A	B	C	D	E	F	G	H	I	J	K
1	DRUG_DRUG	DRUG 1	DRUG 2	OR	L_OR	U_OR	P-VALUE	A	B	C	D
2	H4B W3B	ANTICONVULSANTS	ANTIFUNGAL AGENTS	21.00	2.58	170.69	0.00	7	4502	1	13526
3	H7C W1Q	SEROTONIN-NOREPINEPHRINE REUPTAKE-INHIB (SNRIS)	QUINOLONES	21.00	2.58	170.69	0.00	7	4502	1	13526
4	H6H H7T	SKELETAL MUSCLE RELAXANTS	ANTIPSYCHOTICS,ATYPICAL,DOPAMINE,& SEROTONIN ANTAG	18.00	2.17	149.52	0.01	6	4503	1	13526
5	C4K W2A	HYPOGLYCEMICS, INSULIN-RELEASE STIMULANT TYPE	ABSORBABLE SULFONAMIDES	15.00	1.75	128.40	0.01	5	4504	1	13526
6	H2S H7B	SEROTONIN SPECIFIC REUPTAKE INHIBITOR (SSRIS)	ALPHA-2 RECEPTOR ANTAGONIST ANTIDEPRESSANTS	15.00	1.75	128.40	0.01	5	4504	1	13526
7	H4B J2A	ANTICONVULSANTS	BELLADONNA ALKALOIDS	12.00	1.34	107.37	0.03	4	4505	1	13526
8	H2U H7T	TRICYCLIC ANTIDEPRESSANTS & REL. NON-SEL. RU-INHIB	ANTIPSYCHOTICS,ATYPICAL,DOPAMINE,& SEROTONIN ANTAG	10.50	2.18	50.55	0.00	7	4502	2	13525
9	H2F W1K	ANTI-ANXIETY DRUGS	LINCOSAMIDES	7.50	1.46	38.66	0.02	5	4504	2	13525
10	H2S H7C	SEROTONIN SPECIFIC REUPTAKE INHIBITOR (SSRIS)	SEROTONIN-NOREPINEPHRINE REUPTAKE-INHIB (SNRIS)	7.50	1.46	38.66	0.02	5	4504	2	13525
11	H2D H4B	BARBITURATES	ANTICONVULSANTS	6.00	1.50	23.99	0.01	6	4503	3	13524
12	C4G H7C	INSULINS	SEROTONIN-NOREPINEPHRINE REUPTAKE-INHIB (SNRIS)	6.00	1.10	32.76	0.04	4	4505	2	13525
13	C4K H2U	HYPOGLYCEMICS, INSULIN-RELEASE STIMULANT TYPE	TRICYCLIC ANTIDEPRESSANTS & REL. NON-SEL. RU-INHIB	4.50	2.02	10.02	0.00	15	4494	10	13517

Appendix VIII. Table 3B. (Continued)

	A	B	C	D	E	F	G	H	I	J	K
1	**DRUG_DRUG**	**DRUG 1**	**DRUG 2**	**OR**	**L_OR**	**U_OR**	**P-VALUE**	**A**	**B**	**C**	**D**
14	H7T Z2A	ANTIPSYCHOTICS,ATYPICAL,DOP AMINE,& SEROTONIN ANTAG	ANTIHISTAMINES	4.20	1.33	13.23	0.01	7	4502	5	13522
15	M9L S2B	ORAL ANTICOAGULANTS, COUMARIN TYPE	NSAIDS, CYCLOOXYGENASE INHIBITOR - TYPE	4.15	2.04	8.48	0.00	18	4491	13	13514
16	H6H W1D	SKELETAL MUSCLE RELAXANTS	MACROLIDES	4.07	2.04	8.12	0.00	19	4490	14	13513
17	H2S W1Q	SEROTONIN SPECIFIC REUPTAKE INHIBITOR (SSRIS)	QUINOLONES	4.00	2.17	7.37	0.00	24	4485	18	13509
18	H2E H4B	SEDATIVE-HYPNOTICS,NON-BARBITURATE	ANTICONVULSANTS	3.92	1.91	8.08	0.00	17	4492	13	13514
19	H3A H7T	ANALGESICS,NARCOTICS	ANTIPSYCHOTICS,ATYPICAL,DOP AMINE,& SEROTONIN ANTAG	3.75	1.48	9.50	0.01	10	4499	8	13519
20	B3J W5A	EXPECTORANTS	ANTIVIRALS, GENERAL	3.75	1.01	13.97	0.05	5	4504	4	13523
21	H7T J7C	ANTIPSYCHOTICS,ATYPICAL,DOP AMINE,& SEROTONIN ANTAG	BETA-ADRENERGIC BLOCKING AGENTS	3.75	1.01	13.97	0.05	5	4504	4	13523
22	H4B H7C	ANTICONVULSANTS	SEROTONIN-NOREPINEPHRINE REUPTAKE-INHIB (SNRIS)	3.67	1.52	8.85	0.00	11	4498	9	13518
23	H2S H3A	SEROTONIN SPECIFIC REUPTAKE INHIBITOR (SSRIS)	ANALGESICS,NARCOTICS	3.64	2.72	4.85	0.00	104	4405	88	13439
24	J5D Z2F	BETA-ADRENERGIC AGENTS	MAST CELL STABILIZERS	3.60	1.10	11.80	0.03	6	4503	5	13522
25	M4E W1K	LIPOTROPICS	LINCOSAMIDES	3.60	1.10	11.80	0.03	6	4503	5	13522
26	M9L W1W	ORAL ANTICOAGULANTS, COUMARIN TYPE	CEPHALOSPORINS - 1ST GENERATION	3.60	1.10	11.80	0.03	6	4503	5	13522
27	H2F H7C	ANTI-ANXIETY DRUGS	SEROTONIN-NOREPINEPHRINE REUPTAKE-INHIB (SNRIS)	3.55	1.59	7.91	0.00	13	4496	11	13516
28	H2F W3B	ANTI-ANXIETY DRUGS	ANTIFUNGAL AGENTS	3.43	1.24	9.45	0.02	8	4501	7	13520
29	H2F H2U	ANTI-ANXIETY DRUGS	TRICYCLIC ANTIDEPRESSANTS & REL. NON-SEL. RU-INHIB	3.40	2.08	5.56	0.00	34	4475	30	13497
30	H2S H7T	SEROTONIN SPECIFIC REUPTAKE INHIBITOR (SSRIS)	ANTIPSYCHOTICS,ATYPICAL,DOP AMINE,& SEROTONIN ANTAG	3.40	1.70	6.81	0.00	17	4492	15	13512
31	A1A A2A	DIGITALIS GLYCOSIDES	ANTIARRHYTHMICS	3.38	1.30	8.75	0.01	9	4500	8	13519
32	C4N H2S	HYPOGLYCEMICS, INSULIN-RESPONSE ENHANCER (N-S)	SEROTONIN SPECIFIC REUPTAKE INHIBITOR (SSRIS)	3.30	1.40	7.77	0.01	11	4498	10	13517
33	H6H W1Q	SKELETAL MUSCLE RELAXANTS	QUINOLONES	3.27	1.44	7.42	0.00	12	4497	11	13516

	A	B	C	D	E	F	G	H	I	J	K
1	DRUG_DRUG	DRUG 1	DRUG 2	OR	L_OR	U_OR	P-VALUE	A	B	C	D
34	H2U W1D	TRICYCLIC ANTIDEPRESSANTS & REL. NON-SEL. RU-INHIB	MACROLIDES	3.00	1.39	6.47	0.01	13	4496	13	13514
35	M9L M9P	ORAL ANTICOAGULANTS, COUMARIN TYPE	PLATELET AGGREGATION INHIBITORS	3.00	1.05	8.55	0.04	7	4502	7	13520
36	B3J H2S	EXPECTORANTS	SEROTONIN SPECIFIC REUPTAKE INHIBITOR (SSRIS)	2.96	1.70	5.17	0.00	25	4484	26	13501
37	H4B M9L	ANTICONVULSANTS	ORAL ANTICOAGULANTS, COUMARIN TYPE	2.93	1.39	6.19	0.00	14	4495	15	13512
38	H4B W1D	ANTICONVULSANTS	MACROLIDES	2.80	1.35	5.80	0.01	14	4495	15	13512
39	H2E H3A	SEDATIVE-HYPNOTICS,NON-BARBITURATE	ANALGESICS,NARCOTICS	2.79	1.85	4.20	0.00	45	4464	49	13478
40	H2F H2S	ANTI-ANXIETY DRUGS	SEROTONIN SPECIFIC REUPTAKE INHIBITOR (SSRIS)	2.71	2.02	3.64	0.00	85	4424	94	13433
41	C4L H2S	HYPOGLYCEMICS, BIGUANIDE TYPE (NON-SULFONYLUREAS)	SEROTONIN SPECIFIC REUPTAKE INHIBITOR (SSRIS)	2.68	1.40	5.16	0.00	17	4492	19	13508
42	A1A R1F	DIGITALIS GLYCOSIDES	THIAZIDE AND RELATED DIURETICS	2.67	1.03	6.91	0.04	8	4501	9	13518
43	A9A H7E	CALCIUM CHANNEL BLOCKING AGENTS	SEROTONIN-2 ANTAGONIST/REUPTAKE INHIBITORS (SARIS)	2.63	1.28	5.38	0.01	14	4495	16	13511
44	H2S M9L	SEROTONIN SPECIFIC REUPTAKE INHIBITOR (SSRIS)	ORAL ANTICOAGULANTS, COUMARIN TYPE	2.57	1.19	5.56	0.02	12	4497	14	13513
45	H2U W1Q	TRICYCLIC ANTIDEPRESSANTS & REL. NON-SEL. RU-INHIB	QUINOLONES	2.45	1.02	5.92	0.05	9	4500	11	13516
46	C4K H2S	HYPOGLYCEMICS, INSULIN-RELEASE STIMULANT TYPE	SEROTONIN SPECIFIC REUPTAKE INHIBITOR (SSRIS)	2.44	1.39	4.29	0.00	22	4487	27	13500
47	H2F W1D	ANTI-ANXIETY DRUGS	MACROLIDES	2.42	1.36	4.31	0.00	21	4488	26	13501
48	H2F J5D	ANTI-ANXIETY DRUGS	BETA-ADRENERGIC AGENTS	2.36	1.41	3.95	0.00	26	4483	33	13494
49	H2S H3F	SEROTONIN SPECIFIC REUPTAKE INHIBITOR (SSRIS)	ANTIMIGRAINE PREPARATIONS	2.35	1.27	4.35	0.01	18	4491	23	13504
50	H2U H3A	TRICYCLIC ANTIDEPRESSANTS & REL. NON-SEL. RU-INHIB	ANALGESICS,NARCOTICS	2.34	1.62	3.39	0.00	50	4459	64	13463
51	P5A W1D	GLUCOCORTICOIDS	MACROLIDES	2.31	1.51	3.55	0.00	37	4472	48	13479

Appendix VIII. Table 3B. (Continued)

	A	B	C	D	E	F	G	H	I	J	K
1	**DRUG_DRUG**	**DRUG 1**	**DRUG 2**	**OR**	**L_OR**	**U_OR**	**P-VALUE**	**A**	**B**	**C**	**D**
52	C4L H2U	HYPOGLYCEMICS, BIGUANIDE TYPE (NON-SULFONYLUREAS)	TRICYCLIC ANTIDEPRESSANTS & REL. NON-SEL. RU-INHIB	2.29	1.11	4.72	0.02	13	4496	17	13510
53	C4G D4K	INSULINS	GASTRIC ACID SECRETION REDUCERS	2.21	1.32	3.70	0.00	25	4484	34	13493
54	H2F W1Q	ANTI-ANXIETY DRUGS	QUINOLONES	2.20	1.27	3.81	0.00	22	4487	30	13497
55	C7A D4K	HYPERURICEMIA TX - PURINE INHIBITORS	GASTRIC ACID SECRETION REDUCERS	2.12	1.01	4.46	0.05	12	4497	17	13510
56	C4K W1D	HYPOGLYCEMICS, INSULIN-RELEASE STIMULANT TYPE	MACROLIDES	2.05	1.06	3.94	0.03	15	4494	22	13505
57	A9A D4K	CALCIUM CHANNEL BLOCKING AGENTS	GASTRIC ACID SECRETION REDUCERS	1.77	1.35	2.33	0.00	85	4424	145	13382
58	C4K D4K	HYPOGLYCEMICS, INSULIN-RELEASE STIMULANT TYPE	GASTRIC ACID SECRETION REDUCERS	1.75	1.13	2.73	0.01	31	4478	53	13474
59	H2S M4E	SEROTONIN SPECIFIC REUPTAKE INHIBITOR (SSRIS)	LIPOTROPICS	1.75	1.33	2.32	0.00	79	4430	136	13391
60	B3J Z2A	EXPECTORANTS	ANTIHISTAMINES	1.74	1.06	2.86	0.03	25	4484	43	13484
61	M4E W1Q	LIPOTROPICS	QUINOLONES	1.55	1.02	2.34	0.04	34	4475	66	13461
62	C4K C4L	HYPOGLYCEMICS, INSULIN-RELEASE STIMULANT TYPE	HYPOGLYCEMICS, BIGUANIDE TYPE (NON-SULFONYLUREAS)	1.44	1.13	1.85	0.00	94	4415	196	13331
63	A4D A9A	HYPOTENSIVES, ACE INHIBITORS	CALCIUM CHANNEL BLOCKING AGENTS	1.31	1.03	1.66	0.03	100	4409	230	13297

Appendix VIII. Table 4A. Odds Ratios for Drug Disease Interactions

DISEASE_DRUG	DRUG	DISEASE	OR	L_OR	U_OR	P-VALUE	A	B	C	D
30000 P5A	GLUCOCORTICOIDS	ANXIETY STATE UNSPEC	15.00	1.75	128.40	0.01	5	4504	1	13526
07054 H3A	ANALGESICS,NARCOTICS	CHR HEPATITIS C WOCOMA	12.00	1.34	107.37	0.03	4	4505	1	13526
4019 H2V	ANTI-NARCOLEPSY/ANTI-HYPERKINESIS, STIMULANT-TYPE	UNS HYPERTENSION	12.00	1.34	107.37	0.03	4	4505	1	13526
4160 J5D	BETA-ADRENERGIC AGENTS	PRIMARY PULMONARY HYPERTENSION	9.00	0.94	86.53	0.06	3	4506	1	13526

DISEASE_DRUG	DRUG	DISEASE	OR	L_OR	U_OR	P-VALUE	A	B	C	D
5715 H3A	ANALGESICS,NARCOTICS	CIRRHOSIS LIVER WO ALCOHOL	9.00	0.94	86.53	0.06	3	4506	1	13526
7802 C4L	HYPOGLYCEMICS, BIGUANIDE TYPE (NON-SULFONYLUREAS)	SYNCOPE/COLLAPSE	9.00	0.94	86.53	0.06	3	4506	1	13526
4254 J7A	ALPHA/BETA-ADRENERGIC BLOCKING AGENTS	OTH PRIMARY CARDIOMYOPATHIES	7.50	1.46	38.66	0.02	5	4504	2	13525
7802 A9A	CALCIUM CHANNEL BLOCKING AGENTS	SYNCOPE/COLLAPSE	7.00	1.81	27.07	0.00	7	4502	3	13524
7802 A4D	HYPOTENSIVES, ACE INHIBITORS	SYNCOPE/COLLAPSE	6.75	2.08	21.92	0.00	9	4500	4	13523
07051 R1M	LOOP DIURETICS	AC/UNS HEPATITIS C WOCOMA	6.00	0.54	66.17	0.14	2	4507	1	13526
07054 H2S	SEROTONIN SPECIFIC REUPTAKE INHIBITOR (SSRIS)	CHR HEPATITIS C WOCOMA	6.00	0.54	66.17	0.14	2	4507	1	13526
25040 A4D	HYPOTENSIVES, ACE INHIBITORS	DIABETES RENAL MANIF TYPE II	6.00	0.54	66.17	0.14	2	4507	1	13526
25040 C4G	INSULINS	DIABETES RENAL MANIF TYPE II	6.00	0.54	66.17	0.14	2	4507	1	13526
25050 A4F	HYPOTENSIVES,ANGIOTENSIN RECEPTOR ANTAGONIST	DIABETES EYE MANIF TYPE II	6.00	0.54	66.17	0.14	2	4507	1	13526
29620 P5A	GLUCOCORTICOIDS	DEPRESSIVE TYPE PSYCHOSIS	6.00	0.54	66.17	0.14	2	4507	1	13526
29622 P5A	GLUCOCORTICOIDS	MAJ DEPRESS DIS SGL EPI MODERATE	6.00	0.54	66.17	0.14	2	4507	1	13526
29690 Z2A	ANTIHISTAMINES	UNS AFFECTIVE PSYCHOSIS	6.00	0.54	66.17	0.14	2	4507	1	13526
3004 P5A	GLUCOCORTICOIDS	NEUROTIC DEPRESSION	6.00	0.54	66.17	0.14	2	4507	1	13526
34510 Z2A	ANTIHISTAMINES	GRAND MALY WO INTRACT EPILEPSY	6.00	0.54	66.17	0.14	2	4507	1	13526
4011 J5G	BETA-ADRENERGICS AND GLUCOCORTICOIDS COMBINATION	BENIGN HYPERTENSION	6.00	0.54	66.17	0.14	2	4507	1	13526
40290 S2B	NSAIDS, CYCLOOXYGENASE INHIBITOR - TYPE	HYPERTENSIVE HEART DIS UNSPEC	6.00	0.54	66.17	0.14	2	4507	1	13526
4254 M9L	ORAL ANTICOAGULANTS, COUMARIN TYPE	OTH PRIMARY CARDIOMYOPATHIES	6.00	1.10	32.76	0.04	4	4505	2	13525

Appendix VIII. Table 4A. (Continued)

DISEASE_DRUG	DRUG	DISEASE	OR	L_OR	U_OR	P-VALUE	A	B	C	D
4289 J7C	BETA-ADRENERGIC BLOCKING AGENTS	UNS HEART FAILURE	6.00	0.54	66.17	0.14	2	4507	1	13526
49390 H3E	ANALGESIC/ANTIPYRETICS,NON-SALICYLATE	UNS ASTHMA WOSTATUS ASTHMATICUS	6.00	0.54	66.17	0.14	2	4507	1	13526
5715 C4G	INSULINS	CIRRHOSIS LIVER WO ALCOHOL	6.00	0.54	66.17	0.14	2	4507	1	13526
585 H2S	SEROTONIN SPECIFIC REUPTAKE INHIBITOR (SSRIS)	CHRONIC RENAL FAILURE	6.00	0.54	66.17	0.14	2	4507	1	13526
25000 A4B	HYPOTENSIVES,SYMPATHOLYTIC	DIABETES UNCOMPL TYPE II	4.50	1.60	12.64	0.00	9	4500	6	13521
25001 J7C	BETA-ADRENERGIC BLOCKING AGENTS	DIABETES UNCOMPL TYPE I	3.67	1.52	8.85	0.00	11	4498	9	13518
4011 J5D	BETA-ADRENERGIC AGENTS NSAIDS, CYCLOOXYGENASE	BENIGN HYPERTENSION	3.20	1.58	6.47	0.00	16	4493	15	13512
4011 S2B	INHIBITOR - TYPE	BENIGN HYPERTENSION	3.16	2.03	4.92	0.00	40	4469	38	13489
07044 H3A	ANALGESICS,NARCOTICS	CHR HEPATITIS C W COMA	3.00	0.19	47.96	0.44	1	4508	1	13526
07051 R1H	POTASSIUM SPARING DIURETICS	AC/UNS HEPATITIS C WOCOMA	3.00	0.19	47.96	0.44	1	4508	1	13526
07054 H4B	ANTICONVULSANTS	CHR HEPATITIS C WOCOMA	3.00	0.19	47.96	0.44	1	4508	1	13526
25000 A4Y	HYPOTENSIVES,MISCELLANEOUS	DIABETES UNCOMPL TYPE II	3.00	0.42	21.30	0.27	2	4507	2	13525
25002 A4B	HYPOTENSIVES,SYMPATHOLYTIC	DIABETES UNCOMP TYPE II UNCONTRD	3.00	0.19	47.96	0.44	1	4508	1	13526
25040 A4F	HYPOTENSIVES,ANGIOTENSIN RECEPTOR ANTAGONIST	DIABETES RENAL MANIF TYPE II	3.00	0.19	47.96	0.44	1	4508	1	13526
25040 J7C	BETA-ADRENERGIC BLOCKING AGENTS	DIABETES RENAL MANIF TYPE II	3.00	0.19	47.96	0.44	1	4508	1	13526
25040 R1M	LOOP DIURETICS	DIABETES RENAL MANIF TYPE II	3.00	0.19	47.96	0.44	1	4508	1	13526
25041 A4D	HYPOTENSIVES, ACE INHIBITORS	DIABETES RENAL MANIF TYPE I	3.00	0.42	21.30	0.27	2	4507	2	13525
25041 R1F	THIAZIDE AND RELATED DIURETICS	DIABETES RENAL MANIF TYPE I	3.00	0.19	47.96	0.44	1	4508	1	13526
25041 W1Q	QUINOLONES	DIABETES RENAL MANIF TYPE I	3.00	0.19	47.96	0.44	1	4508	1	13526

DISEASE_DRUG	DRUG	DISEASE	OR	L_OR	U_OR	P-VALUE	A	B	C	D
25042 C4G	INSULINS	DIABETES RENAL MANIF TYPE II UNC	3.00	0.19	47.96	0.44	1	4508	1	13526
25062 J7C	BETA-ADRENERGIC BLOCKING AGENTS	DIABETES NEUR MANIF TYPE II UNCN	3.00	0.19	47.96	0.44	1	4508	1	13526
2930 H2F	ANTI-ANXIETY DRUGS	ACUTE DELIRIUM	3.00	0.19	47.96	0.44	1	4508	1	13526
29650 H2M	ANTI-MANIA DRUGS	BIPOLAR AFFECT DIS DEPRESS UNS	3.00	0.19	47.96	0.44	1	4508	1	13526
29680 H2M	ANTI-MANIA DRUGS	UNS MANIC DEPRESSIVE PSYCHOSIS	3.00	0.19	47.96	0.44	1	4508	1	13526
29690 H2E	SEDATIVE-HYPNOTICS, NON- BARBITURATE	UNS AFFECTIVE PSYCHOSIS	3.00	0.19	47.96	0.44	1	4508	1	13526
29690 H2S	SEROTONIN SPECIFIC REUPTAKE INHIBITOR (SSRIS)	UNS AFFECTIVE PSYCHOSIS	3.00	0.42	21.30	0.27	2	4507	2	13525
29690 H4B	ANTICONVULSANTS	UNS AFFECTIVE PSYCHOSIS	3.00	0.42	21.30	0.27	2	4507	2	13525
3090 P5A	GLUCOCORTICOIDS	ADJUST REAC BRIEF DEPRESSIVE	3.00	0.19	47.96	0.44	1	4508	1	13526
34500 P5A	GLUCOCORTICOIDS	PETIT MAL WO INTRACT EPILEPSY	3.00	0.19	47.96	0.44	1	4508	1	13526
34500 Z2A	ANTIHISTAMINES	PETIT MAL WO INTRACT EPILEPSY	3.00	0.19	47.96	0.44	1	4508	1	13526
34510 H2S	SEROTONIN SPECIFIC REUPTAKE INHIBITOR (SSRIS)	GRAND MALY WO INTRACT EPILEPSY	3.00	0.19	47.96	0.44	1	4508	1	13526
34510 P5A	GLUCOCORTICOIDS	GRAND MALY WO INTRACT EPILEPSY	3.00	0.19	47.96	0.44	1	4508	1	13526
34590 R1M	LOOP DIURETICS	UNS EPILEPSY WO INTRACT EPILEPSY	3.00	0.19	47.96	0.44	1	4508	1	13526
40291 J5D	BETA-ADRENERGIC AGENTS	HYPERTEN HEART DIS W CHF	3.00	0.19	47.96	0.44	1	4508	1	13526
40291 J7C	BETA-ADRENERGIC BLOCKING AGENTS	HYPERTEN HEART DIS W CHF	3.00	0.19	47.96	0.44	1	4508	1	13526
40391 C4G	INSULINS	RENAL HYPERT UNSPEC/FAILURE	3.00	0.19	47.96	0.44	1	4508	1	13526
40391 H4B	ANTICONVULSANTS	RENAL HYPERT UNSPEC/FAILURE	3.00	0.19	47.96	0.44	1	4508	1	13526

Appendix VIII. Table 4A. (Continued)

DISEASE_DRUG	DRUG	DISEASE	OR	L_OR	U_OR	P-VALUE	A	B	C	D
4280 J7A	ALPHA/BETA-ADRENERGIC BLOCKING AGENTS	CONGESTIVE HEART FAILURE	3.00	0.97	9.30	0.06	6	4503	6	13521
4281 A1A	DIGITALIS GLYCOSIDES	LEFT HEART FAILURE	3.00	0.19	47.96	0.44	1	4508	1	13526
4281 C4G	INSULINS	LEFT HEART FAILURE	3.00	0.19	47.96	0.44	1	4508	1	13526
4281 M9L	ORAL ANTICOAGULANTS, COUMARIN TYPE	LEFT HEART FAILURE	3.00	0.19	47.96	0.44	1	4508	1	13526
4293 J5D	BETA-ADRENERGIC AGENTS	CARDIOMEGALY	3.00	0.42	21.30	0.27	2	4507	2	13525
49121 H2E	SEDATIVE-HYPNOTICS, NON- BARBITURATE	OBSTRUCT CHRON BRONCHITIS W EXAC	3.00	0.19	47.96	0.44	1	4508	1	13526
4928 J7C	BETA-ADRENERGIC BLOCKING AGENTS	OTH EMPHYSEMA	3.00	0.19	47.96	0.44	1	4508	1	13526
49390 J7C	BETA-ADRENERGIC BLOCKING AGENTS	UNS ASTHMA WOSTATUS ASTHMATICUS	3.00	0.97	9.30	0.06	6	4503	6	13521
5716 H3A	ANALGESICS,NARCOTICS	BILIARY CIRRHOSIS	3.00	0.19	47.96	0.44	1	4508	1	13526
5716 P5A	GLUCOCORTICOIDS	BILIARY CIRRHOSIS	3.00	0.19	47.96	0.44	1	4508	1	13526
5718 H2F	ANTI-ANXIETY DRUGS	OTH CHRONIC NONALCOHOLIC LIVER DIS	3.00	0.19	47.96	0.44	1	4508	1	13526
5728 H3A	ANALGESICS,NARCOTICS	OTH SEQUELAE CHRONIC LIVER DISEASE	3.00	0.19	47.96	0.44	1	4508	1	13526
5733 M4E	LIPOTROPICS	UNS HEPATITIS	3.00	0.19	47.96	0.44	1	4508	1	13526
5733 S2B	NSAIDS, CYCLOOXYGENASE INHIBITOR - TYPE	UNS HEPATITIS	3.00	0.19	47.96	0.44	1	4508	1	13526
5739 J7C	BETA-ADRENERGIC BLOCKING AGENTS	UNS DISORDER LIVER	3.00	0.19	47.96	0.44	1	4508	1	13526
5739 P5A	GLUCOCORTICOIDS	UNS DISORDER LIVER	3.00	0.19	47.96	0.44	1	4508	1	13526
5739 R1M	LOOP DIURETICS	UNS DISORDER LIVER	3.00	0.19	47.96	0.44	1	4508	1	13526
5849 A4D	HYPOTENSIVES, ACE INHIBITORS	UNS ACUTE RENAL FAILURE	3.00	0.19	47.96	0.44	1	4508	1	13526
5849 R1L	POTASSIUM SPARING DIURETICS IN COMBINATION	UNS ACUTE RENAL FAILURE	3.00	0.19	47.96	0.44	1	4508	1	13526
585 C4L	HYPOGLYCEMICS, BIGUANIDE TYPE (NON-SULFONYLUREAS)	CHRONIC RENAL FAILURE	3.00	0.19	47.96	0.44	1	4508	1	13526
585 H4B	ANTICONVULSANTS	CHRONIC RENAL FAILURE	3.00	0.19	47.96	0.44	1	4508	1	13526
585 W1Q	QUINOLONES	CHRONIC RENAL FAILURE	3.00	0.42	21.30	0.27	2	4507	2	13525

DISEASE_DRUG	DRUG	DISEASE	OR	L_OR	U_OR	P-VALUE	A	B	C	D
586 A4D	HYPOTENSIVES, ACE INHIBITORS	UNS RENAL FAILURE	3.00	0.19	47.96	0.44	1	4508	1	13526
7802 A1A	DIGITALIS GLYCOSIDES	SYNCOPE/COLLAPSE	3.00	0.19	47.96	0.44	1	4508	1	13526
7802 C4G	INSULINS	SYNCOPE/COLLAPSE	3.00	0.19	47.96	0.44	1	4508	1	13526
7802 H2E	SEDATIVE-HYPNOTICS,NON-BARBITURATE	SYNCOPE/COLLAPSE	3.00	0.19	47.96	0.44	1	4508	1	13526
7802 H7T	ANTIPSYCHOTICS,ATYPICAL,DOPAMINE,& SEROTONIN ANTAG	SYNCOPE/COLLAPSE	3.00	0.19	47.96	0.44	1	4508	1	13526
V420 C4G	INSULINS	KIDNEY REPLACED BY TRANSPLANT	3.00	0.19	47.96	0.44	1	4508	1	13526
V451 C4G	INSULINS	RENAL DIALYSIS STATUS	3.00	0.19	47.96	0.44	1	4508	1	13526
V451 H3A	ANALGESICS,NARCOTICS	RENAL DIALYSIS STATUS	3.00	0.19	47.96	0.44	1	4508	1	13526
4019 S2B	NSAIDS, CYCLOOXYGENASE INHIBITOR - TYPE	UNS HYPERTENSION	2.54	1.83	3.53	0.00	66	4443	78	13449
4019 J5D	BETA-ADRENERGIC AGENTS	UNS HYPERTENSION	2.45	1.32	4.58	0.00	18	4491	22	13505
311 P5A	GLUCOCORTICOIDS	DEPRESSIVE DISORDER NEC	2.40	0.64	8.94	0.19	4	4505	5	13522
585 A4D	HYPOTENSIVES, ACE INHIBITORS	CHRONIC RENAL FAILURE	2.40	0.64	8.94	0.19	4	4505	5	13522
5715 R1M	LOOP DIURETICS	CIRRHOSIS LIVER WO ALCOHOL	2.25	0.50	10.05	0.29	3	4506	4	13523
586 H3A	ANALGESICS,NARCOTICS	UNS RENAL FAILURE	2.25	0.50	10.05	0.29	3	4506	4	13523
7802 H2S	SEROTONIN SPECIFIC REUPTAKE INHIBITOR (SSRIS)	SYNCOPE/COLLAPSE	2.25	0.50	10.05	0.29	3	4506	4	13523
4011 Z4B	LEUKOTRIENE RECEPTOR ANTAGONISTS	BENIGN HYPERTENSION	2.00	0.56	7.09	0.28	4	4505	6	13521
4280 H2S	SEROTONIN SPECIFIC REUPTAKE INHIBITOR (SSRIS)	CONGESTIVE HEART FAILURE	2.00	0.71	5.62	0.19	6	4503	9	13518
25000 A4F	HYPOTENSIVES,ANGIOTENSIN RECEPTOR ANTAGONIST	DIABETES UNCOMPL TYPE II	1.91	1.10	3.30	0.02	21	4488	33	13494
25001 A4F	HYPOTENSIVES,ANGIOTENSIN RECEPTOR ANTAGONIST	DIABETES UNCOMPL TYPE I	1.91	0.74	4.92	0.18	7	4502	11	13516
25000 J7A	ALPHA/BETA-ADRENERGIC BLOCKING AGENTS	DIABETES UNCOMPL TYPE II	1.80	0.43	7.53	0.42	3	4506	5	13522
25002 J7C	BETA-ADRENERGIC BLOCKING AGENTS	DIABETES UNCOMP TYPE II UNCONTRD	1.80	0.65	4.95	0.26	6	4503	10	13517

Appendix VIII. Table 4A. (Continued)

DISEASE_DRUG	DRUG	DISEASE	OR	L_OR	U_OR	P-VALUE	A	B	C	D
4280 C4K	HYPOGLYCEMICS, INSULIN-RELEASE STIMULANT TYPE	CONGESTIVE HEART FAILURE	1.80	0.65	4.95	0.26	6	4503	10	13517
585 H3A	ANALGESICS,NARCOTICS	CHRONIC RENAL FAILURE	1.80	0.43	7.53	0.42	3	4506	5	13522
4254 A1A	DIGITALIS GLYCOSIDES	OTH PRIMARY CARDIOMYOPATHIES	1.71	0.50	5.86	0.39	4	4505	7	13520
4280 M9L	ORAL ANTICOAGULANTS, COUMARIN TYPE	CONGESTIVE HEART FAILURE	1.69	0.75	3.82	0.21	9	4500	16	13511
4280 J5D	BETA-ADRENERGIC AGENTS	CONGESTIVE HEART FAILURE	1.64	0.61	4.42	0.33	6	4503	11	13516
25001 J7A	ALPHA/BETA-ADRENERGIC BLOCKING AGENTS	DIABETES UNCOMPL TYPE I	1.50	0.14	16.54	0.74	1	4508	2	13525
25002 A4F	HYPOTENSIVES,ANGIOTENSIN RECEPTOR ANTAGONIST	DIABETES UNCOMP TYPE II UNCONTRD	1.50	0.38	6.00	0.57	3	4506	6	13521
25040 C4K	HYPOGLYCEMICS, INSULIN-RELEASE STIMULANT TYPE	DIABETES RENAL MANIF TYPE II	1.50	0.14	16.54	0.74	1	4508	2	13525
25061 J7C	BETA-ADRENERGIC BLOCKING AGENTS	DIABETES NEURO MANIF TYPE I	1.50	0.14	16.54	0.74	1	4508	2	13525
4019 Z4B	LEUKOTRIENE RECEPTOR ANTAGONISTS	UNS HYPERTENSION	1.50	0.27	8.19	0.64	2	4507	4	13523
40210 S2B	NSAIDS, CYCLOOXYGENASE INHIBITOR - TYPE	BENIGN HYPERTEN HEART DIS UNSPEC	1.50	0.14	16.54	0.74	1	4508	2	13525
4280 C4N	HYPOGLYCEMICS, INSULIN-RESPONSE ENHANCER (N-S)	CONGESTIVE HEART FAILURE	1.50	0.38	6.00	0.57	3	4506	6	13521
4280 S2B	NSAIDS, CYCLOOXYGENASE INHIBITOR - TYPE	CONGESTIVE HEART FAILURE	1.50	0.45	4.98	0.51	4	4505	8	13519
4280 Z4B	LEUKOTRIENE RECEPTOR ANTAGONISTS	CONGESTIVE HEART FAILURE	1.50	0.14	16.54	0.74	1	4508	2	13525
4292 H2S	SEROTONIN SPECIFIC REUPTAKE INHIBITOR (SSRIS)	UNS CARDIOVASCULAR DISEASE	1.50	0.14	16.54	0.74	1	4508	2	13525
49121 J7C	BETA-ADRENERGIC BLOCKING AGENTS	OBSTRUCT CHRON BRONCHITIS W EXAC	1.50	0.14	16.54	0.74	1	4508	2	13525
5733 A9A	CALCIUM CHANNEL BLOCKING AGENTS	UNS HEPATITIS	1.50	0.14	16.54	0.74	1	4508	2	13525
5733 H3A	ANALGESICS,NARCOTICS	UNS HEPATITIS	1.50	0.14	16.54	0.74	1	4508	2	13525
5739 H3A	ANALGESICS,NARCOTICS	UNS DISORDER LIVER	1.50	0.14	16.54	0.74	1	4508	2	13525

DISEASE_DRUG	DRUG	DISEASE	OR	L_OR	U_OR	P-VALUE	A	B	C	D
5849 H3A	ANALGESICS,NARCOTICS	UNS ACUTE RENAL FAILURE	1.50	0.14	16.54	0.74	1	4508	2	13525
585 C4K	HYPOGLYCEMICS, INSULIN-RELEASE STIMULANT TYPE	CHRONIC RENAL FAILURE	1.50	0.14	16.54	0.74	1	4508	2	13525
585 C4N	HYPOGLYCEMICS, INSULIN-RESPONSE ENHANCER (N-S)	CHRONIC RENAL FAILURE	1.50	0.14	16.54	0.74	1	4508	2	13525
585 R1M	LOOP DIURETICS	CHRONIC RENAL FAILURE	1.50	0.38	6.00	0.57	3	4506	6	13521
586 C4G	INSULINS	UNS RENAL FAILURE	1.50	0.27	8.19	0.64	2	4507	4	13523
586 C4K	HYPOGLYCEMICS, INSULIN-RELEASE STIMULANT TYPE	UNS RENAL FAILURE	1.50	0.14	16.54	0.74	1	4508	2	13525
V420 J7C	BETA-ADRENERGIC BLOCKING AGENTS	KIDNEY REPLACED BY TRANSPLANT	1.50	0.14	16.54	0.74	1	4508	2	13525
4280 A1A	DIGITALIS GLYCOSIDES	CONGESTIVE HEART FAILURE	1.39	0.72	2.69	0.32	13	4496	28	13499
25000 J7C	BETA-ADRENERGIC BLOCKING AGENTS	DIABETES UNCOMPL TYPE II	1.38	0.91	2.08	0.13	33	4476	72	13455
585 C4G	INSULINS	CHRONIC RENAL FAILURE	1.25	0.44	3.55	0.68	5	4504	12	13515
4280 H2U	TRICYCLIC ANTIDEPRESSANTS & REL. NON-SEL. RU-INHIB	CONGESTIVE HEART FAILURE	1.20	0.23	6.19	0.83	2	4507	5	13522
7802 A7B	VASODILATORS,CORONARY	SYNCOPE/COLLAPSE	1.20	0.23	6.19	0.83	2	4507	5	13522
585 J7C	BETA-ADRENERGIC BLOCKING AGENTS	CHRONIC RENAL FAILURE	1.13	0.30	4.24	0.86	3	4506	8	13519
07051 H2E	SEDATIVE-HYPNOTICS,NON-BARBITURATE	AC/UNS HEPATITIS C WOCOMA	1.00	0.10	9.61	1.00	1	4508	3	13524
07051 H3A	ANALGESICS,NARCOTICS	AC/UNS HEPATITIS C WOCOMA	1.00	0.10	9.61	1.00	1	4508	3	13524
25040 C4L	HYPOGLYCEMICS, BIGUANIDE TYPE (NON-SULFONYLUREAS)	DIABETES RENAL MANIF TYPE II	1.00	0.10	9.61	1.00	1	4508	3	13524
25041 C4G	INSULINS	DIABETES RENAL MANIF TYPE I	1.00	0.10	9.61	1.00	1	4508	3	13524
4254 J7C	BETA-ADRENERGIC BLOCKING AGENTS	OTH PRIMARY CARDIOMYOPATHIES	1.00	0.20	4.95	1.00	2	4507	6	13521
4289 A1A	DIGITALIS GLYCOSIDES	UNS HEART FAILURE	1.00	0.10	9.61	1.00	1	4508	3	13524
49390 H3D	ANALGESIC/ANTIPYRETICS, SALICYLATES	UNS ASTHMA WOSTATUS ASTHMATICUS	1.00	0.10	9.61	1.00	1	4508	3	13524

Appendix VIII. Table 4A. (Continued)

DISEASE_DRUG	DRUG	DISEASE	OR	L_OR	U_OR	P-VALUE	A	B	C	D
496 J7C	BETA-ADRENERGIC BLOCKING AGENTS	CHRONIC AIRWAY OBSTRUCTION NEC	1.00	0.43	2.35	1.00	7	4502	21	13506
586 R1M	LOOP DIURETICS	UNS RENAL FAILURE	1.00	0.10	9.61	1.00	1	4508	3	13524
7802 J7C	BETA-ADRENERGIC BLOCKING AGENTS	SYNCOPE/COLLAPSE	1.00	0.27	3.69	1.00	3	4506	9	13518
4280 C4L	HYPOGLYCEMICS, BIGUANIDE TYPE (NON-SULFONYLUREAS)	CONGESTIVE HEART FAILURE	0.90	0.25	3.27	0.87	3	4506	10	13517
496 H2E	SEDATIVE-HYPNOTICS,NON-BARBITURATE	CHRONIC AIRWAY OBSTRUCTION NEC	0.86	0.18	4.13	0.85	2	4507	7	13520
4280 C4G	INSULINS	CONGESTIVE HEART FAILURE	0.82	0.23	2.93	0.76	3	4506	11	13516
2765 S2B	NSAIDS, CYCLOOXYGENASE INHIBITOR - TYPE	VOLUME DEPLETION DISORDER	0.75	0.08	6.71	0.80	1	4508	4	13523
4254 C4K	HYPOGLYCEMICS, INSULIN-RELEASE STIMULANT TYPE	OTH PRIMARY CARDIOMYOPATHIES	0.75	0.08	6.71	0.80	1	4508	4	13523
4280 M9P	PLATELET AGGREGATION INHIBITORS	CONGESTIVE HEART FAILURE	0.75	0.16	3.53	0.72	2	4507	8	13519
5715 R1H	POTASSIUM SPARING DIURETICS	CIRRHOSIS LIVER WO ALCOHOL	0.75	0.08	6.71	0.80	1	4508	4	13523
4280 J7C	BETA-ADRENERGIC BLOCKING AGENTS	CONGESTIVE HEART FAILURE	0.43	0.10	1.89	0.26	2	4507	14	13513

Appendix VIII. Table 4B. Odds Ratios for Drug Disease Interactions

	A	B	C	D	E	F	G	H	I	J	K
1	DISEASE_DRUG	DRUG	DISEASE	OR	L_OR	U_OR	P-VALUE	A	B	C	D
2	30000 P5A	GLUCOCORTICOIDS	ANXIETY STATE UNSPEC	15.00	1.75	128.40	0.01	5	4504	1	13526
3	07054 H3A	ANALGESICS,NARCOTICS	CHR HEPATITIS C WOCOMA	12.00	1.34	107.37	0.03	4	4505	1	13526
4	4019 H2V	ANTI-NARCOLEPSY/ANTI-HYPERKINESIS, STIMULANT-TYPE	UNS HYPERTENSION	12.00	1.34	107.37	0.03	4	4505	1	13526
5	4254 J7A	ALPHA/BETA-ADRENERGIC BLOCKING AGENTS	OTH PRIMARY CARDIOMYOPATHIES	7.50	1.46	38.66	0.02	5	4504	2	13525

Appendix VIII. Table 4B. (Continued)

	A	B	C	D	E	F	G	H	I	J	K
1	DISEASE_DRUG	DRUG	DISEASE	OR	L_OR	U_OR	P-VALUE	A	B	C	D
6	7802 A9A	CALCIUM CHANNEL BLOCKING AGENTS	SYNCOPE/COLLAPSE	7.00	1.81	27.07	0.00	7	4502	3	13524
7	7802 A4D	HYPOTENSIVES, ACE INHIBITORS	SYNCOPE/COLLAPSE	6.75	2.08	21.92	0.00	9	4500	4	13523
8	4254 M9L	ORAL ANTICOAGULANTS, COUMARIN TYPE	OTH PRIMARY CARDIOMYOPATHIES	6.00	1.10	32.76	0.04	4	4505	2	13525
9	25000 A4B	HYPOTENSIVES,SYMPATHOLYTIC	DIABETES UNCOMPL TYPE II	4.50	1.60	12.64	0.00	9	4500	6	13521
10	25001 J7C	BETA-ADRENERGIC BLOCKING AGENTS	DIABETES UNCOMPL TYPE I	3.67	1.52	8.85	0.00	11	4498	9	13518
11	4011 J5D	BETA-ADRENERGIC AGENTS	BENIGN HYPERTENSION	3.20	1.58	6.47	0.00	16	4493	15	13512
12	4011 S2B	NSAIDS, CYCLOOXYGENASE INHIBITOR - TYPE	BENIGN HYPERTENSION	3.16	2.03	4.92	0.00	40	4469	38	13489
13	4019 S2B	NSAIDS, CYCLOOXYGENASE INHIBITOR - TYPE	UNS HYPERTENSION	2.54	1.83	3.53	0.00	66	4443	78	13449
14	4019 J5D	BETA-ADRENERGIC AGENTS	UNS HYPERTENSION	2.45	1.32	4.58	0.00	18	4491	22	13505
15	25000 A4F	HYPOTENSIVES,ANGIOTENSIN RECEPTOR ANTAGONIST	DIABETES UNCOMPL TYPE II	1.91	1.10	3.30	0.02	21	4488	33	13494

Appendix IX. Example Profiles

Patient ID: 5702AAAAAAACBMGK, Year of Birth: 1935, Gender: Female, Trigger Date: 02/20/2001

Date	Type	Code	Diagnosis	Procedure	Rx	Days Supply
01/06/2001	DIAG	25000	DIABETES UNCOMPL TYPE II			
01/06/2001	DIAG	27800	OBESITY UNSPEC			
01/06/2001	DIAG	4019	UNS HYPERTENSION			
01/06/2001	DIAG	41090	AMI UNS SITE UNS EOC			
01/06/2001	DIAG	4111	INTERMEDIATE CORONARY SYNDROME			
01/06/2001	DIAG	78650	UNSPEC CHEST PAIN			
01/06/2001	DIAG	78651	PRECORDIAL PAIN			
01/06/2001	DIAG	78701	NAUSEA W VOMITING			
01/22/2001	DRUG	00378020801			FUROSEMIDE	
01/22/2001	DRUG	59762372704			GLYBURIDE	
01/23/2001	DRUG	00005321943			ATENOLOL	
01/29/2001	DRUG	00378034505			DIAZEPAM	
01/29/2001	DRUG	00378104901			DOXEPIN HCL	
01/30/2001	DIAG	25000	DIABETES UNCOMPL TYPE II			
01/30/2001	DIAG	78050	UNS SLEEP DISTURBANCE			
02/01/2001	DRUG	00087607005			METFORMIN HCL	
02/03/2001	DRUG	00069306075			AZITHROMYCIN	
02/03/2001	DRUG	00258365401			BENZONATATE	
02/06/2001	DRUG	00002314460			NIZATIDINE	
02/08/2001	DIAG	4660	ACUTE BRONCHITIS			
02/08/2001	CPT4	99213		OFFICE/OUTPATIENT VISIT, EST		
02/09/2001	DRUG	00026851251			CIPROFLOXACIN HCL	
02/10/2001	DRUG	61570007201			ESTROGENS,ESTERIFIED	
02/17/2001	DRUG	00085045803			LORATADINE	
02/19/2001	DRUG	61570007201			ESTROGENS,ESTERIFIED	

66 YO FEMALE WITH A HX OF DM II, SLEEP DISTURBANCE, CHEST PAIN, HYPERTENSION, IS TAKING GLYBURIDE, DOXEPIN, FUROSEMIDE, ATENOLOL, DIAZEPAM, DOXEPIN, METFORMIN, AND NIZATIDINE. THE DOXEPIN AND FUROSEMIDE AFFECT BLOOD SUGAR CONTROL. THE DIAZEPAM, NIZATIDINE, BENZONATATE, AND DOXEPIN INTERACT TO INCREASE DROWSINESS. THE METFORMIN AND GLYBURIDE MAY CAUSE EXCESSIVE HYPOGLYCEMIA. THE ATENOLOL MAY MASK THE SIGNS OF HYPOGLYCEMIA IN DIABETIC PATIENTS. DOXEPIN HAS BEEN ASSOCIATED WITH SYNCOPE AND FALLS IN OLDER PATIENTS. DIAZEPAM IS A LONG-ACTING BENZODIAZEPINE AND MAY PRODUCE PROLONGED SEDATION AND INCREASE THE RISK OF FALLS.

Date	Type	Code	Diagnosis	Procedure	Rx	Days Supply
02/20/2001	DIAG	E8199	MVA UNS INJURING UNS PERSON			
02/20/2001	DIAG	7231	CERVICALGIA			
02/20/2001	DIAG	8470	SPRAIN/STRAIN OF NECK			
02/20/2001	DIAG	8470	SPRAIN/STRAIN OF NECK			
02/20/2001	DRUG	00406035705			HYDROCODONE BIT/ACETAMINOPHEN	
02/20/2001	DRUG	52544080601			METHOCARBAMOL	

Patient ID: 5401AAAAAAABIYSO, Year of Birth: 1922, Gender: Male, Trigger Date: 11/11/1999

Date Supply	Type	Code	Diagnosis	Procedure	Rx	Days of
09/24/1999	DIAG	4280	CONGESTIVE HEART FAILURE			
09/24/1999	DIAG	78057	OTH/UNS SLEEP APNEA			
09/28/1999	DIAG	25000	DIABETES UNCOMPL TYPE II			
09/29/1999	DRUG	00007414020			CARVEDILOL	
10/04/1999	DRUG	00039022310			GLIMEPIRIDE	
10/05/1999	DRUG	00172423480			BUMETANIDE	
10/07/1999	DIAG	V048	VACCINE FOR INFLUENZA			
10/07/1999	CPT4	90659		FLU VACCINE, WHOLE, IM		
10/08/1999	DRUG	00029315920			ROSIGLITAZONE MALEATE	
10/08/1999	DRUG	00085078701			POTASSIUM CHLORIDE	
10/08/1999	DIAG	4019	UNS HYPERTENSION			
10/08/1999	DIAG	5939	UNS DISORDER KIDNEY/URETER			
10/08/1999	CPT4	99213		OFFICE/OUTPATIENT VISIT, EST		
10/09/1999	DRUG	00006001958			LISINOPRIL	
10/09/1999	DRUG	00781205101			TERAZOSIN HCL	
10/15/1999	DIAG	4280	CONGESTIVE HEART FAILURE			
10/15/1999	DIAG	5939	UNS DISORDER KIDNEY/URETER			
10/18/1999	DRUG	00078023405			FLUVASTATIN SODIUM	
10/18/1999	DRUG	00186045258			FELODIPINE	

77 YO MALE PATIENT WITH A HISTORY OF CONGESTIVE HEART FAILURE, HYPERTENSION, AND DM TYPE II IS TREATED WITH CARVEDILOL, BUMETANIDE, LISINOPRIL FOR CONGESTIVE HEART FAILURE AND HYPERTENSION, GLIMEPIRIDE AND ROSIGLITAZONE FOR DM, FLUVASTATIN FOR HYPERLIPIDEMIA, TERAZOSIN FOR PROSTATIC HYPERTROPHY, FELODIPINE FOR HYPERTENSION, POTASSIUM FOR ELECTROLYTE DEPLETION CAUSED BY THE BUMETANIDE. THE CARVEDILOL MAY POTENTIATE HYPOGLYCEMIA AND MASK ITS SIGNS, IT ALSO CAUSES DIZZINESS. LISINOPRIL MAY CAUSE HYPOTENSION AND DIZZINESS. BUMETANIDE AFFECTS GLUCOSE CONTROL AND CAUSES DIZZINESS. THE HYPOGLYCEMIC DRUGS MAY CAUSE HYPOGLYCEMIA, ESPECIALLY IN COMBINATION WITH CARVEDILOL. ROSIGLITAZONE MAY WORSEN CHF. TERAZOSIN CAN CAUSE DIZZINESS AND HEADACHE AND POSTURAL HYPOTENSION. FELODIPINE SHOULD BE USED WITH CAUTION IN PATIENTS WITH CHF.

Date	Type	Code	Diagnosis			
11/11/1999	DIAG	E8120	MVA COLLISION UNSP DRIVER			
11/11/1999	DIAG	E8199	MVA UNS INJURING UNS PERSON			
11/11/1999	DIAG	4019	UNS HYPERTENSION			
11/11/1999	DIAG	4280	CONGESTIVE HEART FAILURE			
11/11/1999	DIAG	5939	UNS DISORDER KIDNEY/URETER			
11/11/1999	DIAG	7840	HEADACHE			
11/11/1999	DIAG	81200	FRACTURE UP END HUMERUS UNSP CLOS			
11/11/1999	DIAG	81220	FRACTURE HUMERUS UNSP CLOSED			
11/11/1999	DIAG	8180	FRACTURE ARM MULT/UNSP CLOSED			

11/11/1999	DIAG	87320	OPEN WOUND OF UNSPECE UNSPEC				
11/11/1999	DIAG	87342	OPEN WOUND OF FOREHEAD				
11/11/1999	DIAG	8738	OPEN WOUND OF HEAD OT				
11/11/1999	DIAG	95901	UNS HEAD INJURY				
11/11/1999	DIAG	9591	OTH/UNS INJURY TRUNK				

Patient ID: d510AAAAAAGHBJQL, Year of Birth: 1917, Gender: Female, Trigger Date: 09/13/2000

Date	Type	Code	Diagnosis	Procedure	Rx	Days of Supply
05/09/2000	DIAG	7804	DIZZINESS/GIDDINESS			0
05/26/2000	DIAG	25000	DIABETES UNCOMPL TYPE II			0
05/26/2000	DIAG	25000	DIABETES UNCOMPL TYPE II			0
06/05/2000	DIAG	1101	DERMATOPHYTOSIS NAIL			0
06/05/2000	CPT4	11721		DEBRIDE NAIL, 6 OR MORE		0
07/06/2000	DRUG	00049156066			GLIPIZIDE 30	
07/06/2000	DRUG	00087606005			METFORMIN HCL 30	
07/06/2000	DRUG	00378265010			AMITRIPTYLINE HCL 30	
07/06/2000	DRUG	55953054435			RANITIDINE HCL 90	
08/01/2000	DIAG	53081	ESOPHAGEAL REFLUX			
08/07/2000	DIAG	36616	NUCLEAR SCLEROSIS			
08/07/2000	CPT4	92014		EYE EXAM & TREATMENT		
08/21/2000	DIAG	68111	ONYCHIA/PARONYCHIA TOE			
08/21/2000	CPT4	10060		DRAINAGE OF SKIN ABSCESS		
08/22/2000	DIAG	78650	UNSPEC CHEST PAIN			
08/28/2000	DRUG	00049156066			GLIPIZIDE 30	
08/28/2000	DRUG	00087606005			METFORMIN HCL	
08/28/2000	DRUG	00378265010			AMITRIPTYLINE HCL	

83 YO FEMALE WITH DM II, EOSPHAGEAL REFLUX, AND HAS HAD BOUTS OF DIZZINESS/GIDDINESS AND CHEST PAIN, IS RECEIVING GLIPIZIDE, METFORMIN, AND AMITRIPTYLINE. AMITRIPTYLINE AFFECTS GLUCOSE CONTROL AND ALSO CAUSES DROWSINESS. RANITIDINE AND AMITRIPTYLINE SHOULD BE USED WITH CAUTION IN ELDERLY PTS BECAUSE OF INCREASED CNS REACTIONS. THE GLIPIZIDE AND METFORMIN MAY CAUSE EXCESSIVE HYPOGLYCEMIA.

09/13/2000	DIAG	E8120	MVA COLLISION UNSP DRIVER			
09/13/2000	CPT4	99283		EMERGENCY DEPT VISIT		
09/13/2000	DIAG	25000	DIABETES UNCOMPL TYPE II			
09/13/2000	DIAG	78650	UNSPEC CHEST PAIN			
09/13/2000	DIAG	92411	CONTUSION OF KNEE			
09/13/2000	DIAG	9248	CONTUSION OF MULTIPLE SITES NEC			

Patient ID: e810AAAAAAAKECPD, Year of Birth: 1931, Gender: Female, Trigger Date: 09/04/1999

Date	Type	Code	Diagnosis	Procedure	Rx	Days Supply
07/16/1999	DRUG	00002861501			INSULIN ZINC EXTEND HUMAN REC	30
07/16/1999	DRUG	00049156066			GLIPIZIDE	30
07/16/1999	DRUG	00087607005			METFORMIN HCL	30
07/16/1999	DRUG	00378262510			AMITRIPTYLINE HCL	30
07/16/1999	DRUG	59762738002			IBUPROFEN	30
07/16/1999	DIAG	25001	DIABETES UNCOMPL TYPE I			
07/16/1999	DIAG	2810	PERNICIOUS ANEMIA			
07/16/1999	DIAG	3579	UNS INFLAMMATORY/TOXIC NEUROPATHY			
07/16/1999	DIAG	71690	UNS ARTHROPATHY SITE UNS			
07/16/1999	DIAG	7291	UNS MYALGIA/MYOSITIS			
08/31/1999	DIAG	25001	DIABETES UNCOMPL TYPE I			
08/31/1999	DIAG	486	PNEUMONIA ORGANISM UNS			
08/31/1999	DIAG	78650	UNSPEC CHEST PAIN			

68 YO FEMALE WITH A HX OF DM II, PNEUMONIA, ARTHROPATHY, MYALGIA, NEUROPATHY IS BEING TREATED WITH IBUPROFEN FOR PAINFUL CONDITIONS. GLIPIZIDE, METFORMIN, INSULIN IS BEING USED FOR THE DM II. THESE HYPOGLYCEMIC DRUGS MAY CAUSE EXCESSIVE HYPOGLYCEMIA. THE AMITRIPTYLINE AFFECTS BLOOD SUGAR LEVEL CONTROL AND CAUSES DROWSINESS.

Date	Type	Code	Diagnosis	Procedure	Rx	Days Supply
09/04/1999	DIAG	E8129	MVA COLLIS UNSP PERS UNSPEC			
09/04/1999	DRUG	52544034905			HYDROCODONE BIT/ACETAMINOPHEN	2
09/04/1999	DIAG	8409	SPRAIN/STRAIN SHOULDER/ARM UNSPEC			
09/04/1999	DIAG	8470	SPRAIN/STRAIN OF NECK			
09/04/1999	DIAG	95909	INJURY FACE/NECK			
09/04/1999	DIAG	9592	OTH/UNS INJURY SHOULDER/UPPER ARM			

Patient ID: e810AAAAAACGLKBK, Year of Birth: 1927, Gender: Male, Trigger Date: 08/19/2000

Date	Type	Code	Diagnosis	Procedure	Rx	Days Supply
06/14/2000	DIAG	25000	DIABETES UNCOMPL TYPE II			
06/19/2000	DIAG	3659	UNS GLAUCOMAS			
06/19/2000	DIAG	36616	NUCLEAR SCLEROSIS			

Date	Type	Code	Diagnosis	Procedure	Rx	Days Supply
06/26/2000	DRUG	50111036603			AMITRIPTYLINE HCL	30
06/30/2000	DIAG	3659	UNS GLAUCOMAS			
06/30/2000	DIAG	3659	UNS GLAUCOMAS			
06/30/2000	CPT4	92083		VISUAL FIELD EXAMINATION(S)		
06/30/2000	CPT4	99212		OFFICE/OUTPATIENT VISIT, EST		
07/11/2000	DIAG	25000	DIABETES UNCOMPL TYPE II			
007/11/2000	DIAG	7038	OTHER DISEASES NAIL			
08/11/2000	DRUG	00078017605			FLUVASTATIN SODIUM	30
08/11/2000	DRUG	55953034480			GLYBURIDE	30

73 YO MALE WITH DM II AND GLAUCOMA IS TREATED FOR THE DM WITH GLYBURIDE AND IS ALSO RECEIVING AMITRIPTYLINE WHICH AFFECTS BLOOD SUGAR LEVELS, WORSENS GLAUCOMA, AND CAUSES DROWSINESS. GLYBURIDE AND AMITRIPTYLINE SHOULD BE USED WITH CAUTION IN ELDERLY PTS.

Date	Type	Code	Diagnosis	Procedure	Rx	Days Supply
08/19/2000	DIAG	E8130	MVA OT VEH COLLISION DRIVER			
08/19/2000	DIAG	7242	LUMBAGO			
08/19/2000	DIAG	7245	UNS BACKACHE			
08/19/2000	DIAG	8479	SPRAIN/STRAIN OF BACK UNSPEC			

Patient ID: h702AAAAAAAHCBCG, Year of Birth: 1921, Gender: Male, Trigger Date: 04/17/1999

Date	Type	Code	Diagnosis	Procedure	Rx	Days Supply
02/10/1999	DIAG	25000	DIABETES UNCOMPL TYPE II			
02/10/1999	DIAG	3569	UNS IDIOPATHIC PERIPH NEUROPATHY			
02/12/1999	DRUG	38245043310			GLYBURIDE	30
02/17/1999	DRUG	00597005801			TAMSULOSIN HCL	30
02/17/1999	DRUG	55953054470			RANITIDINE HCL	30
02/19/1999	DRUG	50924055350			BLOOD SUGAR DIAGNOSTIC	25
02/24/1999	DRUG	00364250801			NORTRIPTYLINE HCL	30
02/25/1999	DRUG	00228271311			ISOSORBIDE MONONITRATE	30
03/05/1999	DRUG	00006007231			FINASTERIDE	30
03/05/1999	DRUG	00088179730			DILTIAZEM HCL	30
03/05/1999	DRUG	00093074101			PROPOXYPHENE HCL	30
03/08/1999	DRUG	38245043310			GLYBURIDE	30
03/15/1999	DRUG	00228205210			DIAZEPAM	30
03/15/1999	DRUG	08881602018			LANCETS	20
03/15/1999	DRUG	55953054470			RANITIDINE HCL	30
03/16/1999	DRUG	00597005801			TAMSULOSIN HCL	30
03/22/1999	DIAG	41401	ATHEROSCLER NATIVE CORONARY ART			
03/22/1999	DIAG	V4581	AORTOCORONARY BYPASS STATUS			
03/22/1999	CPT4	99213		OFFICE/OUTPATIENT VISIT, EST		
03/24/1999	DRUG	00364250801			NORTRIPTYLINE HCL	30
03/30/1999	DRUG	50924055350			BLOOD SUGAR DIAGNOSTIC	25
04/05/1999	DRUG	00006007231			FINASTERIDE	30

Date	Type	Code	Diagnosis	Procedure	Rx	Days Supply
04/05/1999	DRUG	00088179730			DILTIAZEM HCL	30
04/05/1999	DRUG	00378013001			PROPOXYPHENE HCL/ACETAMINOPHEN	30
04/12/1999	DRUG	38245043310			GLYBURIDE	30
04/12/1999	DRUG	55953054470			RANITIDINE HCL	30

78 YO OLD MALE WITH A HISTORY OF CORONARY ATHEROSCLEROSIS, AORTOCORONARY BYPASS, DIABETES TYPE II, PERIPHERAL NEUROPATHY, AND HEARING LOSS WAS BEING TREATED WITH NORTRIPTYLINE AND PROPOXYPHENE (BOTH WITH CNS EFFECTS). PROPOXYPHENE AND NORTRIPTYLINE SHOULD NOT BE USED IN ELDERLY PATIENTS. THE PATIENT IS ALSO RECEIVING GLYBURIDE WHICH LOWERS BLOOD SUGAR AND MAY CAUSE HYPOGLYCEMIA, ESPECIALLY IN THE ELDERLY. RANITIDINE AND DILTIAZEM INTERACT TO INCREASE THE HYPOTENSIVE EFFECTS OF DILTIAZEM.

Date	Type	Code	Diagnosis	Procedure	Rx	Days Supply
04/17/1999	DIAG	E8120	MVA COLLISION UNSP DRIVER			
04/17/1999	DIAG	E8495	PLACE OCCURRENCE STREET/HIGHWAY			
04/17/1999	DIAG	E8495	PLACE OCCURRENCE STREET/HIGHWAY			
04/17/1999	DIAG	71941	PAIN IN JOINT SHOULDER			
04/17/1999	DIAG	7231	CERVICALGIA			
04/17/1999	DIAG	7248	OTH SYMPTOMS REFERABLE TO BACK			
04/17/1999	DIAG	8470	SPRAIN/STRAIN OF NECK			

Patient ID: h702AAAAAAANXKJG, Year of Birth: 1932, Gender: Female, Trigger Date: 09/21/1998

Date	Type	Code	Diagnosis	Procedure	Rx	Days Supply
07/23/1998	DRUG	00087607005			METFORMIN HCL	30
07/23/1998	DRUG	00781148801			AMITRIPTYLINE HCL	30
07/23/1998	DIAG	4732	CHRONIC ETHMOIDAL SINUSITIS			
07/23/1998	DIAG	4779	ALLERGIC RHINITIS CAUSE UNS			
08/13/1998	DRUG	00087081941			BUSPIRONE HCL	30
08/13/1998	DRUG	00087607005			METFORMIN HCL	30
08/14/1998	DRUG	00006011754			MONTELUKAST SODIUM	30
08/14/1998	DRUG	00049156066			GLIPIZIDE	30
08/14/1998	DRUG	00085061402			ALBUTEROL	2
08/19/1998	DRUG	00049156066			GLIPIZIDE	30
08/19/1998	DRUG	00781148801			AMITRIPTYLINE HCL	30
08/19/1998	DRUG	49502069703			ALBUTEROL SULFATE	30
08/24/1998	DRUG	00536403644			METHYLPREDNISOLONE	30
09/03/1998	DIAG	4720	CHRONIC RHINITIS			
09/10/1998	DRUG	00085061402			ALBUTEROL	2
09/11/1998	DRUG	00075006037			TRIAMCINOLONE ACETONIDE	20
09/11/1998	DRUG	49502069703			ALBUTEROL SULFATE	30
09/16/1998	DRUG	00049156066			GLIPIZIDE	30
09/16/1998	DRUG	00087607005			METFORMIN HCL	30
09/16/1998	DRUG	00536432510			PREDNISONE	30

66 YO FEMALE WITH A HX OF DM II, SINUSITIS AND RHINITIS IS BEING TREATED WITH GLIPIZIDE, METFORMIN AND IS ALSO TAKING AMITRIPTYLINE, ALBUTEROL, THEOPHYLLINE, PREDNISONE, AND MONTELUKAST. THE AMITRIPTYLINE, ALBUTEROL, AND STEROIDS AFFECT BLOOD SUGAR CONTROL. THE ALBUTEROL AND THEOPHYLLINE CAUSE JITTERINESS AND NERVOUSNESS. THE AMITRIPTYLINE CAUSES DROWSINESS.

Date	Type	Code	Diagnosis	Procedure
09/21/1998	DIAG	E8190	MVA UNS INJURING MVA DRIVER	
09/21/1998	DIAG	71941	PAIN IN JOINT SHOULDER	
09/21/1998	DIAG	8409	SPRAIN/STRAIN SHOULDER/ARM UNSPEC	
09/21/1998	CPT4	450		X-RAY EXAM OF SHOULDER
09/21/1998	CPT4	73030		X-RAY EXAM OF SHOULDER
09/21/1998	CPT4	99283		EMERGENCY DEPT VISIT

Patient ID: d510AAAAAAGNKJOQ, Year of Birth: 1922, Gender: Male, Trigger Date: 07/16/1998

Date	Type	Code	Diagnosis	Procedure	Rx	Days Supply
05/13/1998	DRUG	00074632113			ERYTHROMYCIN BASE	10
05/13/1998	DRUG	59762371704			TRIAZOLAM	60
05/19/1998	DRUG	00378045705			LORAZEPAM	30
05/20/1998	DRUG	00029321120			PAROXETINE HCL	90
05/27/1998	DRUG	00056017270			WARFARIN SODIUM	30
06/02/1998	DIAG	42731	ATRIAL FIBRILLATION			0
06/09/1998	DRUG	00065024615			BETAXOLOL HCL	30
06/15/1998	DRUG	00378045705			LORAZEPAM	30
06/23/1998	DIAG	41401	ATHEROSCLER NATIVE CORONARY ART			0
06/23/1998	DIAG	41401	ATHEROSCLER NATIVE CORONARY ART			0
06/23/1998	DIAG	42731	ATRIAL FIBRILLATION			0
			0			
06/24/1998	DRUG	00056017270			WARFARIN SODIUM	90
06/24/1998	DIAG	250				0
06/24/1998	DIAG	V709	UNS GENERAL MEDICAL EXAMINATION			0
07/15/1998	DIAG	42732	ATRIAL FLUTTER			0
07/15/1998	CPT4	85610		PROTHROMBIN TIME		0

77YO MALE WITH A HX OF CORONARY ATHEROSCLEROSIS AND ATRIAL FIBRILLATION/FLUTTER WAS
BEING TREATED WITH THREE CNS AFFECTING DRUGS (TRIAZOLAM, LORAZEPAM, AND PAROXETINE) ALL
OF WHICH ARE SEDATING. THE HEART RHYTHM DISORDER MAY ALSO BE DRIVER IMPAIRING. THE
BETAXOLOL IS A BETA BLOCKER WHICH CAN CAUSE DIZZINESS.

0

Date	Type	Code	Diagnosis	Procedure			0
07/16/1998	CPT4	99284		EMERGENCY DEPT VISIT			0
07/18/1998	DRUG	00781140405					
07/16/1998	DIAG	9223	CONTUSION OF CHEST WALL				
07/16/1998	DIAG	E9120	MVA COLLISION UNSP DRIVER				

Patient ID: d51OAAAAAAG0XTVS, Year of Birth: 1931, Gender: Female, Trigger Date: 04/08/1998

Date	Type	Code	Diagnosis	Procedure	Rx	Days of Supply
02/12/1998	DIAG	29632	MAJ DEPRESS DIS RECURR EPI MOD			
02/17/1998	DIAG	36616	NUCLEAR SCLEROSIS			
02/24/1998	DRUG	00046087502				28
02/24/1998	DRUG	61314032810			FLUOROMETHOLONE	7
03/02/1998	DRUG	00049490066			SERTRALINE HCL	60
03/02/1998	DRUG	00087081841			BUSPIRONE HCL	30
03/02/1998	DRUG	51875034501			HYDROXYZINE HCL	12
03/02/1998	DIAG	6929	CONTACT DERMATITIS UNS CAUSE			0
03/02/1998	DIAG	7089	UNSPEC URTICARIA			0
03/06/1998	DIAG	6160	CERVICITIS/ENDOCERVICITIS			0
03/28/1998	DRUG	00046087502				28
03/28/1998	DRUG	59762371804			TRIAZOLAM	30

67 YO FEMALE WITH DEPRESSION AND VISUAL PROBLEMS WAS TREATED WITH FOUR CNS AFFECTING
MEDICATIONS — SERTRALINE, BUSPIRONE, HYDROXYZINE, AND TRIAZOLAM.

04/08/1998	DIAG	E8199	MVA UNS INJURING UNS PERSON			0
04/08/1998	CPT4	72070		X-RAY EXAM OF THORACIC SPINE		0
04/08/1998	CPT4	72100		X-RAY EXAM OF LOWER SPINE		0
04/08/1998	CPT4	73560		X-RAY EXAM OF KNEE, 1 OR 2		0

Date	Type	Code	Diagnosis	Procedure	Rx	Days Supply
04/08/1998	CPT4	73620		X-RAY EXAM OF FOOT		0
04/08/1998	CPT4	99283		EMERGENCY DEPT VISIT		0
04/08/1998	CPT4	99283		EMERGENCY DEPT VISIT		
04/08/1998	DIAG	71945	PAIN IN JOINT PELVIS/THIGH			0
04/08/1998	DIAG	71946	PAIN IN JOINT LOWER LEG			0
04/08/1998	DIAG	71947	PAIN IN JOINT ANKLE/FOOT			0
04/08/1998	DIAG	7242	LUMBAGO			0
04/08/1998	DIAG	9599	INJURY UNS SITE			0

Patient ID: e810AAAAAABAOSFG. Year of Birth: 1928. Gender: Female. Trigger Date: 03/08/2001

Date	Type	Code	Diagnosis	Procedure	Rx	Days Supply
01/09/2001	DIAG	4619	UNS ACUTE SINUSITIS			
01/09/2001	DIAG	7840	HEADACHE			
01/17/2001	DRUG	00603388128			HYDROCODONE BIT/ACETAMINOPHEN	15
01/24/2001	DRUG	00228205950			LORAZEPAM	12
01/25/2001	DRUG	00364233701			CLINDAMYCIN HCL	7
01/30/2001	DRUG	00603388128			HYDROCODONE BIT/ACETAMINOPHEN	5
01/31/2001	DRUG	00456404001			CITALOPRAM HYDROBROMIDE	30
02/13/2001	DRUG	00228205950			LORAZEPAM	12
02/13/2001	DRUG	00378262510			AMITRIPTYLINE HCL	20
02/13/2001	DIAG	29633	MAJ DEPRESS DIS RECUR EPI SEV			
02/13/2001	DIAG	3039				
02/13/2001	DIAG	7245	UNS BACKACHE			
02/13/2001	DIAG	73300	OSTEOPOROSIS UNSPEC			
02/28/2001	DRUG	00069306075			AZITHROMYCIN	5
03/04/2001	DRUG	00228205950			LORAZEPAM	12
03/04/2001	DRUG	00456404001			CITALOPRAM HYDROBROMIDE	30

73 YO FEMALE WITH A HX OF MAJOR DEPRESSION, BACKACHE, OSTEOPOROSIS, HEADACHE, SINUSITIS, IS TREATED WITH FOUR CNS AFFECTING MEDICATIONS –HYDROCODONE, LORAZEPAM, CITALOPRAM, AND AMITRIPTYLINE. LORAZEPAM, HYDROCODONE, AND AMITRIPTYLINE SHOULD BE USED WITH CAUTION IN OLDER PATIENTS BECAUSE THEY CAN CAUSE SOMNOLENCE AND DIZZINESS.

Date	Type	Code	Diagnosis	Procedure	Rx	Days Supply
03/08/2001	DIAG	E8130	MVA OT VEH COLLISION DRIVER			
03/08/2001	DIAG	E8130	MVA OT VEH COLLISION DRIVER			
03/08/2001	CPT4	324				
03/08/2001	CPT4	450				
03/08/2001	CPT4	71020		CHEST X-RAY		
03/08/2001	CPT4	99283		EMERGENCY DEPT VISIT		
03/08/2001	DIAG	7840	HEADACHE			

Date	Type	Code			

03/08/2001 DRUG 00603388128 HYDROCODONE BIT/ACETAMINOPHEN 1
03/08/2001 DIAG 78650 UNSPEC CHEST PAIN
03/08/2001 DIAG 78652 PAINFUL RESPIRATION
03/08/2001 DIAG 9221 CONTUSION OF CHEST WALL
03/08/2001 DIAG 9591 OTH/UNS INJURY TRUNK

Patient ID: 5401AAAAAAAVJRBF, Year of Birth: 1921, Gender: Female, Trigger Date: 05/24/1999

Date Supply	Type	Code	Diagnosis	Procedure	Rx	Days of
03/23/1999	DRUG	00603107558			GUAIFENESIN/CODEINE PHOS	
03/30/1999	CPT4	84702		CHORIONIC GONADOTROPIN TEST		
03/31/1999	DRUG	00603242621			BENZONATATE	
03/31/1999	DRUG	49884056905			AMOXICILLIN TRIHYDRATE	
03/31/1999	DIAG	4619	UNS ACUTE SINUSITIS			
03/31/1999	DIAG	490	BRONCHITISACUTE/CHRONIC			
04/12/1999	DRUG	00182127405			ACETAMINOPHEN/CAFFEINE/BUTALB	
04/19/1999	DIAG	70219	OTH SEBORRHEIC KERATOSIS			
04/19/1999	DIAG	70909	OTHER DYSCHROMIA			
05/03/1999	DRUG	00597008130			IPRATROPIUM BROMIDE	
05/03/1999	DRUG	49884056905			AMOXICILLIN TRIHYDRATE	
05/03/1999	DIAG	4619	UNS ACUTE SINUSITIS			
05/17/1999	DRUG	00048105005			LEVOTHYROXINE SODIUM	
05/22/1999	DIAG	42742	VENTRICULAR FLUTTER			

78 YO FEMALE WITH VENTRICULAR FLUTTER AND ACUTE BRONCHITIS/SINUSITIS IS BEING TREATED
WITH AMOXICILLIN AND BENZONATATE AND GUIFENESIN WITH CODEINE FOR COUGH AND ACETAMINOPHEN
WITH CAFFEINE AND BUTALBITAL FOR PAIN. THE TWO MEDICINES FOR COUGH AND THE PAIN
MEDICINE CAN CAUSE SEDATION, DIZZINESS, AND MENTAL CONFUSION. IPRATROPIUM IS USED FOR
BRONCHITIS BUT IT CAN CAUSE PALPITATIONS, NERVOUSNES, AND DIZZINESS. LEVOTHYROXINE,
PARTICULARLY IN THE ELDERLY, CAN CAUSE TACHYCARDIA, ARRHYTHMIAS.

05/24/1999 DIAG E8190 MVA UNS INJURING MVA DRIVER

Patient ID: 4001AAAAAAAIGEWV, Year of Birth: 1920, Gender: Female, Trigger Date: 09/03/1999

Date	Type	Code	Diagnosis	Procedure	Rx	Days Supply
06/28/1999	DRUG	00378003210			METOPROLOL TARTRATE	
06/28/1999	DRUG	38245022520			POTASSIUM CHLORIDE	
06/29/1999	DIAG	42731	ATRIAL FIBRILLATION			
06/29/1999	DIAG	V5861	ENCOUNTER LONG TERM ANTICOAGULANT			
06/29/1999	CPT4	85610		PROTHROMBIN TIME		
07/13/1999	DRUG	00228222296			HYDROCHLOROTHIAZIDE	
07/13/1999	DRUG	00310013034			LISINOPRIL	
07/24/1999	DIAG	42731	ATRIAL FIBRILLATION			
07/24/1999	DIAG	4280	CONGESTIVE HEART FAILURE			
07/24/1999	DIAG	V5861	ENCOUNTER LONG TERM ANTICOAGULANT			
07/24/1999	CPT4	80054				
07/24/1999	CPT4	85610		PROTHROMBIN TIME		
08/13/1999	DRUG	00173024975			DIGOXIN	
08/13/1999	DRUG	00555087402			WARFARIN SODIUM	
08/31/1999	DIAG	42731	ATRIAL FIBRILLATION			
08/31/1999	DIAG	V5861	ENCOUNTER LONG TERM ANTICOAGULANT			
08/31/1999	CPT4	85610		PROTHROMBIN TIME		
08/31/1999	HCPCS	G0001		ROUTINE VENIPUNCT CLCT SPECI		

79 YO FEMALE WITH A HISTORY OF ATRIAL FIBRILLATION, CONGESTIVE HEART FAILURE, AND CATARACT IS BEING TREATED WITH DIGOXIN, WARFARIN, HYDROCHLOROTHIAZIDE, LISINOPRIL, METOPROLOL, AND POTASSIUM. OLDER ADULTS MAY DEVELOP EXAGGERATED SERUM/TISSUE CONCENTRATIONS OF DIGOXIN WHICH CAN CAUSE VISUAL DISTURBANCES, DIZZINESS, AND HEART RHYTHM DISTURBANCES. LISINOPRIL CAN CAUSE HYPOTENSION ESPECIALLY IN DEHYDRATED PTS WITH CONGESTIVE HEART FAILURE AND IT CAN ALSO CAUSE DIZZINESS. HYDROCHLOROTHIAZIDE CAN CAUSE DIZZINESS. METOPROLOL CAN CAUSE DROWSINESS.

Date	Type	Code	Diagnosis	Procedure	Rx	Days Supply
09/03/1999	DIAG	E8120	MVA COLLISION UNSP DRIVER			
09/03/1999	DIAG	8500	CONCUSSION WO COMA			
09/03/1999	DIAG	85400	INTRACRANIAL INJURY OT			
09/03/1999	DIAG	8602	TRAUMATIC HEMOTHORAX WO OPEN WD			
09/03/1999	DIAG	86121	LUNG CONTUSION WO OPEN WOUND			

Patient ID: d510AAAAAAFKWQLT, Year of Birth: 1931, Gender: Female, Trigger Date: 01/08/2001

Date Days of Supply	Type	Code	Diagnosis	Procedure	Rx	
12/19/2000	DRUG	00555003302			CHLORDIAZEPOXIDE HCL	30
12/20/2000	DIAG	1121	CANDIDIASIS VULVA/VAGINA			0
12/20/2000	DIAG	25000	DIABETES UNCOMPL TYPE II			0
12/29/2000	DIAG	61610	UNS VAGINITIS/VULVOVAGINITIS			0
01/01/2001	DRUG	00025152531			CELECOXIB	30
01/01/2001	DRUG	00172290880			FUROSEMIDE	30
01/01/2001	DRUG	00186074231			OMEPRAZOLE	30
01/01/2001	DRUG	00245004015			POTASSIUM CHLORIDE	30
01/01/2001	DRUG	00378021001			CHLORPROPAMIDE	30
01/01/2001	DRUG	00406053201			OXYCODONE HCL/ACETAMINOPHEN	20
01/04/2001	DIAG	61610	UNS VAGINITIS/VULVOVAGINITIS			0
01/04/2001	CPT4	99213		OFFICE/OUTPATIENT VISIT, EST		0
01/05/2001	DRUG	00062535001			TERCONAZOLE	7
01/05/2001	DRUG	49158020007			HYDROCORTISONE	7

70 YO FEMALE WITH A HISTORY OF DM TYPE II AND PREVIOUS FRACTURE IS BEING TREATED WITH CELECOXIB AND OXYCODONE FOR PAIN. CHLORPROPAMIDE FOR THE DM. CHLORPROPAMIDE IN OLDER PATIENTS IS PARTICULARLY PRONE TO CAUSING HYPOGLYCEMIA AND DIZZINESS. FUROSEMIDE AFFECTS BLOOD SUGAR CONTROL AND ATENOLOL MAY ALSO AFFECT GLUCOSE CONTROL AND MASK SIGNS OF HYPOGLYCEMIA. OXYCODONE AND CHLORDIAZEPOXIDE SHOULD ALSO BE USED WITH CAUTION IN OLDER PTS AND MAY CAUSE EXCESSIVE SEDATION, DIZZINESS, AND CONFUSION.

Date	Type	Code	Diagnosis	Procedure	Rx	
01/08/2001	DIAG	E8120	MVA COLLISION UNSP DRIVER	01/08/2001 DRUG 00093310905 AMOXICILLIN TRIHYDRATE		2
01/08/2001	DIAG	25000	DIABETES UNCOMPL TYPE II			0
01/08/2001	DIAG	4019	UNS HYPERTENSION			0
01/08/2001	DIAG	71597	OSTEOARTHROSIS UNSP ANKLE/FOOT			0
01/08/2001	DIAG	71887	OTH JOINT DERANGEMENT OT ANKLE/FOOT			0
01/08/2001	DIAG	71887	OTH JOINT DERANGEMENT OT ANKLE/FOOT			0
01/08/2001	DIAG	92420	CONTUSION OF FOOT			0
01/08/2001	DIAG	92420	CONTUSION OF FOOT			0
01/08/2001	CPT4	73630		X-RAY EXAM OF FOOT		0
01/08/2001	CPT4	99283		EMERGENCY DEPT VISIT		0
01/08/2001	HCPCS	A0390		ALS MILEAGE		0
01/08/2001	HCPCS	A0427		AMB SERV ADV LIFE SUPPORT ER		0
01/17/2001	DRUG	00555003302				

Patient ID: 5401AAAAAAATBPWG, Year of Birth: 1927, Gender: Male, Trigger Date: 06/20/1999

Date Supply	Type	Code	Diagnosis	Procedure	Rx	Days of
05/12/1999	DRUG	00378021610			FUROSEMIDE	
05/12/1999	DIAG	78650	UNSPEC CHEST PAIN			
05/27/1999	DRUG	00093314505			CEPHALEXIN MONOHYDRATE	
05/27/1999	DRUG	00185072001			INDOMETHACIN	
05/29/1999	CPT4	85610		PROTHROMBIN TIME		
06/03/1999	DIAG	4011	BENIGN HYPERTENSION			
06/03/1999	DIAG	4280	CONGESTIVE HEART FAILURE			
06/08/1999	DRUG	00555083402			WARFARIN SODIUM	
06/10/1999	DRUG	00078017605			FLUVASTATIN SODIUM	

72 YO MALE WITH HYPERTENSION AND CONGESTIVE HEART FAILURE IS TREATED WITH WARFARIN, FLUVASTATIN, INDOMETHACIN, FUROSEMIDE. INDOMETHCAIN AND FLUVASTATIN INTERACT WITH WARFARIN TO CAUSE BLEEDING. INDOMETHACIN CAN ALSO CAUSE HEADACHES AND CONFUSION. INDOMETHCAIN SHOULD BE USED WITH CAUTION IN PTS WITH CHF. FUROSEMIDE CAN CAUSE HYPOTENSION AND DIZZINESS.

Date Supply	Type	Code	Diagnosis	Procedure	Rx	Days of
06/20/1999	DIAG	E8120	MVA COLLISION UNSP DRIVER			
06/20/1999	DIAG	E8120	MVA COLLISION UNSP DRIVER			
06/20/1999	CPT4	99284		EMERGENCY DEPT VISIT		
06/20/1999	DIAG	8470	SPRAIN/STRAIN OF NECK			
06/20/1999	DIAG	8471	SPRAIN/STRAIN THORACIC REGION			
06/20/1999	DIAG	8479	SPRAIN/STRAIN OF BACK UNSPEC			

6

Patient ID: h702AAAAAAAIOFCJ, Year of Birth: 1922, Gender: Male, Trigger Date: 02/13/1999

Date Supply	Type	Code	Diagnosis	Procedure	Rx	Days of

Date	Type	Code	Description	Service	Drug	Qty
12/02/1998	DRUG	00056017270			WARFARIN SODIUM	30
12/02/1998	DRUG	00088179642			DILTIAZEM HCL	30
12/02/1998	DRUG	00173024975			DIGOXIN	30
01/02/1999	DRUG	00056017270			WARFARIN SODIUM	30
01/02/1999	DRUG	00088179642			DILTIAZEM HCL	30
01/02/1999	DRUG	00173024975			DIGOXIN	30
01/13/1999	DIAG	4280	CONGESTIVE HEART FAILURE			
01/13/1999	DIAG	4280	CONGESTIVE HEART FAILURE			
01/13/1999	DIAG	4280	CONGESTIVE HEART FAILURE			
01/13/1999	CPT4	99232		SUBSEQUENT HOSPITAL CARE		
01/13/1999	CPT4	99233		SUBSEQUENT HOSPITAL CARE		
01/13/1999	CPT4	99254		INITIAL INPATIENT CONSULT		
01/16/1999	DIAG	4280	CONGESTIVE HEART FAILURE			
01/20/1999	DRUG	00093310905			AMOXICILLIN TRIHYDRATE	9
01/20/1999	DRUG	00472001116			GUAIFENESIN/P-EPHED HCL/COD	8
01/20/1999	DIAG	4659	ACUTE UPPER RESP INFECTIONS UNS			
01/20/1999	CPT4	99212		OFFICE/OUTPATIENT VISIT, EST		
02/02/1999	DRUG	00088179642			DILTIAZEM HCL	30
02/02/1999	DRUG	00172290780			FUROSEMIDE	30
02/02/1999	DRUG	00173024975			DIGOXIN	30
02/04/1999	DRUG	00056017270			WARFARIN SODIUM	30

77 YO MALE PT WITH CONGETIVE HEART FAILURE. TREATED FOR CONGESTIVE HEART FAILURE WITH DIGOXIN AND FUROSEMIDE. RECEIVING DILTIAZEM FOR HEART RHYTHM DISORDERS AND WARFARIN FOR ATRIAL FIBRILLATION. RECENT TREATMENT WITH A COUGH MEDICINE WITH CODEINE FOR AN ACUTE URI. OLDER ADULTS MAY DEVELOP EXAGGERATED SERUM/TISSUE CONCENTRATIONS OF DIGOXIN WHICH CAN CAUSE VISUAL DISTURBANCES, DIZZINESS, AND HEART RHYTHM DISTURBANCES. DILTIAZEM AGGRAVATES CHF AND CAUSES DIZZINESS AND HYPOTENSION. THE CODEINE IN THE COUGH MEDICINE MAY CAUSE DROWSINESS. FUROSEMIDE MAY CAUSE DIZZINESS AND HYPOTENSION. THIS PATIENT IS NOT RECEIVING ANY POTASSIUM SUPPLEMENTS.

Date	Type	Code	Description	Service
02/13/1999	DIAG	E8230	OT COLLISION STNDNG OBJ DRIV	
02/13/1999	DIAG	2930	ACUTE DELIRIUM	
02/13/1999	DIAG	3013	EXPLOSIVE PERSONALITY DISORDER	
02/13/1999	DIAG	4590	UNS HEMORRHAGE	
02/13/1999	DIAG	78002	TRANSIENT ALTERATION AWARENESS	
02/13/1999	DIAG	920	CONTUSION FACE/SCALP/NCK	
02/13/1999	CPT4	99221		INITIAL HOSPITAL CARE

Date Supply	Type	Code	Diagnosis	Procedure	Rx	Days of
03/28/2000	DIAG	2449	UNS HYPOTHYROIDISM			0
03/28/2000	DIAG	25000	DIABETES UNCOMPL TYPE II			0
03/28/2000	CPT4	85025		AUTOMATED HEMOGRAM		0
03/29/2000	DRUG	00071015523			ATORVASTATIN CALCIUM	30
03/29/2000	DRUG	00087607111			METFORMIN HCL	30
03/29/2000	DRUG	00378265010			AMITRIPTYLINE HCL	30
03/31/2000	DRUG	00013830304			LATANOPROST	30
03/31/2000	DRUG	00023866510			BRIMONIDINE TARTRATE	30
03/31/2000	DRUG	00048113003			LEVOTHYROXINE SODIUM	30
03/31/2000	DRUG	00310013210			LISINOPRIL	30
04/25/2000	DRUG	00071015523			ATORVASTATIN CALCIUM	30
04/25/2000	DRUG	00087607111			METFORMIN HCL	30
04/25/2000	DRUG	00378265010			AMITRIPTYLINE HCL	30
05/08/2000	DIAG	25000	DIABETES UNCOMPL TYPE II			0
05/08/2000	DIAG	2725	LIPOPROTEIN DEFICIENCIES			0
05/08/2000	CPT4	99213		OFFICE/OUTPATIENT VISIT, EST		0
05/17/2000	DRUG	00048113003			LEVOTHYROXINE SODIUM	30
05/17/2000	DRUG	00310013210			LISINOPRIL	30

68 YO FEMALE WITH A HX OF HYPOTHYROIDISM, DM II. TAKES AMITRIPTYLINE WHICH CAUSES DROWSINESS AND AFFECTS BLOOD SUGAR CONTROL.
THE PATIENT IS ALSO BEING TREATED WITH METFORMIN FOR DM, LEVOTHYROXINE FOR HYPOTHYROIDISM, ATORVASATIN FOR HYPERLIPIDEMIA, LISINOPRIL FOR HYPERTENSION.

Date Supply	Type	Code	Diagnosis	Procedure	Rx	Days of
06/04/2000	DIAG	E8130	MVA OT VEH COLLISION DRIVER			
06/04/2000	DIAG	2449	UNS HYPOTHYROIDISM			0
06/04/2000	DIAG	25000	DIABETES UNCOMPL TYPE II			0
06/04/2000	DIAG	25091	DIABETES W COMPL UNSP TYPE I			0
06/04/2000	DIAG	71949	PAIN IN JOINT MULT SITES			0
06/04/2000	DIAG	72981	SWELLING LIMB			0
06/04/2000	DIAG	78900	ABDOMINAL PAIN UNS SITE			0
06/04/2000	DIAG	9221	CONTUSION OF CHEST WALL			0
06/04/2000	DIAG	9222	CONTUSION OF ABDOMINAL WALL			0
06/04/2000	DIAG	92411	CONTUSION OF KNEE			0

Date	Type	Code	Diagnosis	Procedure	Rx	Days Supply
10/07/1999	DRUG	00006010658			LISINOPRIL	
10/07/1999	DRUG	00049491066			SERTRALINE HCL	
10/07/1999	DRUG	00078017605			FLUVASTATIN SODIUM	
10/07/1999	DRUG	00085078701			POTASSIUM CHLORIDE	
10/07/1999	DRUG	00093067005			GEMFIBROZIL	
10/07/1999	DRUG	00781148810			AMITRIPTYLINE HCL	
10/07/1999	DRUG	52544048701			ESTRADIOL	
11/05/1999	DRUG	00006010658			LISINOPRIL	
11/05/1999	DRUG	00049491066			SERTRALINE HCL	
11/05/1999	DRUG	00085078701			POTASSIUM CHLORIDE	
11/05/1999	DRUG	00093067005			GEMFIBROZIL	
11/05/1999	DRUG	00781148810			AMITRIPTYLINE HCL	
11/05/1999	DRUG	52544048701			ESTRADIOL	
11/08/1999	CPT4	80061		LIPID PANEL		
11/09/1999	DRUG	00078017605			FLUVASTATIN SODIUM	
11/22/1999	DRUG	00005312931			DIAZEPAM	
11/22/1999	DRUG	00085092402			CLOTRIMAZOLE/BETAMET DIPROP	
11/22/1999	DRUG	00781196610			FUROSEMIDE	
11/22/1999	DIAG	4019	UNS HYPERTENSION			
11/22/1999	CPT4	99213		OFFICE/OUTPATIENT VISIT, EST		
11/24/1999	DIAG	7291	UNS MYALGIA/MYOSITIS			
11/28/1999	DRUG	00006010658			LISINOPRIL	
11/28/1999	DRUG	00049491066			SERTRALINE HCL	
11/28/1999	DRUG	00085078701			POTASSIUM CHLORIDE	
11/28/1999	DRUG	00093067005			GEMFIBROZIL	
11/28/1999	DRUG	00781148810			AMITRIPTYLINE HCL	
11/28/1999	DRUG	52544048701			ESTRADIOL	

68 YO FEMALE HAS A HX OF HYPERTENSION AND MYALGIA/MYOSITIS. INTERESTING TO NOTE THAT GEMFIBROZIL AND FLUVASTATIN INTERACT TO CAUSE MYALGIA AND MYOPATHY. CNS IMPAIRING DRUGS PRESCRIBED ARE SERTRALINE, DIAZEPAM, AND AMITRIPTYLINE. PATIENT HAS ALSO BEEN PRESCRIBED LISINOPRIL AND FUROSEMIDE FOR HYPERTENSION.

| 12/01/1999 | DIAG | E8120 | MVA COLLISION UNSP DRIVER | | | |
| 12/01/1999 | DIAG | E8199 | MVA UNS INJURING UNS PERSON | | | |

Patient ID: d510AAAAAACNBMHX, Year of Birth: 1925, Gender: Male, Trigger Date: 08/08/1999

Date	Type	Code	Diagnosis	Procedure	Rx	Days Supply
06/09/1999	DRUG	00045152550			LEVOFLOXACIN	10
06/09/1999	DRUG	51285029504			GUAIFENESIN/PPA HCL	15
06/16/1999	DRUG	59930150008			ALBUTEROL SULFATE	37
06/30/1999	DRUG	00029321120			PAROXETINE HCL	30
06/30/1999	DRUG	00078017605			FLUVASTATIN SODIUM	30
07/14/1999	DRUG	00007411713			FAMCICLOVIR	7
07/14/1999	DIAG	0539	HERPES ZOSTER WO COMPLICATION			0
07/24/1999	DRUG	59930150008			ALBUTEROL SULFATE	37
07/31/1999	DRUG	00029321120			PAROXETINE HCL	30
07/31/1999	DRUG	00078017605			FLUVASTATIN SODIUM	30

74 YO MALE WITH A HX OF CHRONIC AIRWAY OBSTRUCTION AND HERPES ZOSTER, WAS PRESCRIBED LEVOFLOXACIN AND PAROXETINE WHICH MAY CAUSE CNS EFFECTS. PAROXETINE AND ALBUTEROL BOTH MAY CAUSE JITTERINESS. FLUVASTATIN MAY CAUSE HEADACHE AND DIZZINESS.

						0
08/08/1999	DIAG	9591	OTH/UNS INJURY TRUNK			0
08/08/1999	DIAG	E8190	MVA UNS INJURING MVA DRIVER			
08/08/1999	DIAG	71944	PAIN IN JOINT HAND			0
08/08/1999	DIAG	7231	CERVICALGIA			0
08/08/1999	DIAG	7840	HEADACHE			0
08/08/1999	DIAG	9190	ABRASION OT			0
08/08/1999	DIAG	95909	INJURY FACE/NECK			0

Patient ID: e810AAAAAABBWDOA, Year of Birth: 1930, Gender: Female, Trigger Date: 01/17/2002

Date	Type	Code	Diagnosis	Procedure	Rx	Days of Supply
12/10/2001	DRUG	00378077201			VERAPAMIL HCL	30

Date	Type	Code	Diagnosis	Procedure	Rx	Days Supply
12/10/2001	DRUG	00555087702			FLUOXETINE HCL	30
12/10/2001	DRUG	61570007301			ESTROGENS,ESTERIFIED	30
12/11/2001	DRUG	00781140405			LORAZEPAM	30
12/17/2001	DIAG	4359	UNS TRANSIENT CEREBRAL ISCHEMIA			
12/17/2001	CPT4	351				
12/17/2001	CPT4	70450		CT HEAD/BRAIN W/O DYE		
01/01/2002	DRUG	00781140410			LORAZEPAM	30
01/02/2002	DRUG	00071015523			ATORVASTATIN CALCIUM	30
01/02/2002	DIAG	2724	OTH/UNS HYPERLIPIDEMIA			
01/02/2002	DIAG	4019	UNS HYPERTENSION			
01/02/2002	DIAG	4359	UNS TRANSIENT CEREBRAL ISCHEMIA			
01/02/2002	DIAG	70219	OTH SEBORRHEIC KERATOSIS			
01/02/2002	CPT4	99214		OFFICE/OUTPATIENT VISIT, EST		
01/09/2002	DRUG	00378077201			VERAPAMIL HCL	30
01/09/2002	DRUG	00555087702			FLUOXETINE HCL	30
01/09/2002	DRUG	61570007301			ESTROGENS,ESTERIFIED	30
01/11/2002	DIAG	71513	OSTEOARTHROSIS LOCAL PRIM FOREARM			
01/11/2002	DIAG	9593	OTH/UNS INJURY ELBOW FOREARM/WRIST			
01/11/2002	CPT4	73110		X-RAY EXAM OF WRIST		

6

72 YO FEMALE WITH A HX OF HYPERTENSION AND TRANSIENT CEREBRAL ISCHEMIA AND OSTEOARTHROSIS IS PRESCRIBED TWO CNS AFFECTING DRUGS —LORAZEPAM AND FLUOXETINE. SHE IS ALSO PRESCRIBED VERAPAMIL FOR HYPERTENSION AND ATORVASTATIN FOR HYPERLIPIDEMIA. VERAPAMIL INTERACTS WITH ATORVASTATIN TO INCREASE THE BLOOD LEVEL OF ATORVASTATIN. VERAPAMIL ALSO MAY CAUSE DIZZINESS.

Date	Type	Code	Diagnosis	Procedure	Rx	Days Supply
01/17/2002	DIAG	E8120	MVA COLLISION UNSP DRIVER			
01/17/2002	DRUG	55370014108			NAPROXEN	30
01/17/2002	DRUG	00591565810			CYCLOBENZAPRINE HCL	30
01/17/2002	DIAG	72190	SPONDYLOSIS UNS SITE WOMYELOPATHY			
01/17/2002	DIAG	7226	DEGENERATION IV DISC SITE UNS			
01/17/2002	DIAG	7231	CERVICALGIA			
01/17/2002	DIAG	7295	PAIN IN LIMB			
01/17/2002	DIAG	9598	INJURY OTHER SITES INC MULT SITES			

Patient ID: a302AAAAAAAS0IOZ, Year of Birth: 1929, Gender: Male, Trigger Date: 05/04/1999

Date	Type	Code	Diagnosis	Procedure	Rx	Days Supply
04/05/1999	DRUG	00007413920			CARVEDILOL	30

Date	Type	Code	Description		Drug	Qty
04/05/1999	DRUG	00904773240			GEMFIBROZIL	30
04/07/1999	DRUG	00005356331			METHOCARBAMOL	12
04/09/1999	DIAG	4280	CONGESTIVE HEART FAILURE			
04/09/1999	DIAG	71590	OSTEOARTHROSIS UNSP SITE			
04/12/1999	DRUG	00049490066			SERTRALINE HCL	30
04/14/1999	DRUG	00093089005			PROPOXYPHENE/ACETAMINOPHEN	16
04/19/1999	DRUG	00005356331			METHOCARBAMOL	12
04/19/1999	DRUG	00310013510			LISINOPRIL	66
04/20/1999	DRUG	00093310905			AMOXICILLIN TRIHYDRATE	1
04/20/1999	DRUG	00172290970			HYDROXYZINE PAMOATE	30
04/20/1999	DIAG	4280	CONGESTIVE HEART FAILURE			
04/20/1999	DIAG	4280	CONGESTIVE HEART FAILURE			
04/22/1999	DIAG	71590	OSTEOARTHROSIS UNSP SITE			
04/22/1999	HCPCS	J1885		INJ KETOROLAC TROMETHAMINE P		
04/23/1999	DIAG	72400	SPINAL STENOSIS UNS NONCERVICAL			
04/23/1999	DIAG	78057	OTH/UNS SLEEP APNEA			
04/23/1999	HCPCS	E1403				
04/28/1999	DIAG	53010	UNS ESOPHAGITIS			
04/28/1999	CPT4	99214		OFFICE/OUTPATIENT VISIT, EST		
05/03/1999	DRUG	00071035323			TROGLITAZONE	30
05/03/1999	DRUG	00228208550			PROPOXYPHENE/ACETAMINOPHEN	7

70 YO MALE WITH CHF, OSTEOARTHROSIS, SPINAL STENOSIS, AND SLEEP APNEA IS TREATED WITH CARVEDILOL, LISINOPRIL, AND GEMFIBROZIL FOR CARDIOVASCULAR DISORDERS. THE PROPOXYPHENE AND METHOCARBAMOL IS FOR THE OSTEOARTHROSIS AND SPINAL STENOSIS. SERTRALINE IS AN SSRI ANTIDEPRESSANT. HYDROXYZINE IS AN ANTIHISTAMINE. HYDROXYZINE, METHOCARBAMOL, AND PROPOXYPHENE HAVE INCREASED CNS EFFECTS IN OLDER PTS. THESE INCLUDE SEDATION, CONFUSION, DIZZINESS. SERTRALINE MAY CAUSE NERVOUSNESS. LISINOPRIL AND CARVEDILOL MAY CAUSE HYPOTENSION. THE SLEEP APNEA MAY HAVE MORE DAYTIME SEDATION ASSOCIATED WITH IT.

13

Date	Type	Code	Description
05/04/1999	DIAG	E8120	MVA COLLISION UNSP DRIVER

Date	Type	Code	Diagnosis	Procedure	Rx	
Days of Supply						

Date	Type	Code	Diagnosis	Procedure	Rx	
03/04/2001	DRUG	00378075101			CYCLOBENZAPRINE HCL	30
03/24/2001	DRUG	00005321943			ATENOLOL	30
03/24/2001	DRUG	59911581201			LORAZEPAM	30
03/30/2001	DRUG	00378075101			CYCLOBENZAPRINE HCL	30
04/13/2001	DRUG	00300304613			LANSOPRAZOLE	30
04/18/2001	DIAG	4019	UNS HYPERTENSION			
04/18/2001	CPT4	99214		OFFICE/OUTPATIENT VISIT, EST		
04/26/2001	DRUG	00005321943			ATENOLOL	30
04/26/2001	DRUG	00046086781			ESTROGENS,CONJUGATED	90
04/29/2001	DRUG	00378075101			CYCLOBENZAPRINE HCL	30
04/30/2001	DRUG	00071015623			ATORVASTATIN CALCIUM	30
05/04/2001	DRUG	59911581201			LORAZEPAM	30
05/14/2001	DRUG	00300304613			LANSOPRAZOLE	30

66 YO FEMALE HAS HYPERTENSION. SHE IS RECEIVING ATENOLOL TO TREAT THE
HYPERTENSION. SHE IS TAKING CONJUGATED ESTROGENS, ATORVASTATIN, AND LANSOPRAZOLE.
SHE IS ALSO RECEIVING TWO CNS AFFECTING DRUGS —CYCLOBENZAPRINE AND LORAZEPAM.
ATENOLOL MAY CAUSE HYPOTENSION, DIZZINESS, INSOMNIA, AND CONFUSION.

Date	Type	Code	Diagnosis			
05/24/2001	DIAG	E8190	MVA UNS INJURING MVA DRIVER			
05/24/2001	DIAG	E8495	PLACE OCCURRENCE STREET/HIGHWAY			
05/24/2001	DIAG	7809	OTH GENERAL SYMPTOMS			
05/24/2001	DIAG	8470	SPRAIN/STRAIN OF NECK			
05/24/2001	DIAG	9529	SPINAL CORD INJURY UNS SITE			

Patient ID: h702AAAAAAAMTNBC, Year of Birth: 1928, Gender: Female, Trigger Date: 06/28/1999

Date	Type	Code	Diagnosis	Procedure	Rx	
Days Supply						

05/07/1999 DRUG	00083006330				BENAZEPRIL HCL	30
05/11/1999 DRUG	00406036105				HYDROCODONE BIT/ACETAMINOPHEN	30
05/22/1999 DRUG	00049490066				SERTRALINE HCL	30
06/01/1999 DRUG	00364047505				CARISOPRODOL	3
06/01/1999 DIAG	7245	UNS BACKACHE				
06/04/1999 DRUG	00025138131				OXAPROZIN	10
06/11/1999 DRUG	00083006330				BENAZEPRIL HCL	30
06/11/1999 DRUG	00087606010				METFORMIN HCL	30
06/17/1999 DRUG	00406036105				HYDROCODONE BIT/ACETAMINOPHEN	3
06/24/1999 DRUG	00364047505				CARISOPRODOL	3

71 YO FEMALE PT WITH A HX OF BACKACHE. SHE IS TAKING FOUR DRUGS THAT AFFECT THE
CNS -HYDROCODONE, SERTRALINE, OXAPROZIN, AND CARISOPRODOL. THEY CAUSE DIZZINESS,
DROWSINESS, CONFUSION, BLURRED VISION. BENAZEPRIL CAN ALSO CAUSE DIZZINESS AND
HYPOTENSION.

06/28/1999 DIAG	E8139	MVA OT VEH COLLISION PERS UNSP
06/28/1999 DIAG	E8495	PLACE OCCURRENCE STREET/HIGHWAY
06/27/1999 DIAG	4590	UNS HEMORRHAGE
06/27/1999 DIAG	9598	INJURY OTHER SITES INC MULT SITES
06/28/1999 DIAG	8470	SPRAIN/STRAIN OF NECK
06/28/1999 DIAG	95200	C1 C4 INJ W UNS SPINAL CORD INJ
06/28/1999 DIAG	9591	OTH/UNS INJURY TRUNK

11
Patient ID: d510AAAAAAFKWQLT, Year of Birth: 1931, Gender: Female, Trigger Date: 01/08/2001

| Date | Type | Code | Diagnosis | Procedure | Rx | |
Days of Supply						
12/19/2000 DRUG		00555003302			CHLORDIAZEPOXIDE HCL	30
12/20/2000 DIAG		1121	CANDIDIASIS VULVA/VAGINA			0
12/20/2000 DIAG		25000	DIABETES UNCOMPL TYPE II			0
12/29/2000 DIAG		61610	UNS VAGINITIS/VULVOVAGINITIS			0
12/29/2000 CPT4		76075		US EXAM, ABDOM, LIMITED		0
12/29/2000 CPT4		99213		OFFICE/OUTPATIENT VISIT, EST		0
01/01/2001 DRUG		00025152531			CELECOXIB	30
01/01/2001 DRUG		00172290880			FUROSEMIDE	30
01/01/2001 DRUG		00186074231			OMEPRAZOLE	30

Date	Type	Code			
01/01/2001	DRUG	00245004015		POTASSIUM CHLORIDE	30
01/01/2001	DRUG	00378021001		CHLORPROPAMIDE	30
01/01/2001	DRUG	00406053201		OXYCODONE HCL/ACETAMINOPHEN	20
01/04/2001	CPT4	99213	OFFICE/OUTPATIENT VISIT, EST		0
01/05/2001	DRUG	00062535001		TERCONAZOLE	7
01/05/2001	DRUG	49158020007		HYDROCORTISONE	7

70 YO FEMALE WITH A HISTORY OF DM TYPE II AND PREVIOUS FRACTURE IS BEING TREATED WITH CELECOXIB AND OXYCODONE FOR PAIN. CHLORPROPAMIDE FOR THE DM. CHLORPROPAMIDE IN OLDER PATIENTS IS PARTICULARLY PRONE TO CAUSING HYPOGLYCEMIA AND DIZZINESS. FUROSEMIDE AFFECTS BLOOD SUGAR CONTROL AND ATENOLOL MAY ALSO AFFECT GLUCOSE CONTROL AND MASK SIGNS OF HYPOGLYCEMIA. OXYCODONE AND CHLORDIAZEPOXIDE SHOULD ALSO BE USED WITH CAUTION IN OLDER PTS AND MAY CAUSE EXCESSIVE SEDATION, DIZZINESS, AND CONFUSION.

Date	Type	Code	Diagnosis	Rx	
01/08/2001	DIAG	92420	CONTUSION OF FOOT		0
01/08/2001	DIAG	E8120	MVA COLLISION UNSP DRIVER		
01/08/2001	DRUG	00093310905		AMOXICILLIN TRIHYDRATE	2
01/08/2001	DIAG	25000	DIABETES UNCOMPL TYPE II		0
01/08/2001	DIAG	4019	UNS HYPERTENSION		0
01/08/2001	DIAG	71597	OSTEOARTHROSIS UNSP ANKLE/FOOT		0
01/08/2001	DIAG	71887	OTH JOINT DERANGEMENT OT ANKLE/FOOT		0
01/08/2001	DIAG	71887	OTH JOINT DERANGEMENT OT ANKLE/FOOT		0
01/08/2001	DIAG	92420	CONTUSION OF FOOT		0

Patient ID: e810AAAAAABUMGYK, Year of Birth: 1932, Gender: Female, Trigger Date: 10/02/2000

Date Days Supply	Type	Code	Diagnosis	Procedure	Rx	
07/17/2000	DIAG	71941	PAIN IN JOINT SHOULDER			
07/17/2000	DIAG	71941	PAIN IN JOINT SHOULDER			
07/17/2000	CPT4	73030		X-RAY EXAM OF SHOULDER		
07/17/2000	CPT4	99204		OFFICE/OUTPATIENT VISIT, NEW		
07/27/2000	DRUG	00378400301			ALPRAZOLAM	14
08/15/2000	DRUG	00310013234			LISINOPRIL	30
08/15/2000	DRUG	55953034370			GLYBURIDE	30
08/28/2000	DRUG	00378400301			ALPRAZOLAM	14
08/28/2000	DRUG	00456032301			LEVOTHYROXINE SODIUM	30
08/28/2000	DIAG	71591	OSTEOARTHROSIS UNSP SHOULDER			

Date	Type	Code	Diagnosis	Procedure	Rx	
08/28/2000	DIAG	71591	OSTEOARTHROSIS UNSP SHOULDER			
08/28/2000	DIAG	71591	OSTEOARTHROSIS UNSP SHOULDER			
08/28/2000	CPT4	20610		DRAIN/INJECT, JOINT/BURSA		
08/28/2000	CPT4	73030		X-RAY EXAM OF SHOULDER		
08/28/2000	HCPCS	J0702		INJ BETAMETHASONE ACETATE &		
09/18/2000	DRUG	00310013234			LISINOPRIL	30
09/18/2000	DRUG	55953034370			GLYBURIDE	30
09/28/2000	DRUG	00378400301			ALPRAZOLAM	14

68 YO FEMALE HAS A HISTORY OF OSTEOARTHROSIS AND DM II. SHE IS BEING PRESCRIBED ALPRAZOLAM, GLYBURIDE, LISINOPRIL, AND LEVOTHYROXINE. SIDE EFFECTS OF GLYBURIDE ARE HEADACHE AND DIZZINESS. LEVOTHYROXINE CAN CAUSE NERVOUSNESS AND PALPITATIONS. LISINOPRIL CAN CAUSE HYPOTENSION. ALPRAZOLAM CAN CAUSE DROWSINESS, ATAXIA, AND LIGHTHEADEDNESS.

Date	Type	Code	Diagnosis	Procedure	Rx	
10/02/2000	DIAG	E8130	MVA OT VEH COLLISION DRIVER			
10/02/2000	DIAG	71941	PAIN IN JOINT SHOULDER			
10/02/2000	DIAG	7231	CERVICALGIA			
10/02/2000	DIAG	8470	SPRAIN/STRAIN OF NECK			

Patient ID: h702AAAAAAALNJXR, Year of Birth: 1933, Gender: Male, Trigger Date: 12/16/1999

Date Days Supply	Type	Code	Diagnosis	Procedure	Rx	
10/18/1999	DRUG	59772691001			POTASSIUM CHLORIDE	30
10/18/1999	DIAG	25000	DIABETES UNCOMPL TYPE II			
10/18/1999	DIAG	25000	DIABETES UNCOMPL TYPE II			
10/18/1999	CPT4	99212		OFFICE/OUTPATIENT VISIT, EST		
10/18/1999	HCPCS	J1820		INJ INSULIN TO 100 UNITS		
10/21/1999	DRUG	00049276066			DOXAZOSIN MESYLATE	30
10/28/1999	DRUG	00002871501			INSUL NPH HU REC/INS RG HU REC	30
11/03/1999	DRUG	00378020810			FUROSEMIDE	30
11/15/1999	DRUG	52544024001			LORAZEPAM	30
11/16/1999	DIAG	V048	VACCINE FOR INFLUENZA			
11/16/1999	CPT4	90782		INJECTION, SC/IM		
11/16/1999	HCPCS	G0008		ADMIN FLU VIRUS VAC-NO MD FE		
11/19/1999	DRUG	59772691001			POTASSIUM CHLORIDE	30
12/06/1999	DRUG	00378020810			FUROSEMIDE	30
12/07/1999	DRUG	00002871501			INSUL NPH HU REC/INS RG HU REC	30

66 YO MALE IS A TYPE II DIABETIC. HE IS TREATED WITH INSULIN. FUROSEMIDE MAY CAUSE
HYPERGLYCEMIA AND CAUSE DIZZINESS. DOXAZOSIN CAN CAUSE MARKED HYPOTENSION AND
SYNCOPE. AS WELL AS SOMNOLENCE AND FATIGUE. GREATER THAN 10% OF PATIENTS EXPERIENCE
SEDATION WITH LORAZEPAM.

Date	Type	Code	Description
12/16/1999	DIAG	E8120	MVA COLLISION UNSP DRIVER
12/16/1999	DIAG	E8495	PLACE OCCURRENCE STREET/HIGHWAY
12/16/1999	DIAG	7231	CERVICALGIA
12/16/1999	DIAG	8470	SPRAIN/STRAIN OF NECK
12/16/1999	DIAG	8472	SPRAIN/STRAIN LUMBAR REGION

REFERENCES

Beers, M. H. (1997). Explicit Criteria for Determining Potentially Inappropriate Medication Use by the Elderly: An Update. *Archives of Internal Medicine, 157*, 1531-1536.

Carr, D. B. (2000). Cardiovascular Medicine Update: The Older Adult Driver. *American Family Physician,* Jan; 61(1).

Chan, M., Nicklason, F. & Vial, J. H. (2001). Adverse drug events as a cause of hospital admission in the elderly. *Intern Med J.,* May-Jun;*31*(4),199-205

Curtis, L. H., Ostbye, T., Sendersky, V., Hutchison, S., Dans, P. E., Wright, A., Woosley, R. L. & Schulman, K. A. (2004). Inappropriate prescribing for elderly Americans in a large outpatient population. *Arch Intern Med.*, Aug 9-23;*164*(15),1621-5.

Edwards, J. G. (1995). Depression, antidepressants, and accidents. Editorial. *BMJ, 311*, 887 - 888.

Ellenhorn's Medical Toxicology, 2nd ed

Federal Interagency Forum on Aging Related Statistics, 2000.

Federspiel, C. F., Ray, W. A. & Schaffner, W. (1976). Medicaid records as a valid data source: the Tennessee experience. *Med Care.* Feb;*14*(2),166-72

Fick, D. M., et al. Updating the Beers Criteria for Potentially Inappropriate Medication Use in Older Adults. *Arch Intern Med,163*, Dec 8/22/2003.

Foley, D. J., et al. Risk factors for motor vehicle crashes among older drivers in a rural community. *J Am Geriatr Soc.* 1995 Jul, *43(7)*, 776-781.

Gresset, J. & Meyer, F. (1994). Risk of automobile accidents among elderly drivers with impairments or chronic diseases. *Can J Public Health.* Jul-Aug, *85(4)*, 282-5.

Hanlon, J. T., Schmader, K. E. & Koronkowski, M. J. (1997). et.al., Adverse drug events in high risk older outpatients. *J Am Geriatr Soc.* Aug, *45(8)*, 945-8

Hemmelgarn, B. (1997). et al. *Benzodiazepine use and the risk of motor vehicle crash in the elderly.* JAMA Jul2, *278(1)*, 27-31.

Hennessy, S., Bilker, W. B., Weber, A. & Strom, B. L. (2003). Descriptive analyses of the integrity of a US Medicaid claims database, *Pharmacoepidemiol Drug Saf.* Mar, *12(2)*, 103-11

Hohl, C., Dankoff, J., Colacone, A. & Afilalo, M. (2001). Polypharmacy, adverse drug-related events, and potential adverse drug interactions in elderly patients presenting to an emergency department. *Ann Emerg Med,38*, 666-671

Hu, P. S. (1998). et al. Crash risks of older drivers: a panel data analysis. *Accid Anal Prev* Sep, *30(5)*, 569-81.

Jacobs, P., Lier, D. & Schopflocher, D. (1999). Long term medical costs of motor vehicle casualties in Alberta: a population - based, incidence approach. *Accid Anal Prev.* 2004 Nov, *36(6)*, 1099-103

Kelly, R., Warke, T. & Steele, I. (1999). "Medical restrictions to driving: the awareness of patients and doctors" *Postgrad. Med. J.*, September 1, *75(887)*, 537 - 539.

Koepsell, T. D., et al. (1994). Medical conditions and motor vehicle collision injuries in older adults. *J Am Geriatr Soc.* Jul, *42(7)*, 695-700.

Leveille, S. G., et al. (1994). Psychoactive medications and injurious motor vehicle collisions involving older drivers. *Epidemiology*, Nov, *5(6)*, 591-598.

Li, G., Braver, E. R., et al. (2003). "Fragility versus excessive crash involvement as determinants of high death rates per vehicle-mile of travel among older drivers." *Accid Anal Prev 35(2)*, 227-35.

Lyman, J. M., et al. (2001). Factors related to driving difficulty and habits in older drivers. *Accid Anal Prev.* May, *33(3)*, 413-21.

Masa, J. F., et al. (2000). Habitually sleepy drivers have a high frequency of automobile crashes associated with respiratory disorders during sleep. *Am J Respir Crit Care Med.* Oct, *162(4 Pt1)*, 1407-12.

McGwin, G. Jr., Sims, R. V., Pulley, L. & Roseman, J. M. (2000). Relations among chronic medical conditions, medications, and automobile crashes in the elderly: a population-based case-control study. *Am J Epidemiol.* Sep 1, *152(5)*, 424-31.

McGwin. G., et al. (1999). Diabetes and automobile crashes in the elderly. A population-based case-control study. *Diabetes Care.* Feb, *22(2)*, 220-7.

Millar, W. J. (1999). *"Older Drivers: A Complex Public Health Issue"*, Health Reports, Autumn 1999, *Vol. 11*, No.2.

Morgan, R. & King, D. (1995). The older driver: A review. *Postgrad Med J, 71(839)*, 525-528.

Morse, M. L. (1991). "Detecting Adverse Drug Reactions: The Record-Linkage System—A Duality of Purpose." *International Journal of Risk and Safety in Medicine* 2:51-56.

National Center for Health Statistics, *Centers for Disease Control and Prevention.* (1998). 1998 NAMCS Micro-data file Documentation.

National Center for Health Statistics, *Centers for Disease Control and Prevention.* (1999). 1999 NAMCS Micro-data file Documentation.

National Center for Health Statistics, *Centers for Disease Control and Prevention.* (2000). 2000 NAMCS Micro-data file Documentation.

Noble: *Textbook of Primary Care Medicine*, (2005). 3rd Ed Oak Ridge National Laboratory.

Owsley, C. (1994). *Vision and driving in the elderly.* Optom Vis Sci, 71, 727-35

Owsley, C., McGwin G. Jr., Sloane, M., Wells, J., Stalvey, B. T. & Gauthreaux S. (2002). Impact of Cataract Surgery on Motor Vehicle Crash Involvement by Older Adults *JAMA*, August 21, *288(7)*, 841 - 849

Quan, H., Parsons, G. A. & Ghali, W. A. (2002). Validity of information on comorbidity derived from ICD-9-CCM administrative data, *Med Care.* Aug, *40(8)*, 675-85.

Ray, W. A., Fought, R. L., Decker, M. D. (1992). Psychoactive drugs and the risk of injurious motor vehicle crashes in elderly drivers, *Am J Epidemiol.* Oct 1, *136(7)*, 873-83

Roos, L. L., Walld, R., Wajda, A., Bond, R. & Hartford, K. (1996). Record linkage strategies, outpatient procedures, and administrative data. *Med Care.* Jun, *34(6)*, 570-82

Sims, R. V., et al. (2001).Mobility impairments in crash-involved older drivers. *J Aging Health* Aug, *13(3)*, 430-8.

Sims, R. V., et al. (2000). Exploratory study of incident vehicle crashes among older drivers. *J Gerontol A Biol Sci Med Sci.* Jan, *55(1)*, M22-27.

Strom, B. L. & Morse, M. L. (1988). "*Use of Computerized Databases to Survey Drug Utilization in Relation to Diagnoses.*" *Acta Med Scand Suppl., 721*,13-20.

Strom, B. L., Carson, J. L., Morse, M. L. & Soper, K. A. (1984). "A Novel Approach to a Long-Term Post-Marketing Surveillance Study, Using Medicaid Billing Data." *Clinical Pharmacology and Therapeutics*, *35*, 278.

US Department of Transportation. *The Changing Face of Transportation.* 2000 http://www.bts.gov/publications/the_ changing_face_of_ transportation chapter_03. html. Accessed March 2005.

Walker, A. M. (2001). Pattern recognition in health insurance claims databases. *Pharmacoepidemiol Drug Saf.* Aug-Sep, *10(5)*, 393-7

Wilchesky, M., Tamblyn, R. M. & Huang, A. (2004). Validation of diagnostic codes within medical services claims. *J Clin Epidemiol.* Feb, *57(2)*, 131-41

Willcox, S. M., et al. (1994). *Inappropriate Drug Prescribing for the Community-Dwelling Elderly. JAMA, 272*, 292-296.

Worth, R. M. & Mytinger, R. E. (1996). Medical insurance claims as a source of data for research: accuracy of diagnostic coding. *Hawaii Med J.* Jan, *55(1)*, 9-11.

End Notes

[1] The set of factors that contribute to the occurrence of a disease.

[2] Study subjects taking barbiturates and mast cell stabilizers had the highest Odds Ratios. However, there are only ten cases and four controls taking barbiturates and seven cases and seven controls taking mast cell stabilizers. The Odds Ratios for those two drugs need to be confirmed by further studies. The remaining drug classes exhibited larger numbers of study subjects taking these drugs.

[3] The study design methodology attempted to rule out head trauma as a result of an MVC by employing temporal sequence and date of service screens. The resulting risk was a measure of subjects with existing head trauma, who subsequently experienced an MVC.

[4] Therapeutic conflicts between medications and existing diseases and other drugs were determined using a proprietary set of clinical rules used in the RxWise™ adverse drug event detection system

[5] Co-linearity with the underlying diseases cannot be ruled out by our study methodology

[6] This may be clinically reasonable due to the fact that the efficacy of some common anticonvulsants are potentiated by barbiturates used in smaller doses than those doses used for sedation alone

[7] Goodness-of-fit statistics examine the difference between the observed frequency and the expected frequency for groups of patients. The statistic can be used to determine if the model provides a good fit for the data. If the P-value is large, then the model is well calibrated and fits the data well; if the P-value is small (smaller than alpha), then the model is not well calibrated. One such statistic is the Hosmer-Lemeshow goodness-of-fit statistic.

In: Older Drivers Impaired by Multiple Medications
Editors: Lisa M. Perkins and Danielle J. White

ISBN: 978-1-61209-374-1
© 2011 Nova Science Publishers, Inc.

Chapter 2

A PILOT STUDY TO TEST MULTIPLE MEDICATION USAGE AND DRIVING FUNCTIONING*

National Highway Safety Traffic Administration

ACKNOWLEDGMENTS

The authors wish to thank the following individuals and their organizations for their invaluable contributions to this project (in alphabetical order): Patricia Alderson, Rehab Services manager, Cokesbury Village Continuing Care Retirement Community; Dr. Nicole Brandt, consultant (pharmacy/medication reviews); Tom Difilippo, manager of Rehabilitation Services, Oak Crest Erickson Retirement Community; Dr. Laura Finn, consultant (pharmacy/medication reviews); Arlene Klapproth, OTR, Oak Crest Erickson Retirement Community; Dr. Scott Masten, CA DMV (statistical support); Michael Mercadante, consultant (video systems specialist); Matthew J. Narrett, M.D. (executive vice president and chief medical officer for Erickson Retirement Communities); Dr. John Parrish, executive director, the Erickson Foundation; Rose Phung, consultant (instrumented vehicle video coding); Debbie Racosky, manager of Rehabilitation Services, Charlestown Erickson Retirement Community; Dr. Yu-Ling Shao, research coordinator, the Erickson Foundation; Dr. Jane Stutts, consultant (epidemiology/research design); Mary Wagner, National Director of Rehabilitation Services, Erickson Retirement Communities; and Kim White, OT/CDRS, consultant (on-road driving evaluations).

LIST OF ACRONYMS AND ABBREVIATIONS

ACE	Angiotensin-Converting Enzyme
ADR	Adverse Drug Reaction

---

* This is an edited, reformatted and augmented edition of a National Highway Traffic Safety Administration publication.

AHRQ	Agency for Healthcare Research and Quality
ARCI	Addiction Research Center Inventory
ASF	Advanced Systems Format
BRT	Brake Reaction Time
CAPI	Computer-Assisted Personal Interviewing
CCRC	Continuing Care Retirement Center
CERTs	Centers for Education and Research on Therapeutics
CDRS	Certified Driver Rehabilitation Specialist
CMS	Centers for Medicare & Medicaid Services
CNS	Central Nervous System
COX	Cyclooxygenase
CRO	Controlled-Release Oxycodone
CSH	Carotid Sinus Hypersensitivity
CVS	Cardiovascular System
d.f.	Degrees of Freedom
DC	Direct Current
DHI	DrivingHealth® Inventory
DSS	Decision Support System
DSST	Digit Symbol Substitution Test
DUA	Data Use Agreement
EEG	Electroencephalogram
FARS	Fatality Analysis Reporting System
FRIDS	Fall-Risk-Increasing Drugs
GPRD	General Practice Research Database
GPS	Global Positioning System
HCUP	Healthcare Cost and Utilization Project
HIPAA	Health Insurance Portability and Accountability Act
HMG/COA	5-Hydroxy-3-Methylglutaryl-Coenzyme A
HMO	Health Maintenance Organization
Hz	Hertz
IRB	Institutional Review Board
ICD-9-CM	International Classification of Diseases, Ninth Revision, Clinical Modification
KML	Keyhole Markup Language
LCD	Liquid Crystal Display
MAX	Medicaid Analytic eXtract
MCBS	Medicare Current Beneficiary Survey
MHRA	Medicines & Healthcare Products Regulatory Agency
MSIS	Medicaid Statistical Information System
MSS	Musculoskeletal System
NaSSA	Noradrenergic and Specific Serotonergic Antidepressant
NDC	National Drug Code
NHS	National Health Service
NHTSA	National Highway Traffic Safety Administration
NIS	Nationwide Inpatient Sample
NMEA	NationalMarine Electronics Association

NRAR	Norwegian Road Accident Registry
NSAIDs	Non-Steroidal Anti-Inflammatory Drugs
OBD	On-Board Diagnostic
OCME	Office of the Chief Medical Examiner
OH	Orthostatic Hypotension
OR	Odds Ratio
OT	Occupational Therapist
OTC	Over the Counter
PBM	Pharmacy Benefits Management
PDI	Potentially Driver Impairing
PI	Principal Investigator
PIP	Potentially Inappropriate Prescription
RT	Reaction Time
Rx	Prescription
SDLP	Standard Deviation of Lateral Positioning
SIR	Standardized Incidence Ratio
SMRFs	State Medicaid Research Files
SNRI	Serotonin-Norepinephrine Reuptake Inhibitor
SSN	Social Security Number
SSRI	Selective Serotonin Reuptake Inhibitor
TCA	Tricyclic Antidepressant
TOVA	Test of Variables of Attention
TRB	Transportation Research Board
VHA	Veteran's Health Administration
VVC	Vasovagal Collapse
X^2	Chi-Square Test Statistic

EXECUTIVE SUMMARY

The number of older licensed drivers in the United States is growing at a rate faster than the overall population. As people age, they are more likely to take one or more potentially driver-impairing (PDI) medications. TransAnalytics, LLC, completed a pilot study to gain a better understanding of the safety impact on older drivers of taking multiple PDI medications, providing an update on the prevalence of prescription medications in the older population, and the effects on driving of specific drugs/drug classes. Research activities included a literature review; a data mining exercise; the prioritization of other databases for future data mining; and a field study including on-road evaluations of older drivers who take multiple PDI medications by an occupational therapist, and associated instrumented vehicle observations. The results of this work point to what appear to be relatively stronger, and weaker, strategies for carrying out future studies in this vital area of research.

The literature review in this project examined recently published research to update a prior NHTSA report (Literature Review of Polypharmacy and Older Drivers: Identifying Strategies to Study Drug Usage and Driving Functioning Among Older Drivers, DOT HS 810 558) on the effects of different types of PDI drugs on driving. New information about specific drugs/drug classes and driving is provided for an anti-seizure medication (topiramate) used for migraine prevention and other therapies; acute and stable dosing of opioids; sedating and non-sedating antihistamines; antidepressants; short- and long-half-life sedative-hypnotics; an immediate-release versus extended-release anti-anxiety medication (benzodiazepine); a skeletal muscle relaxant (carisoprodol); and anti-diabetic medications. In addition, this review provided insight into the risk associated with chronic medical conditions versus the effects of the medications that treat these conditions.

This question was examined in the context of studies bearing on the risk of falls; there is evidence that the same medications that mediate falls risk may also mediate motor vehicle crash risk. What emerges in this review is that some geriatric patients experience an increased risk of falling due to cardiovascular adverse effects of sedatives, antihypertensives, and other medications, and that when these fall-risk-increasing drugs are withdrawn there is a resulting, persistent benefit a significant reduction in the occurrence of falls (Van der Velde et al., 2007). At the same time, researchers have found that chronic medical conditions were often more important than medications in causing falls in high-functioning community-dwelling older people (Lee et al., 2006). This underscores a need for NHTSA to sponsor future, periodic updates to remain current with new research. Also, many older people are likely to benefit from an individualized medication review by their pharmacist, with physician follow-up, potentially leading to the withdrawal of selected medications, for selected conditions, and/or their replacement with alternative prescriptions without known PDI (or fall-risk-increasing) effects.

This project defined an ideal database to study the crash involvement of older drivers taking PDI medications— which would contain linked medical, hospital, and pharmaceutical data for each eligible person and would be the *only* provider of services—then evaluated a number of candidates for such work. The "ideal" database, which would capture the complete record of drug utilization for a patient (driver), unfortunately does not presently exist. However, several promising candidates for future NHTSA investigations were identified, in particular, the Ingenix LabRx® database (United Healthcare) and the Veteran's Health Administration Pharmacy Benefits Management Database (VHA/PBM).

In this project, data mining was performed in the Pharmetrics database, a patient-level administrative claims database containing prescription information and E-codes signifying the incidence of motor vehicle injuries to identify drivers who were taking PDI medications and were involved in crashes. The number of PDI drugs taken by crash-involved individuals within the age cohorts from 16 through 49, and within 5-year cohorts from 50 up through 75+, ranged from zero to 16. The use of multiple PDI medications by crash-involved drivers, who are 50 and older, climbs steadily with age, until leveling off at the 65- to 69-year-old cohort. At the same time, one-third to one-half of crash-involved drivers in each of these cohorts were taking no PDI medications. From this exercise, a set of two PDI drug combinations—hypotensives in combination with one or more other classes of PDI medications such as lipotropics, beta blockers, calcium channel blockers, NSAIDS, SSRIs, and gastric acid secretion reducers—emerged as inclusion criteria for a subsequent field study.

Forty-four healthy older drivers between the ages of 57 and 89, who drove 50 miles and/or three days each week, participated in a pilot study to examine their use of PDI medications and driving abilities. A pharmacist collected data on each participant's medication usage via one-on-one "brown bag" medication reviews. Each driver's functional status was measured using a computer-based test battery including high- and low-contrast acuity measures, plus physical and cognitive measures validated as significant predictors of at-fault crashes among seniors in earlier NHTSA research. Then, an occupational therapist/certified driver rehabilitation specialist (OT/CDRS) measured drivers' on-road performance. This included onboard measures of brake response time under alerted and unalerted conditions.

Due to the small sample size relative to the number of drugs and drug classes, logistic regression was unable to significantly associate medication usage with observed differences in functional (cognitive) status, driving evaluation outcomes, or brake response time. It was observed that the drivers who "failed" the OT evaluation were also among the oldest, however. This may be an indication of greater impairment in driving performance due to PDI medications with increasing age, due to a wide range of physiological changes and changes in how these drugs are metabolized. While these results must be regarded as tentative, it appears that ACE inhibitors, generally, and ACE inhibitor/thiazide diuretic combinations may deserve special attention in future research.

The private cars of a sub-sample of 5 individuals who underwent evaluation by the OT/CDRS were equipped with instruments to collect video, GPS and speed recordings, as they drove independently. These same instruments were present during their drives with the OT, which took place on the same roads, at similar times of day and under similar conditions. The goal was to examine the variability in behaviors serving as surrogates of driver attention/distraction, plus speed choice, as a function of driving context. In the aggregate, these drivers spent more time looking down and inside the vehicle and less looking toward the inside rearview mirror when driving independently than when the OT was present, including during intersection negotiation. A case study also revealed that, on common road segments, an 82-year-old study participant was more likely to drive slower on her own than during the OT evaluation, when other traffic was present; but *faster* on her own under "empty road" conditions, where other traffic could not affect speed choice. Such differences between independent driving and (older) peoples' behavior during a driving evaluation may have significant safety implications.

One important conclusion from this pilot study is that small-sample empirical investigations do not appear to be a practical route to a better understanding of (multiple) medications and driving impairment. The prevalence of PDI drugs in any population-based sample works against successfully modeling the predictor-criterion relationships of greatest interest; and, sample recruitment is daunting. At the same time, two promising methods for future research can be recommended. First, databases highlighted in this chapter can be used to mine patient-level information, an approach that may be quite valuable in pinpointing drugs and combinations of drugs to target in future information and education interventions. Further, there is preliminary evidence to recommend monitoring (with consent) drivers' behavior using unobtrusive, affordable, miniature in-car instrumentation packages. This research methodology offers a unique opportunity to measure behavioral variability as a function of driving context, and to determine normative exposure levels to a wide range of hypothesized risk factors.

INTRODUCTION

Project Objectives

This project sought to identify trends in exposure to potentially driver impairing (PDI) medications by seniors and then, using complementary approaches, to improve our understanding about how the use of multiple medications relates to the ability to drive safely. These goals were accomplished by satisfying the following specific objectives:

- Critically review new reports, surveys, and other studies throughout the entire project to continuously update the state-of-the-knowledge concerning older adults who are at risk from exposure to PDI medications.
- Use a proprietary, patient-level database supplied by NHTSA to perform data mining to better characterize drug use among older adults, and in particular, to identify subgroups of drugs and combinations of drugs that are most strongly associated with injurious motor vehicle crashes.
- Design and conduct a pilot study using field data collection procedures to reveal how specific combinations of prescription and over-the-counter medications effect driving behavior under defined observational conditions, using both between- and within-subjects analysis methods.
- Evaluate the feasibility of using large, administrative claims databases to conduct further NHTSA research investigating driver characteristics, medication usage, and crash and injury experience.
- Develop recommendations for a research strategy that is most likely to result in findings that will support future NHTSA efforts to inform individuals, and their pharmacists, physicians and other health care providers, about the impact of medication usage on safe driving.

Background

The number of older, licensed drivers in the United States is growing at a rate faster than the overall population. In 1988, at the time the first TRB Special Report *Transportation in an Aging Society* was published, 12% of the population was 65 or older. By the year 2020, the U.S. Census Bureau projects that roughly 1 in 5 people will be 65 or older, and almost half of those will be 75 or older. At the same time, reliance on the private automobile as the primary means of transportation, either as a driver or passenger, is increasing for this segment of the population. The increasing frailty that comes with advancing age means that older vehicle occupants, if involved in a crash, will suffer more serious injuries and are at significantly greater risk of being killed than their younger counterparts. In 2001-2002, per mile driven, drivers 80 and older had higher rates of passenger vehicle fatal crash involvements than drivers in all other age groups except teenagers, and those 85 and older had the highest rates (Insurance Institute for Highway Safety, 2003). When the driver fatality rate is calculated based on the estimated annual travel, the rate for drivers 85 and older is *ten times higher* than the rate for drivers age 30 to 60.

There are a number of factors that may contribute to the increased crash and fatality rates among older drivers, most notably a range of age-related diminished capabilities documented in related NHTSA projects (Staplin, Gish, and Wagner, 2003). At the same time, the medical conditions that are more prevalent in old age and the medications used to treat them have come under increased scrutiny as the reason for such declines.

In 2004, 37.4% of non-institutionalized people over 65 assessed their heath as excellent or very good; this compared to 65.8% for people 18 to 64 (Administration on Aging, 2004). Most older people have at least one chronic condition and many have multiple conditions. Among the most frequently occurring conditions among older people in 2000-2001 were: hypertension (49.2%), arthritic symptoms (36.1%), all types of heart disease (31.1%), any cancer (20.0), sinusitis (15.1%), and diabetes (15.0).

In a cohort study of nearly 28,000 Medicare+Choice enrollees cared for by a multi-specialty practice (an ambulatory clinic setting) during a 12-month study period between 1999 and 2000, researchers found that 75% of the sample received prescriptions for six or more prescription drugs (Gurwitz, Field, Harrold, Rothchild, Debellis, Seger, Cadoret, Fish, Garber, Kelleher, & Bates, 2003). Residents of long-term care facilities were excluded from the study. The average age of the subjects in the sample was 74.7 (sd=6.7). The age and gender distribution of the sample was similar to that of the U.S. population 65 and older. Forty-nine percent of the sample was prescribed medications in four or more categories. The specific prescription medication categories and percentage of enrollees receiving prescriptions were as follows:

- Cardiovascular (53.2%)
- Antibiotics/anti-infectives (44.5%)
- Diuretics (29.5%)
- Opioids (21.9%)
- Antihyperlipidemic (21.7%)
- Nonopioid analgesics (19.8%)
- Gastrointestinal tract (19.0%)
- Respiratory tract (15.6%)
- Dermatologic (14.8%)
- Antidepressants (13.2%)
- Sedatives/hypnotics (12.9%)
- Nutrients/supplements (12.3%)
- Hypoglycemics (11.5%)
- Steroids (9.7%)
- Ophthalmics (9.6%)
- Thyroid (9.4%)
- Antihistamines (9.2%)
- Hormones (9.1%)
- Anticoagulants (7.0%)
- Muscle relaxants (5.4%)
- Osteoporosis (5.3%)
- Antiseizure (3.4%)
- Antigout (3.2%)

- Antineiplastics (2.8%)
- Antiplatelets (1.3%)
- Antipsychotics (1.2%)
- Antiparkinsonians (0.9%)
- Alzheimer disease (0.9%)
- Immunomodulators (0.04%)

Hébert, Bravo, Korner-Bitensky, and Boyer (1996) found that the consumption of three or more drugs per day increases the risk of functional decline in elderly people by 60% (cited in Allard, Hébert, Rioux, Asselin, & Voyer, 2001). In a recent and comprehensive National survey of U.S. noninstitutionalized adults, Gurwitz (2004) reported that more than 90% of people 65 or older use at least 1 medication per week; more than 40% of this population uses 5 or more different medications per week; and 12% use 10 or more different medications per week. The risks of polypharmacy include an increase in the number of potentially inappropriate prescriptions, cognitive disorders, falls, hip fractures, depression, and incontinence (Gurwitz, Soumerari, & Avorn, 1990). Additionally, the results of a recent NHTSA study have suggested that there is an increased risk of motor vehicle crashes for older drivers who use multiple potentially driver-impairing medications (LeRoy & Morse, 2005).

In Wilkinson and Moskowitz's (2001) review of 11 epidemiological studies of medication use and traffic safety risk (primarily in older drivers) in the United States and Canada between 1991-2000, it was concluded that the prescription drugs most likely to be associated with motor vehicle crashes by older drivers include the same CNS (central nervous system) medications found to increase risk in adults younger than age 65—namely, benzodiazepines (especially long-acting), cyclic antidepressants, and opioid analgesics. Further, they cite a study by Stuck, Beers, Steiner, Aronow, Rubenstein, and Beck (1994) who found that depressed, community-dwelling elderly were eight times as likely as their non-depressed counterparts to be prescribed a long-acting benzodiazepine in addition to their antidepressant medication.

In theory, all psychoactive compounds (depending on dose), may have detrimental effects on psychomotor performance underlying driving skills (Walsh, de Gier, Christopherson, & Verstraete, 2004). Carr (2004) states that in this era of polypharmacy, there are a myriad of sedating medications that could contribute to driving impairment. A simple drug review may identify benzodiazepines, anticholinergics, narcotics, alcohol, or other medications that, once discontinued, may decrease crash risk.

In Leroy and Morse's (2005) case-control analysis using a pharmaceutical claims database with codes indicating services rendered as the result of a motor vehicle crash, higher percentages of crash-involved drivers were prescribed two or more prescriptions than non-crash-involved drivers. Potentially driver-impairing medicines were used by greater percentages of crash-involved drivers than by non-crash-involved drivers (e.g., narcotic analgesics, skeletal muscle relaxants, anti-anxiety medications, NSAIDs and COX inhibitors). The most frequently appearing drug combinations (in descending order of frequency) in the group of crash-involved drivers 50 and older were:

- Narcotics + NSAIDs;

- Skeletal Muscle Relaxants + NSAIDs;
- Narcotics + Skeletal Muscle Relaxants;
- Narcotics + Skeletal Muscle Relaxants + NSAIDs;
- Narcotics + Antibiotics;
- Gastric Acid Secretion Reducers + Narcotics;
- Anti-Anxiety Drugs + Narcotics;
- Selective Serotonin Reuptake Inhibitor (SSRI) Antidepressants + Narcotics;
- Narcotics + NSAIDs + Antibiotics.

Preliminary results of Leroy and Morse's (2005) analysis indicate that 64% of the drivers 50 and older who had a motor vehicle crash had received a prescription for a potentially driver-impairing medication within the prior 60 days. This compares to 54% of the non-crashed-involved drivers 50 and older. To qualify as a PDI medication, the medication had to be associated with known effects on the central nervous system, blood sugar levels, blood pressure, vision, or otherwise have the potential to interfere with driving skills. Possible PDI effects include sedation, hypoglycemia, blurred vision, hypotension, dizziness, fainting (syncope), and loss of coordination (ataxia). Preliminary results are suggestive that the following medications are impairing and related to crash risk: narcotic analgesics, antidepressants, anti-diabetic agents, anti-anxiety agents, antihypertensive agents, and skeletal muscle relaxants.

Together, these facts—much higher numbers of older people in the population, who rely to an overwhelming extent on automobiles, are at exaggerated risk of death or injury in a crash, experience age-related diminished capabilities and medical conditions that affect safe driving performance, and take multiple medicines that alone or in combination are potentially driver impairing—lend urgency to continuing investigations to identify medication use in this population and to determine the effects of (multiple) medications on driving functioning.

DATA MINING OF ADMINISTRATIVE DATABASE

Data Mining Objective

The goal in this project task was to conduct exploratory analyses in a proprietary database that is the property of NHTSA, the PharMetrics Patient-Level Database developed through a prior contract (LeRoy & Morse, 2005), to identify trends in the usage of medications within subgroups of older drivers that could help guide the research design for the present project. In particular, we were seeking to update and refine our understanding about the exposure of seniors to potentially driver-impairing prescription medications, and to prioritize specific combinations of PDI medications for the later pilot study. The database analyses described herein were performed mainly by the Highway Safety Research Center at the University of North Carolina.

The PharMetrics database consists of SAS tables summarizing information about individuals with (cases) and without (controls) motor vehicle crash involvement, who are enrolled in prescription medication insurance plans. It includes ICD-9-CM classification codes for causes of injury ("E-codes") together with entries for patient demographics, number of medications dispensed, patterns of medication combinations, and disease prevalence, for 33,519 "cases" (patients with crashes in the enrollment population) and for 100,557 "controls" (patients without motor vehicle crashes in the enrollment population). A subset of 22,574 cases was selected for the present analyses, as described below. Also, the database includes records for crash-involved drivers *only if* (1) the driver sustained an injury severe enough to result in a hospital treatment and associated insurance payment, and (2) the driver had at least 6 months of continuous insurance coverage prior to the date of the crash/injury. For these reasons, this dataset may not be truly representative of the (older) American population, i.e., biases from these selection factors are certainly plausible. It also may be noted that there is no indication of "fault" for the crashes encompassed in this database.

Analyses reported by LeRoy and Morse provided the starting point for the present work. These researchers examined occurrences of drug-drug conflicts and drug-disease conflicts in the database, performing odds ratio calculations on cases versus controls. The drug classes for which statistically significant relationships were demonstrated are presented in Appendix VIII, Table 1 of their final report; these relationships were used as a selection factor in the present analyses.

Methods and Results

The selected cases included in the database developed by LeRoy and Morse (2005) reflect subsets of E-codes that exclude, for example, collisions with trains; injuries suffered when boarding or alighting from a vehicle (e.g., a bus); and other non-collision-related injuries that are associated with motor vehicle use (e.g., poisoning from exhaust fumes). Crash types included in the database are: E811—*motor vehicle traffic accidents involving re-entrant collision with another vehicle* (e.g., collisions at intersections, or when passing); E812—*other motor vehicle traffic accidents involving collision with a motor vehicle* (e.g., a collision with a parked, stopped, stalled, or disabled vehicle); E813—*motor vehicle traffic accidents involving collision with another [non-motor] vehicle* (e.g., a collision with a cyclist); E814—*motor vehicle traffic accidents involving collision with pedestrian*; E815— *other motor vehicle traffic accidents involving a collision on the highway* (e.g., striking an abutment, animal, or debris); and, E816— *motor vehicle traffic accidents due to loss of control, without a collision on the highway* (e.g., losing control on a curve).

Of particular interest in this research is the medication information for individuals in the database with (selected types of) motor vehicle crashes, as a function of driver age. The analyses conducted by LeRoy and Morse examined only two broad categories—above and below age 50. Our efforts were principally devoted to a finer discrimination among older cohorts of crash-involved drivers, as described in the following pages.

First, our PharMetrics E-code study population was defined as those involved in the six crash types listed above, plus those with "unspecified" (E819) crash types, while continuing to exclude E-codes connoting "sources of external injury" deemed not relevant to the current project goals. Also, E-code suffixes of both "0" and "2" (the 4th digit in the diagnosis code), signifying drivers and motorcycle drivers, respectively, were included. Age was computed by subtracting the year of birth from the year of the E-code diagnosis. Cutpoints were then created at 5-year increments beginning at age 50 and increasing to age 85+, and frequencies

A Pilot Study to Test Multiple Medication Usage and Driving Functioning 273

were tabulated for each cohort. These data are presented in Table 1 for drivers of passenger vehicles and Table 2 for motorcycle drivers.

Another key step in this exercise was to ascertain which medications prescribed for the crash-involved individuals in the PharMetrics database were actually "current" at the time of a crash. Several data elements coded in the database were potentially relevant to this determination – "days supply," "quantity," "amount," and "Rx date." The date of each crash for each person represented in Tables 1 and 2 was also contained in the database.

If the "days supply" entry exceeded the interval between the Rx date and the crash date (allowing for up to three days for Rx overlap and processing delays) the prescription was deemed current. Of course, there is no guarantee that a person's medications were always taken on the prescribed schedule; but, proper compliance was assumed for the purposes of these analyses. Next, because insurance companies require that pharmacies provide the "days supply" information to receive payment for prescriptions, records without such an entry may be questioned. Records where the entry in the "days supply" field was missing or "0" were excluded.

Another crucial step involved the sorting and reclassification of every specific medication entered into the records of the PharMetrics study population—i.e., for which the prescription was current at the time a driver (or motorcycle driver) had a crash—into its "therapeutic drug class." This was necessary because PDI medications are identified at this level. Following LeRoy and Morse (2005), to qualify as a potentially driver-impairing medication, a drug *must be associated with central nervous system side effects, alter blood sugar levels, affect blood pressure, affect vision, or otherwise have the potential to interfere with driving skills.*

With reference to the case-control study reported by LeRoy and Morse, 90 drug classes were identified as potentially driver impairing. As determined in the present analyses, the (mean) number of "current" (at time of crash) PDIs taken by patients in different age groups in the PharMetrics database increased sharply for those 50 and older versus the 16 to 49 group; continued to climb as the patient database was truncated at successively older 5-year cohorts; then leveled off when the "65 and older" threshold was reached. These findings are summarized below for all crash-involved drivers:

For drivers age:	16-49	50+	55+	60+	65+	70+	75+
(n =)	(18,837)	(3,737)	(2,212)	(1,208)	(643)	(474)	(299)
The mean number of PDI meds was:	0.42	1.28	1.43	1.56	1.63	1.66	1.64

Next, we addressed a more specific question: *How many PDI meds were being taken by how many drivers* (assuming compliance with their prescription regimes) *within each age cohort of interest, at the time of their involvem ent in a motor vehicle crash?* With this information, we could consider which specific age cohorts to focus upon in continuing research including actual driver performance measurement; and which drugs (classes) deserve priority in such work, as well. The present analyses yielded the distribution of medications by age cohort displayed in Table 3. As indicated, the number of PDI drugs taken by individuals in the study population ranges from zero to 16 (absent 13 and 14). The proportions taking multiple (two or more) medications are highlighted.

As indicated, the rate of use of multiple PDI medications by crash-involved drivers climbs with age until leveling off at the 65- to 69-year-old cohort. Another perspective on these data is provided by the following graphics, which look more narrowly at the contrast between zero, one, and multiple drug usage. Figure 1 contrasts these relationships in a bar graph, while Figure 2 focuses still more closely on the changes in multiple drug use with driver age, as presently classified.

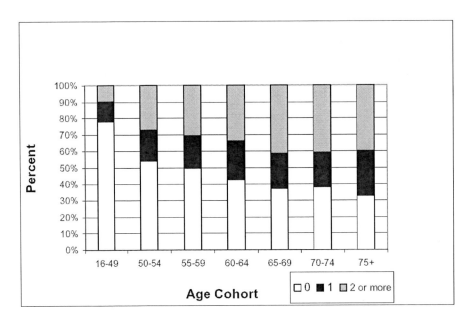

Figure 1. Proportions of crash-involved drivers within each age cohort taking none, versus one, versus multiple (2 or more) PDI medications at time of crash

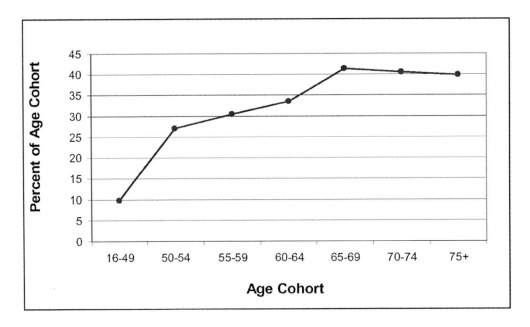

Figure 2. Proportion of crash-involved drivers in each age cohort taking multiple (2 or more) PDI medications at time of crash

Table 1. Age distribution of crash-involved passenger vehicle drivers in E-code study population.

Diagnosis	16-49	50-54	55-59	60-64	65-69	70-74	75-79	80-84	85+
E8110 - *motor vehicle traffic accidents involving re-entrant collision with another vehicle*	41	8	5	0	0	0	2	2	0
E8120 - *other motor vehicle traffic accidents involving collision with a motor vehicle*	9,783	741	529	292	93	95	95	51	20
E8130 - *motor vehicle traffic accidents involving collision with another [non-motor] vehicle*	1,725	156	111	56	18	22	26	19	12
E8140 - *motor vehicle traffic accidents involving collision with pedestrian*	56	9	2	4	0	2	2	1	0
E8150 - *other motor vehicle traffic accidents involving a collision on the highway*	528	42	23	16	6	0	0	0	0
E8160 - *motor vehicle traffic accidents due to loss of control, without a collision on the highway*	1,932	134	702	51	4	9	4	4	5
E8190 – *other; unspecified*	2,889	244	153	97	47	42	37	8	7
Total % (includes all codes within age cohort)	83.3	6.6	4.4	2.5	0.8	0.8	0.8	0.4	0.2
Total	**16,954**	**1,341**	**898**	**518**	**169**	**171**	**166**	**86**	**44**

Table 2. Age distribution of crash-involved motorcycle drivers in E-code study population

Diagnosis	16-49	50-54	55-59	60-64	65-69	70-74	75-79	80-84	85+
E8112 - *motor vehicle traffic accidents involving re-entrant collision with another vehicle*	4	1	0	1	0	0	0	0	0
E8122 - *other motor vehicle traffic accidents involving collision with a motor vehicle*	394	52	26	15	0	1	1	1	2
E8132 - *motor vehicle traffic accidents involving collision with another [non-motor] vehicle*	77	9	4	0	0	0	0	0	0

Table 2. (Continued)

Diagnosis	16-49	50-54	55-59	60-64	65-69	70-74	75-79	80-84	85+
E8142 - *motor vehicle traffic accidents involving collision with pedestrian*	5	0	2	0	0	0	0	0	0
E8152 - *other motor vehicle traffic accidents involving a collision on the highway*	82	9	4	2	0	1	0	0	0
E8162 - *motor vehicle traffic accidents due to loss of control, without a collision on the highway*	682	65	40	19	1	1	0	0	0
E8192 – *other; unspecified*	639	56	34	13	0	2	0	0	0
Total % (includes all codes within age cohort)	83.8	8.6	4.9	2.2	--	--	--	--	--
Total	**1,883**	**192**	**110**	**50**	**1**	**5**	**1**	**1**	**2**

Table 3. Age cohort by number of current prescribed PDI medications, for all crash-involved drivers in PharMetrics database

No. of PDI meds.	Age group													
	16-49		50-54		55-59		60-64		65-69		70-74		75+	
	n	%	n	%	n	%	n	%	n	%	n	%	n	%
0	14,721	78.1	827	54.2	499	49.7	240	42.5	63	37.3	67	38.2	98	32.8
1	2,274	12.1	287	18.8	199	19.8	135	23.9	36	21.3	37	21.1	82	27.4
2	922	4.9	182	11.9	119	11.9	65	11.5	32	18.9	21	12.0	42	14.0
3	437	2.3	106	7.0	72	7.3	48	8.5	20	11.8	22	12.6	29	9.7
4	220	1.2	59	3.9	40	3.9	24	4.2	6	3.6	15	8.6	23	7.7
5	122	0.6	31	2.0	35	3.5	27	4.8	5	2.9	1	0.6	15	5.0
6	67	0.4	15	1.0	16	1.6	9	1.6	2	1.2	5	2.9	4	1.3
7	30	0.2	6	0.4	10	1.0	4	0.7	3	1.8	3	1.7	3	1.0
8	23	0.1	3	0.2	6	0.6	6	1.0	2	1.2	1	0.6	3	1.0
9	5	0.0	2	0.1	5	0.5	3	0.5	0	--	2	1.1	.	.
10	9	0.0	4	0.3	1	0.1	2	0.4	0	--	0	--	.	.

Table 3. (Continued)

No. of PDI meds.	Age group													
	16-49		50-54		55-59		60-64		65-69		70-74		75+	
	n	%	n	%	n	%	n	%	n	%	n	%	n	%
11	6	0.0	0	--	0	--	2	0.4	0	--	1	0.6	.	.
12	.	.	3	0.2	1	0.1	0	--	0	--	0	--	.	.
15	1	0.0	0	--	0	--	0	--	0	--	0	--	.	.
16	.	.	0	--	1	0.1	0	--	0	--	0	--	.	.
2 or more	1,842	9.8	411	27.0	306	30.5	190	33.6	70	41.4	71	40.6	119	39.8
All	18,837		1,525		1,004		565		169		175		299	

278   National Highway Safety Traffic Administration

One question that may be asked with regard to these data is whether the number/proportion of crash-involved drivers taking multiple (two or more) medications increases significantly with increasing age. This may be framed in terms of a chi-square analysis, where the data from the "0', "1', and "2 or more' rows in Table 3 are entered as the observed values. Comparing these to the (calculated) expected values in each cell yields a X^2 test statistic of 1747.12, indicating a difference that is significant at $p < .001$ (d.f. = 12). This profoundly significant test result may be explained by the lower-than-expected use of PDI medications by the 16 to 49 age group and the higher-than-expected use by the older driver cohorts.

Another way of capturing this trend is to display the multipliers that reveal how many more crash-involved drivers than were expected are taking multiple PDI medications, in each group of (increasingly) older drivers:

For drivers aged:	50-54	55-59	60-64	65-69	70-74	75+
The multiplier indicating higher-than-expected use of PDI meds was:	2.02	2.29	2.52	3.11	3.04	2.99

At this point in the data mining exercise, we turned our attention from *how many* drugs were used by older, crash-involved drivers, to *what kind* of drugs. An analysis was performed to identify the top 25 most frequently prescribed therapeutic classes of PDI medications for selected age cohorts. In consideration of the data describing (1) the mean exposure to PDI meds by age group, noted earlier; and (2) the rate of multiple PDI drug use as a function of increasing age, shown above, the 50-and-older and 65-and-older groups were targeted for this analysis. That is, the 50-and-older group marks a clear departure from the data extracted for the 16 to 49 age group, while the data reported here also point to age 65 as a benchmark of sorts, in the changing pattern of PDI drug use (especially multiple PDI drugs) by crash-involved drivers.

The results shown in Tables 4 and 5 indicate that the top 25 therapeutic classes account for 88.7% of the PDI drugs prescribed for drivers 65 and older and 86.4% of the PDI drugs prescribed for 50-and-older drivers in the PharMetrics E-code study population.

The final activity in this task was to attempt to determine which specific *combinations* of PDI medications were most strongly represented among the crash-involved study population. Given the scope of this data mining exercise, it was necessary to narrow our focus to a limited number of age groups and a limited number of drugs-in-combination—while still yielding a result that would be useful to inform the research design for the subsequent pilot testing.

Referring back to Table 3 for a moment, the diminishing cell counts in successively older cohorts of drivers taking multiple (2 or more) medications is, in itself, a limiting factor in these continuing analyses. For example, there were 1,167 drivers in the study population taking multiple medications when the age cutoff is 50, but this number drops to 260 when considering only those individuals 65 and older. When examining the cell counts for 3, 4, 5, etc., PDI medications taken concurrently, the frequencies also decline precipitously under any/all age categories.

Taking these trends into account, our continuing analyses were focused upon the row in Table 3 corresponding to *two PDI medications*. By seeking to identify relationships at this level of analysis, we can encompass as much data as possible that pertains to combinations of drugs associated with crash-involved drivers (i.e., in the PharMetrics E-code study population).

Table 4. Top 25 PDI medications prescribed for crash-involved drivers 65 and older in PharMetrics database where prescription is current at time of crash.

	Therapeutic Drug Class	Frequency	Percent	Cumulative Frequency	Cumulative Percent
	65 and older				
1.	CALCIUM CHANNEL BLOCKING AGENTS	89	8.52	89	8.52
2.	HYPOTENSIVES, ACE INHIBITORS	88	8.42	177	16.94
3.	LIPOTROPICS	79	7.56	256	24.50
4.	BETA-ADRENERGIC BLOCKING AGENTS	59	5.65	315	30.14
5.	GASTRIC ACID SECRETION REDUCERS	56	5.36	371	35.50
6.	NSAIDS, CYCLOOXYGENASE INHIBITOR - TYPE	51	4.88	422	40.38
7.	THYROID HORMONES	50	4.78	472	45.17
8.	ANALGESICS,NARCOTICS	49	4.69	521	49.86
9.	HYPOGLYCEMICS, INSULIN-RELEASE STIMULANT TYPE	49	4.69	570	54.55
10.	LOOP DIURETICS	41	3.92	611	58.47
11.	ANTI-ANXIETY DRUGS	36	3.44	647	61.91
12.	ALPHA-ADRENERGIC BLOCKING AGENTS	30	2.87	677	64.78
13.	DIGITALIS GLYCOSIDES	25	2.39	702	67.18
14.	SELECTIVE SEROTONIN REUPTAKE INHIBITOR (SSRIS)	25	2.39	727	69.57
15.	VASODILATORS,CORONARY	25	2.39	752	71.96
16.	THIAZIDE AND RELATED DIURETICS	22	2.11	774	74.07
17.	TRICYCLIC ANTIDEPRESSANTS & REL. NON-SEL. RU-INHIB	22	2.11	796	76.17
18.	POTASSIUM SPARING DIURETICS IN COMBINATION	21	2.01	817	78.18
19.	HYPOGLYCEMICS, BIGUANIDE TYPE (NON-SULFONYLUREAS)	20	1.91	837	80.10
20.	SEDATIVE-HYPNOTICS,NON-BARBITURATE	20	1.91	857	82.01
21.	ANTICONVULSANTS	15	1.44	872	83.44
22.	BETA-ADRENERGIC AGENTS	15	1.44	887	84.88
23.	SKELETAL MUSCLE RELAXANTS	15	1.44	902	86.32
24.	HYPOTENSIVES,ANGIOTENSIN RECEPTOR ANTAGONIST	13	1.24	915	87.56
25.	HYPERURICEMIA TX - PURINE INHIBITORS	12	1.15	927	88.71

Table 5. Top 25 PDI medications prescribed for crash-involved drivers 50 and older in PharMetrics database where prescription is current at time of crash

	Therapeutic Drug Class	Frequency	Percent	Cumulative Frequency	Cumulative Percent
	50 and older				
1.	LIPOTROPICS	367	7.68	367	7.68
2.	HYPOTENSIVES, ACE INHIBITORS	364	7.62	731	15.30
3.	NSAIDS, CYCLOOXYGENASE INHIBITOR – TYPE	287	6.01	1018	21.30
4.	GASTRIC ACID SECRETION REDUCERS	283	5.92	1301	27.22
5.	CALCIUM CHANNEL BLOCKING AGENTS	281	5.88	1582	33.10
6.	ANALGESICS, NARCOTICS	271	5.67	1853	38.77
7.	BETA-ADRENERGIC BLOCKING AGENTS	242	5.06	2095	43.84
8.	SELECTIVE SEROTONIN REUPTAKE INHIBITORS (SSRIS)	226	4.73	2321	48.57
9.	THYROID HORMONES	208	4.35	2529	52.92
10.	HYPOGLYCEMICS, INSULIN-RELEASE STIMULANT TYPE	175	3.66	2704	56.58
11.	ANTI-ANXIETY DRUGS	173	3.62	2877	60.20
12.	ANTICONVULSANTS	126	2.64	3003	62.84
13.	THIAZIDE AND RELATED DIURETICS	112	2.34	3115	65.18
14.	TRICYCLIC ANTIDEPRESSANTS & REL. NON-SEL. RU-INHIB.	112	2.34	3227	67.52
15.	SKELETAL MUSCLE RELAXANTS	110	2.30	3337	69.83
16.	HYPOGLYCEMICS, BIGUANIDE TYPE (NON-SULFONYLUREAS)	104	2.18	3441	72.00
17.	POTASSIUM SPARING DIURETICS IN COMBINATION	104	2.18	3545	74.18
18.	LOOP DIURETICS	100	2.09	3645	76.27
19.	BETA-ADRENERGIC AGENTS	83	1.74	3728	78.01
20.	ALPHA-ADRENERGIC BLOCKING AGENTS	79	1.65	3807	79.66
21.	HYPOTENSIVES, ANGIOTENSIN RECEPTOR ANTAGONIST	75	1.57	3882	81.23
22.	SEDATIVE-HYPNOTICS, NON-BARBITURATE	70	1.46	3952	82.70
23.	SEROTONIN-2 ANTAGONIST/REUPTAKE INHIBITORS (SARIS)	63	1.32	4015	84.01
24.	DIGITALIS GLYCOSIDES	57	1.19	4072	85.21
25.	INSULINS	57	1.19	4129	86.40

Maintaining a focus on the 65-and-older group is attractive from the standpoint that—based on the present analyses—polypharmacy among crash-involved drivers appears to level off at this age. It also is a widely accepted cutoff for designating "older" drivers in the technical and popular literature on this subject. Inspection of Tables 4 and 5, however, reveals some differences in the prevalence of medications taken by the 65-and-older group versus a group that includes younger (50-and-older) drivers. While the primary anti-hypertensives are second in prevalence among both cohorts, lipotropics (used to lower blood cholesterol) are more prevalent among middle-aged drivers while medications to relieve angina and prevent heart attacks (calcium channel blockers and beta blockers) are more prevalent among drivers 65 and older.

Given these contrasts, it seemed valuable to include both the 50-and-older and the 65-and-older groups in the remaining analyses to determine which specific combinations of PDI medications were most commonly prescribed to crash-involved drivers. The leading combinations follow in Tables 6 and 7, in order of decreasing frequency of database entries (percent calculations rounded to nearest tenth).

The combinations of medications highlighted in Tables 6 and 7 are not exhaustive. Specifically, the combinations of medications listed represent a common fraction of the total 2-PDI counts for both the 65-and-older group (95) and the 50-and-older group (461) -- approximately 40% in each case.

While the numbers and percentages in these lists are small in absolute terms, it should be noted that these values pertain exclusively to the two-drug combinations—not the phenomenon of polypharmacy, more generally—among older, crash-involved drivers in this database. Also, according to the present analyses, from one-third to one-half of crash-involved drivers in each cohort older than 50 were taking no PDI medications at all.

Table 6. Most frequent two-PDI drug combinations for crash-involved drivers 65 and older

Drug Combination	n	%
Hypotensives (Angiotensin-converting enzyme [ACE] Inhibitors) + Antidepressants	4	0.6
Hypotensives (ACE Inhibitors) + Thyroid Hormones	4	0.6
Hypotensives (ACE Inhibitors) + Lipotropics (HMG/COA Reductase Inhibitors)	3	0.5
Hypotensives (ACE Inhibitors) + Non-steroidal anti-inflammatory drugs (NSAIDS)	2	0.3
Diuretics + NSAIDS	2	0.3
Diuretics + Cardiotonic Drugs	2	0.3
Benzodiazepines (Anxiolytic/Sedative/Hypnotic) + Lipotropics (HMG/COA Reductase Inhibitors)	2	0.3
Beta-Adrenergic Blocking Agents + Lipotropics (HMG/COA Reductase Inhibitors)	2	0.3
Benzodiazepines (Anxiolytic/Sedative/Hypnotic) + Beta-Adrenergic Blocking Agents	2	0.3
Hypotensives (ACE Inhibitors) + Beta-Adrenergic Blocking Agents	2	0.3
Hypotensives (ACE Inhibitors) + Selective Serotonin Reuptake Inhibitors (SSRIS)	2	0.3
NSAIDS + Calcium Channel Blocking Agents	2	0.3
Diuretics (Loop) + Digitalis Glycosides	2	0.3
Hypotensives (ACE Inhibitors) + Gastric Acid Secretion Reducers	2	0.3
Hypotensives (ACE Inhibitors) + Calcium Channel Blocking Agents	2	0.3
Analgesic/Narcotics + Gastric Acid Secretion Reducers	2	0.3

Table 7. Most frequent 2-PDI drug combinations for crash-involved drivers 50 and older

Drug Combination	n	%
Hypotensives (ACE Inhibitors) + Calcium Channel Blocking Agents	12	0.3
Diuretics + Beta-Adrenergic Blocking Agents	11	0.3
Hypotensives (ACE Inhibitors) + Antidepressants	10	0.3
Antidepressants + Benzodiazepines (Anxiolytic/Sedative/Hypnotic)	10	0.3
NSAIDS + Opiate Agonists	9	0.2
Analgesic/Narcotics + NSAIDS	9	0.2
Antidepressants + Lipotropics (HMG/COA Reductase Inhibitors)	9	0.2
Hypotensives (ACE Inhibitors) + Beta-Adrenergic Blocking Agents	9	0.2
Hypoglycemics (Biguanide Type) + Hypoglycemics (Sulfonylurea Type)	8	0.2
Opiate Agonists + Skeletal Muscle Relaxants	8	0.2
Hypotensives (ACE Inhibitors) + Dihydropyridines	8	0.2
Analgesic/Narcotics + Skeletal Muscle Relaxants	8	0.2
Hypoglycemics (Insulin Release Stimulant Type) + Hypoglycemics (Non-sulfonylureas)	8	0.2
Lipotropics + Calcium Channel Blocking Agents	7	0.2
Hypotensives (ACE Inhibitors) + Thyroid Hormones	7	0.2
Beta-Adrenergic Blocking Agents + Lipotropics (HMG/COA Reductase Inhibitors)	7	0.2
Hypotensives (ACE Inhibitors) + Lipotropics (HMG/COA Reductase Inhibitors)	7	0.2
Anti-Anxiety Drugs + Selective Serotonin Reuptake Inhibitor (SSRIS)	6	0.2
Diuretics (Potassium Sparing) + Beta-Adrenergic Blocking Agents	6	0.2
Gastric Acid Secretion Reducers + NSAIDS	6	0.2
Hypotensives (ACE Inhibitors) + Hypoglycemics (Insulin Release Stimulant Type)	6	0.2
Antidepressants + Proton-Pump Inhibitors	6	0.2
Beta-Adrenergic Blocking Agents + Dihydropyridines	6	0.2
NSAIDS + Histamine H2-Antagonists	6	0.2
Analgesic/Narcotics + Lipotropics	5	0.1
Hypotensives (ACE Inhibitors) + Gastric Acid Secretion Reducers	5	0.1
Beta-Adrenergic Blocking Agents + Gastric Acid Secretion Reducers	5	0.1
Hypotensives (ACE Inhibitors) + Selective Serotonin Reuptake Inhibitors (SSRIS)	5	0.1
Lipotropics + Selective Serotonin Reuptake Inhibitors (SSRIS)	5	0.1
Antidepressants + Beta-Adrenergic Blocking Agents	5	0.1
Antidepressants + NSAIDS	5	0.1
Antidepressants + Thyroid Agents	5	0.1
Hypotensives (ACE Inhibitors) + Hypoglycemics (Sulfonylureas)	5	0.1
Beta-Adrenergic Blocking Agents + Thyroid Agents	5	0.1
Diuretics + Calcium Channel Blocking Agents	5	0.1
Antidepressants + Opiate Agonists	5	0.1

With these caveats, the results of this project activity supported a decision to concentrate on two-PDI drug combinations in the subsequent data collection activities. It was also concluded that a primary focus on medications to lower blood pressure (the hypotensives) was warranted. In fact, a pilot study examining the effects on driving performance of this drug class in combination with certain other PDI medications represented in the lists above – e.g., lipotropics, beta blockers, calcium channel blockers, NSAIDS, SSRIs, and gastric acid secretion reducers – emerged as the research strategy that comports best with these data, while addressing overall project goals.

PILOT TESTING STRATEGIES TO STUDY POLYPHARMACY AND DRIVING

Research Methods

The pilot study included the collection of data describing sample characteristics for forty-four (44) active, older drivers recruited in residential communities in Delaware and Maryland, including functional status measures and medication usage, followed by driving evaluation measures including an on-road examination by an occupational therapist/certified driver rehabilitation specialist (OT/CDRS) and brake response time measures using an instrumented vehicle. For a subsample of five individuals, video, GPS and speed recordings in their own, private cars were also carried out to examine the variability in selected behaviors—surrogates of driver attention/distraction, plus speed choice—during independent driving versus drives with the OT, under comparable conditions.

Sample Recruitment

The recruitment of study participants took place at the Cokesbury Village Continuing Care Retirement Center in Hockessin, DE, a member of the Peninsula United Methodist Homes network; and at the Oak Crest Village and Charlestown campuses of the Erickson Retirement Communities network, located respectively in Parkville, MD, and Catonsville, MD. As noted in the Acknowledgements section of this chapter, the support of management in these facilities was absolutely essential to successful recruitment and to the conduct of this research. So, too, were the efforts of the Rehabilitation Services managers and staff, not only by engaging and maintaining contact with the participants through the multistage data collection efforts, but also in the actual administration of a computer-based test battery to obtain measures of visual, physical, and cognitive function for the study sample.

Following review and approval of planned recruitment methods by the Institutional Review Board at the University of North Carolina, Chapel Hill, flyers were distributed at the residential facilities announcing the research opportunity, outlining inclusion criteria for the study, and providing a point of contact for more information. An "active" driver was defined as a person who drivers at least 50 miles and/or 3 days or more per week. The combinations of medications sought among the study sample—reflecting the earlier data mining activity in this project—included an antihypertensive agent *and* a drug from any *one* of these classes:

SSRIs; gastric acid secretion reducers; lipotropics (non-statins; mainly prescribed for obesity); HMG-COA inhibitors (statins; mainly prescribed to lower cholesterol); or NSAIDs (prescribed for pain). The point of contact during recruitment for more information about study participation was the *TransAnalytics* Principal Investigator (PI). Examples of recruitment material are shown in Appendix A.

In addition, a small number of controls were sought as study participants, who were not taking *any* prescribed drugs that have been identified as PDI medications; the use of non-PDI prescription drugs and/or over-the-counter remedies (vitamins, herbals, etc.) did not disqualify individuals from participation in this group. Despite protracted efforts, only four individuals (of the total of 44 study participants) meeting the criteria for controls could be enlisted in the study.

In fact, there was considerable difficulty in recruiting older drivers taking the medication classes of interest in this research. After fewer than a dozen individuals responded to the first "wave" of flyers distributed in residents' mailboxes, a later questionnaire was distributed by residential community staff, to attempt to learn the reasons for the low response rate, so a follow up effort might be more successful. This questionnaire is shown in Appendix B.

Anonymous feedback was requested. The questionnaire provided 11 potential reasons for non-participation, plus space to write in any other reasons. Residents were asked to check all reasons that pertained to their decision to decline participation and to list any other reasons they chose not to participate. A total of 81 residents completed and returned the survey. The number and percentage of respondents who chose each reason is presented in Table 8 below.

Table 8. CCRC residents' reasons for not participating in this research study

Reason	Frequency (and percent) of respondents (n=81)
I did not qualify for the study based on the medications I am taking.	16 (19.8%)
I do not drive enough to qualify for the study.	25 (30.9%)
I was out of town.	3 (3.7%)
I was too busy; I did not want to commit to the time required for study participation (3 hours).	13 (16%)
I did not feel the incentive payment ($100) offered for study participation was enough.	2 (2.5%)
I did not want to reveal my medication usage or medication history.	1 (1.2%)
I did not want to drive with a stranger (for the driving evaluation part of the study).	1 (1.2%)
I did not want to drive an unfamiliar car (for the evaluation part of the study).	7 (8.6%)
I did not want instrumentation that would record my driving behavior to be installed in my car.	8 (9.9%)
I did not trust that the results of my driving evaluation would remain confidential.	2 (2.5%)
I was worried that the results of my driving evaluation would be reported to the DMV	2 (2.5%)
Other	38 (46.9%)

A Pilot Study to Test Multiple Medication Usage and Driving Functioning

Table 9. CCRC residents' comments explaining reasons for non-participation

Comments related to lack of interest in study (n=4)	
3	Not interested.
1	My available time is too uncertain. Also, my interest in taking such a test was nil regardless of any monetary incentive.
Comments related to not owning a car or driving anymore (n=6)	
1	I do not own a car. My daughter drives me where I need to go.
1	I sold my car and allowed license to lapse before moving here.
1	I gave my car away six years ago. One of my sons needed it more than I did. I have not driven since then and now have a license but husband says I no longer drive.
1	I stopped driving in March 2002 due to poor hearing and wet macular degeneration in both eyes.
1	I don't have a car. I don't drive anymore.
1	Have macular degeneration in my right eye. It came all at once. I decided myself I might be a risky driver so I gave my car [away] and no longer drive. I felt I should practice what I have always preached. I am 92 years old.
Other issues surrounding driving (n=1)	
1	I thought the test would be given on a computer rather than actual driving.
Comments related to not being informed about the study/not receiving a flyer (n=11)	
4	No flyer received. *or* I do not remember getting the flyer.
1	Just never heard of it
1	Don't recall receiving questionnaire
1	We were not asked to participate in the study as we did not live here.
1	We cannot recall receiving this flyer.
1	I did not receive the flyer asking me to join the study. Most likely I would have joined.
1	I did not have full information. Also I do not have the extra time right now.
1	Did not feel original explanation explained enough. Unclear what the benefit was.
Comments relating to lack of follow-up in recruiting (n=2)	
1	Nobody bothered to answer my volunteer.
1	I think I did sign up for this but it has been several months since that moment. Sorry you haven't gotten a good response, as evidenced by the need for this follow-up.
Medication related comments (n=4)	
1	We do not take any medications on a regular basis, then only when absolutely needed.
1	I originally signed up, but was told my medication might disqualify me. When I didn't hear anything for a long time, I assumed I would not qualify by then we had made plans to go on some visits and were very busy so I had to turn down the offer to participate
1	I am not on medication--was that a condition for participation?
1	I don't take medications.
Conflicts with other activities (n=3)	
1	This may have happened as I was moving in and trying to get acclimated. It took awhile to settle in and find my way about.
1	I have too many dentist/doctor/surgeon appointments! Surgery scheduled Jan '07.
1	I was involved with some personal family matters at that time.
Unknown/non-specific reasons for not participating (n=7)	

The 38 "other" reasons provided by CCRC residents for not participating in the study are presented in Table 9 on the next page, grouped into similar response types.

Follow up recruitment efforts were initiated, including an appeal by the PI in a "village meeting" at the Cokesbury Village CCRC. At the Erickson communities, a vigorous, coordinated effort by the Erickson Research Foundation and the Rehabilitation Services department was undertaken to "get the word out." As a result of these efforts, study recruitment goals for drivers using multiple medications in the drug classes of interest were met, and data collection activities were subsequently carried out during the summer and fall of 2006 at Cokesbury Village, and during the spring and summer of 2007 at the Erickson communities.

Data collection was accomplished only through the dedicated efforts of the Rehab Services staff at each residential community, complemented by the specific expertise of a visiting pharmacist who conducted medication reviews, and an occupational therapist/ certified driving rehabilitation specialist (OT/CDRS) who performed on-road driving evaluations as a consultant to this project. Across each participating facility, a common, prescribed series of steps were followed: pre-qualification, functional testing, medication review, and behind-the-wheel evaluation. These activities are described in more detail below.

Pre-qualification

Each prospective study participant was pre-qualified by verbally reviewing his/her current prescriptions in relation to a prepared list of desired drug classes, and common brands within class, through initial telephone contact with the PI; *or,* the initial contact for some participants was with the Rehab manager, onsite at the residential facility, who evaluated their suitability for the study using the same reference list.

Those who were enrolled in the study were advised that they would be required to (a) read a detailed informed consent agreement and agree to the study procedures described therein, if they wished to enroll in the study; (b)complete a set of tests and exercises administered on a computer, requiring approximately one-half hour (but not requiring familiarity with how to use a computer per se); (c) complete a review of all medications they are currently taking, via consultation with a registered pharmacist who would come to their residence, and also request a printout of their current prescriptions from their own pharmacist; (d)complete a behind-the-wheel examination by an occupational therapist in a dual-brake-equipped, mid-size passenger vehicle (Ford Taurus), conducted on streets/highways in the vicinity of their residence; and (e) optionally, to allow the research team to install instrumentation in their own vehicles that would be small and unobtrusive, but would capture on video a record of when, where, and how they drove. All prospective study participants were given a strict assurance of confidentiality, whereby no results would be shared with state government officials or any other parties unless required by law (e.g., in the event of a crash); and of anonymity, whereby participants would be identified via codes instead of names, and driving evaluation data would be reported only in the aggregate.

All questions about the study were answered, and the offer of $100 compensation for study participation, as stated in the recruitment flyers, was reiterated at this time.

Functional Testing

After receiving the prequalification information, the people who remained interested in study defined the participant list for each facility. This list was maintained and updated by the rehab manager in cooperation with the PI. Working from this list, the rehab manager first contacted each participant to arrange a convenient time for him/her to complete the computer-based functional tests in the offices of the Rehab Services unit in each facility.

The functional tests applied in this research were carried out on a PC using a screening program, the DrivingHealth Inventory. The DHI includes measures of physical ability (head/neck mobility, leg strength/mobility/balance) and cognitive ability (visual search/divided attention, visuospatial ability/visual closure, visual information processing speed/divided attention, working memory) validated as at-fault crash predictors in prior research sponsored by NHTSA (see Staplin, Lococo, Gish, & Decina, 2003); plus, two vision measures (high- and low-contrast static acuity) suggested by existing license policy in the United States and by other research (Janke, 1991).

The PI provided on-site training to each facility's Rehab Manager and staff in the use of the DHI computer program. Functional status data for each older driver enrolled in the study were stored on the facilities' PCs until removed by the PI for analysis after data collection was completed. Performance on the measures of functional ability had no bearing on continued study participation; all participants who completed this activity continued to the next stage (medication review).

Medication Review

After completing the functional testing, each participant was introduced (or made aware of a pending contact from) the consulting pharmacist, by the facility Rehab manager. The instructions participants received about the medication review specified that all prescription medications, all over-the-counter medications, and any vitamins or supplements were to be placed in a "brown bag" and brought for pharmacist review at an appointed time. It was stated that these should include, *"every over-the-counter and prescription medication, including pills, liquids, drops, creams/lotions, and inhalants."* It was further specified that participants should, *"include medicines that you take for any medical condition that the doctor gave you or you got from a pharmacy with a prescription, or any other prescription medication that you use and got from a friend or family member. Also, put medications in the bag that you use that were bought at a drug store, grocery store, convenience store, etc., without a prescription, or other nonprescription medication that you use that you got from a friend or family member."*

Each participant brought his/her bag of medications to the appointed time/place for review by the visiting pharmacist, who inquired whether the medications in the bag were still being taken, confirmed the precise regime (dose and schedule information), and entered all information on a prepared form (see Appendix C). The pharmacist provided immediate feedback to the participant if perceived to be in his/her best interest, or if requested at that time; otherwise, participants were provided with individualized feedback on their medication reviews at the conclusion of the project.

Behind-the-Wheel Driving Evaluation

The behind-the-wheel driving evaluation was scheduled by the OT/CDRS with each participant after completion of his/her medication review. At the appointed time, the OT/CDRS met the participant at an agreed-upon location at the residential community, confirmed that he/she held a valid driver's license, and recorded (based on self-report) what medications had been taken within the previous 12 hours. The individual's past medical history, plus driving history and driving restrictions, were also queried. This information, plus the date, time, and road/weather conditions during the evaluation, was recorded on a form developed by the OT/CDRS to score the evaluation outcomes (see Appendix D).

This form included varying numbers of items; each was scored individually as appropriate to behaviors observed under the categories of *vehicle entry, initiating driving/starting procedures, general driving, controlled intersections, uncontrolled intersections, turns, visual skills,* and *lot parking.* An overall rating was also assigned, and any/all interventions required by the OT/CDRS for safety during the driving evaluation were noted. At the end of the form, two items were included to record participants' ratings (7-point bipolar scale) of familiarity with, and frequency of exposure to, the roads traveled on during the driving evaluation. The OT/CDRS added comments and suggestions for improved driving habits on a separate page; these were reviewed with the individual after returning safely to the residential community.

The participant and evaluator proceeded to a parking lot on the premises for familiarization with the test vehicle, and to allow the OT/CDRS to perform a "closed course" evaluation of basic driving skills before leaving the grounds to drive in traffic. The test vehicle, a dual-brake-equipped 1996 Ford Taurus sedan, was loaned to TransAnalytics by NHTSA for this data collection activity.

Additional modifications and instrumentation of the test vehicle were carried out (1) to provide for the safety of the evaluator and examinee, and (2) to collect data to be used in comparing the attention of drivers during the evaluation versus driving alone in their own cars. In the first case, this included a second, inside rear-view mirror installed at the upper right of the windshield, so the OT/CDRS could monitor traffic behind the vehicle when riding in the passenger seat during an on-road evaluation. Special instrumentation included a camera box, with a driver (face) camera and forward road camera, plus a GPS receiver that was attached via suction cups in the center of the windshield just below and behind the rearview mirror. A lockable metal box containing a digital video recorder, a video processor, a DC-DC converter, and a voltage-controlled switch, was placed behind or under the front seat.

Figure 3 presents photos of the vehicle used for on-road testing, plus the items of equipment noted above. The upper left quadrant in Figure 3 shows the test vehicle.

The right half of Figure 3 contains a view of the camera box installed on the windshield (upper right) and of the inside of this enclosure (lower right). The GPS antenna is located in the top left of the camera box, the face camera is located underneath the antenna, and the road camera is to the right. The lower left quadrant shows a picture of the inside of the recording box with digital video recorder, video processor, a power converter, and voltage-controlled switch (to activate the recorder).

The photo above of the camera box mounted below the inside rearview mirror shows how this unit appeared to each older driver evaluated in this study. Participants reported that this device did not obstruct their view or distract them during the driving evaluation. The photos of the components within the camera and recording boxes also show the appearance of these units (during fabrication; not as seen by study participants) but do not clearly reveal their interconnections or functionality. For this information, refer to the schematic drawings in Figures 4 and 5 on the following page.

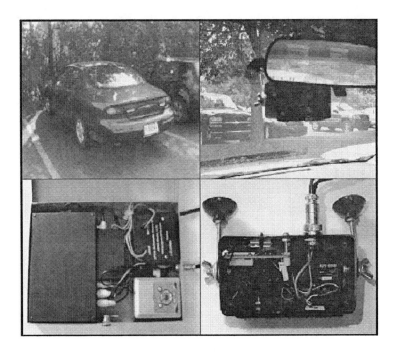

Figure 3. Test vehicle, face and road camera box, and video recording equipment.

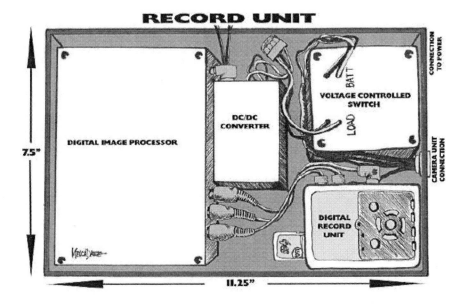

Figure 4. Video recording unit for the driver and road cameras in the test vehicle.

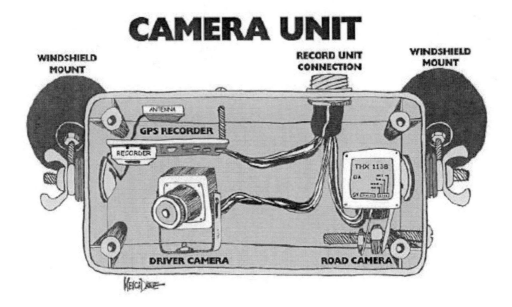

Figure 5. Driver and road camera, plus GPS unit, behind translucent faceplate.

The vehicle instrumentation described above was integrated with one additional data stream, namely, a continuous recording of speed, and brake and throttle position obtained through the on-board diagnostic (OBD) port that is available on all post-1995 vehicles sold in the United States. A commercially-available "car chip" was plugged into this port on the Ford Taurus test vehicle during the OT/CDRS driving evaluations.

Thus, the test vehicle instrumentation system, powered from a 12V DC adapter plugged into the cigarette lighter, was designed to record three types of data, as follows:

- Video: ASF format with 704x496 resolution and 12 Hz frame rate. Each trip is recorded into 10- to 100-second snippets (depending on the amount of motion in the video) which are later combined and rendered in post-processing to produce single clips for subsequent video coding analysis. The recorders were set to start recording automatically when powered on and stop recording when no motion was detected in the driver face view camera for at least 30 seconds.
- GPS: Standard NMEA sentences ($GPGGA for GPS time, latitude, longitude, heading, and $GPVTG for speed) were logged. The lat/long coordinates can be converted to KML format for display on Google Maps.
- OBD: Using the on-board diagnostics capability, the test vehicle speed (at 1 Hz sample rate), throttle position (1 sample every 5 seconds), and engine speed (1 sample every 5 seconds) were logged. The date/time was recorded at the beginning and end of each trip, requiring intermediate times to be interpolated.

These data sources were manually linked using date and time stamps common to each source. Video and OBD times were synchronized to an Internet time server prior to data collection; GPS time was logged directly from GPS satellites.

The OT/CDRS checked to see that all on-board equipment was functioning before meeting the examinees each day. As discussed later, the reliability of some components – the GPS unit, in particular – was not as good as the others, however, and this affected (but did not rule out) the planned comparisons of selected individuals' driving habits when in their own cars versus when driving the test vehicle with the evaluator riding in the passenger seat. It should be noted that *the function of the on-board instrumentation did not impact the OT/CDRS evaluation data in any way*; this outcome was based solely on the scores assigned on the evaluation form during the on-road test.

To begin the behind-the-wheel evaluation, the OT/CDRS typically drove the test vehicle to a location near the residential community that marked the beginning of a pre-planned route, which would be followed by every study participant from a given facility. After moving to the passenger seat, the OT/CDRS provided verbal driving directions for the remainder of the test route. Test routes were designed to include an initial segment of low-demand, residential driving, where a brake response time task (described below) was performed; this lead to driving on arterial routes where participants would encounter stop-sign- and signal-controlled intersections and the potential for conflict with other vehicles would increase significantly. One test route was developed in the Hockessin, DE, vicinity and another in the Parkville, MD, vicinity. Figures 6 and 7 show the roads in each route, including those segments designated for brake response time trials.

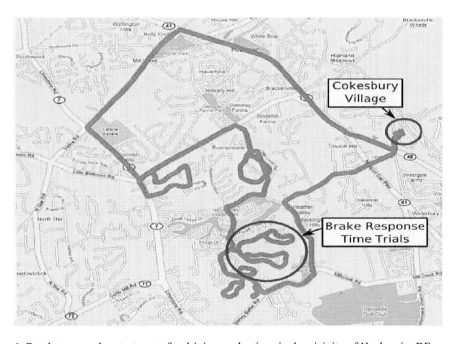

Figure 6. Roads traversed on test route for driving evaluations in the vicinity of Hockessin, DE.

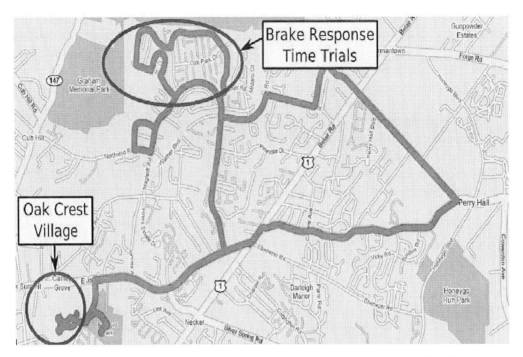

Figure 7. Roads traversed on test route for driving evaluations in the vicinity of Parkville, MD.

The brake response time trials were designed to provide an objective measure of performance (and possible differentiator among the study participants) to complement the driving evaluation scores. This was obtained by placing a small (4 in wide x 3 in high x 3 in deep) enclosure on the dashboard at the A-pillar, in the lower left corner of the windshield. An LCD faced the driver from the inside back of this enclosure. This display, which was connected to an onboard computer, was otherwise blank. But when triggered by the OT/CDRS in the passenger seat, via a button-push mechanism that was out of the driver's sight, one of two images would appear on the display: A "stop ahead" warning sign (MUTCD W3-1), or a stop sign (MUTCD R1-1), as shown below:

The OT/CDRS previewed these displays to each study participant, explaining that these displays would appear unexpectedly as he/she was driving in the residential area. In some cases, only the stop sign would appear, while in other cases the warning sign would appear first with the stop sign following a few seconds later. Participants were instructed to remove their right foot from the accelerator and press the brake as quickly as possible *only when the stop sign appeared*. On trials when the warning sign appeared, their instructions were to wait to respond until the stop sign was in view. A relay was installed on the brake switch circuit to record the RT data using the onboard computer.

W3-1

R1-1

It was hypothesized that (multiple) medication usage might affect the ability to inhibit a planned response, as well as having an effect on the actual brake response time to the stop sign presentation. Thus, both the number of errors (inappropriate brake responses to warning sign stimulus) and the brake RT on the un-alerted trials were scored. A photo of the (stop sign) display as seen by a study participant is shown in Figure 8.

Six practice trials were allowed while the test vehicle was parked, including an equal mix of "alerted" (warning sign followed by stop sign) and "un-alerted" (stop sign only) stimulus presentations. When confident that the study participant understood the instructions, the test drive resumed in the residential neighborhood, and the OT/CDRS triggered 3 more un-alerted and 3 more un-alerted trials while the driver was navigating through the neighborhood. Trial order was pre-programmed into the onboard computer. The OT/CDRS sought to trigger the stimulus presentations at the same exact locations for each study participant, but could alter the protocol if needed due to an unusual event, such as a homeowner backing out of a driveway in potential conflict with the test vehicle. All stimulus presentations for the brake response trials took place on the same streets, in the same residential neighborhoods (i.e., specific to each source community), and under the same conditions of weather (clear and dry) and traffic (none).

After completing the brake response time trials, the OT/CDRS provided verbal directions to the study participant that lead him/her out of the residential neighborhood, onto streets where speed limits were higher, a wider range of traffic control devices were present and maneuvers (e.g., turns) was required, and where there was a progressively higher probability of encounters (and potential conflicts) with other traffic. Throughout each driving evaluation, the OT/CDRS continuously noted scored participants' behavior as per the form included in Appendix D.

Each test drive lasted approximately 45 minutes, from the time the OT/CDRS and a study participant left the residential community, drove to the residential neighborhood and changed positions in the test vehicle, practiced and completed the brake response time trials, then proceeded with the behind-the-wheel evaluation and eventually arrived back at the CCRC, either Cokesbury Village or Oak Crest Village. At that time, the driving evaluator reviewed the individual's results with him/her, providing suggestions and recommendations as appropriate. For selected study participants, a tentative appointment was made at this time to equip the individual's own, personal vehicle with the instrumentation package to be used for the remaining data collection activity.

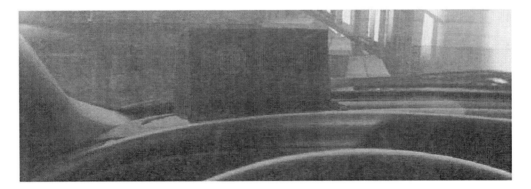

Figure 8. LCD display on dashboard, used for brake response time measure

294 National Highway Traffic Safety Administration

Instrumented Vehicle Comparison of Independent Driving and a Driving Evaluation

The instrumented vehicle portion of the study was designed to acquire 2-3 hours of additional time, location, and driving speed data, obtained over a period of up to one week, for each of five study participants (two males, three females). These individuals did not receive any additional compensation for this activity. This was an exploratory effort, essentially a "proof of concept" that (older) individuals would allow the installation of unobtrusive recording equipment in their own vehicles, and that an instrument package sufficient to the present data needs could be affordably integrated from off-the-shelf electronics and would work reliably – without intervention or maintenance – for an extended period.

The instrumentation package included the same components identified earlier – a video recorder box (under seat) and two-camera enclosure (mounted on windshield under the insider rearview mirror), plus the "car chip" plugged into the OBD2 port to sample vehicle speed once every second. A GPS unit was also placed inside the camera box. As before, a 12V adapter plugged into the cigarette lighter powered these devices, using a motion sensitive switch to ensure that they were in operation only when the vehicle was driven to protect the battery. Connecting cables were tucked under molding, carpet, etc., in participants' vehicles. The cost of each instrument package was under $800, and it required approximately 30 minutes to install and test the components for use in an individual's private car.

As noted earlier, the goal in this data collection activity was to permit a comparison of an (older) driver's behavior when he/she is driving in a test vehicle, with an evaluator, to that same individual's behavior and habits when driving in the same milieu in his/her own vehicle, without an evaluator in the car. To that end, the five study participants were asked to drive according to their normal habits and patterns while their cars were instrumented, with the understanding that such driving could but was not required to include roads in common with the test route they had driven on during their evaluations with the OT/CDRS.

After five to seven days, by appointment, the instrumentation was removed from each participant's car and was returned to TransAnalytics' offices, to offload speed (car chip), location (GPS), and video data for later analysis. An inspection of each participant's vehicle was conducted to ensure that no damage had resulted from the installation of the instrument package.

Data Analysis

Two sets of analyses were conducted in this study. The **primary** analyses, which included the entire sample of older drivers taking known *potentially drive- impairing* medications, were designed to reveal the extent to which driver characteristics—including medication usage—could account for categorical differences in (1) an on-road driving evaluation based on scores assigned by an Occupation Therapist/ Certified Driver Rehabilitation Specialist (OT/CDRS); (2) objective measures of brake reaction time (BRT); and (3) functional status measures using a computer-based battery of tests validated as

A Pilot Study to Test Multiple Medication Usage and Driving Functioning 295

significant predictors of at-fault crash risk in previous NHTSA research. These were between-subjects analyses.

Secondary analyses were performed for the subset of the study sample for whom an instrumentation package was installed in their personal vehicles for a week to unobtrusively monitor their driving habits. These analyses examined differences in attentional behavior—operationally defined as glance direction—as a function of the level of demand of the road/traffic situation, when an individual was driving independently in his/her own car compared to during the on-road evaluation with the OT/CDRS. These analyses relied heavily on the video recordings of the driver's face and the external roadway scene, and entailed an extensive data reduction/coding effort, described below. The secondary analyses were focused on within-subject differences.

Primary Analyses: Effects of Driver Characteristics/Medications

Analysis technique. A total of 21 analyses spanning three different types of dependent measures are described below. These explored the relationships between medication usage and/or other characteristics that distinguish the older drivers in the test sample, and the behaviors used as outcome measures in this research. Outcomes included measures of driving performance and driver functioning, which were scored in terms of broad, categorical differences between study participants. Certain measures (e.g., driving evaluation scores) were recorded only as categorical data; while other measures (brake reaction time) that were initially recorded as continuous data were re-coded as categories of performance. This approach may be justified both in terms of the exploratory nature of this research, and the prolific number of combinations of medications examined herein coupled with the modest effect that can be expected for any particular types of drugs among a group of generally healthy, active seniors. The goal in each analysis was to identify the combination of medications (and/or other driver characteristics) that could best separate study participants according to the classifications of behavior used for a given outcome variable. A linear modeling approach, Logistic Regression, was chosen for these analyses.

Independent/predictor variables. The driver characteristics of greatest interest in these analyses were the prescription drugs, both PDI and non-PDI medications, plus over-the-counter drugs taken by the study participants. All medications identified during the pharmacist reviews were logged according to their *therapeutic class*, not their brand or generic name. In some cases multiple *subclasses* of drugs—though directed at a common therapeutic intervention (e.g., to control high blood pressure)—were distinguished by their metabolic or pharmacological action. These are shown in Table 10 and Table 11.

Other driver characteristics aside from medication usage serving as independent/predictor variables in these analyses included driver age (years); gender; residence (CCRC) location; the study participant's level of familiarity with the driving evaluation route; and the frequency of exposure to all or part of the driving evaluation route in his/her everyday travel. The latter were integer ratings, from "1" to "7" on a bipolar scale where "1" was the lowest score (least familiar; least often traveled) and "7" was the highest score (most familiar; most often traveled).

Table 10. Classes and subclasses of prescription drugs represented in the study sample.

Drug Class and Subclass	Drug Class and Subclass
Antihypertensive Alpha 1 Adrenergic Blocker Beta Blocker ACE Inhibitor Calcium Channel Blocker Combo Calcium Channel Blocker – ACE Inhibitor Angiotensin II Receptor Antagonist Loop Diuretics Potassium Sparing Diuretic Thiazide Diuretic Combination Diuretic	Antidiabetic Sulfonylurea Biguanide Alpha Glucosidase Inhibitor Thiazolidine Dipeptidyl peptidase 4
	Osteoporosis Calcitonin Hormone Bisphosphonate
	Cholesterol Lowering HMG-COA Reductase Inhibitor Antilipemic
Antidepressants	Antianxiety
SSRI	Benzodiazepine
SNRI	Anti-Anxiety Non-BZD
Asthma	Nasal Spray
	Antihistamine
Beta Adrenergic Agents	Anticholinergic
Inhaled Steroid	Steroid
Anticoagulant (Coumadin Type)	Immunomodulator
Antiarrhthmic	Antibiotic
5 Alpha Reductase Inhibitor	Antihistamines - Non Sedating
Antipsychotic	Corticosteroid
Anti Mania	Phosphodiesterase 5 Enzyme Inhibitor
Anti Convulsant	Thyroid Supplement
Aromatase Inhibitor	Potassium Supplement
Cholinesterase Inhibitor	Selective Estrogen Receptive Modulator
Dopamine Agonist	Hormone Replacement Topical Cream
CNS Stimulant	Topical Antibiotic
Proton Pump Inhibitor	Glaucoma Drops
Antispasmodics GU	Steroid Eye Drops
NSAID	Opiate Agonist

Table 11. Classes and subclasses of OTC medications represented in the study sample

Drug Class and Subclass	Drug Class and Subclass
OTC Analgesic	OTC Antacid
OTC Antihistamine (Sedating)	OTC H2 Blocker
OTC Analgesic Antihistamine (Combination)	OTC Cough Drops
OTC Topical Analgesic	OTC Vitamin/Mineral
OTC Antiplatelet	OTC Laxative

A Pilot Study to Test Multiple Medication Usage and Driving Functioning 297

Table 11. (Continued)

Drug Class and Subclass	Drug Class and Subclass
OTC/Joint Supplement	OTC Saline Nasal Spray
OTC Eye Tears	OTC/Fish Oil Supplement
OTC/Eye Supplement	OTC Antiflatulant
OTC/Herbal	OTC Antifungal Topical

Initially, all 72 of the medication classes and subclasses shown in Tables 10 and 11 were included in the present analyses. For every entry in these tables, a "0" or a "1" was entered in each study participant's data file to denote whether s/he was or was not using the medication in question. However, an initial run using PROC LOGISTIC in SAS revealed a number of problems with this analysis approach. Usage data for eight medications was constant; it was necessary to discard these from the model, as things that do not vary cannot be useful predictors. The data for 23 other predictors was completely collinear — that is, these values were totally predicted by some linear combination of other variables in the model. These problems were addressed by combining drugs with related therapeutic applications into a reduced number – 16 – of categories, to allow entry of the medication usage data into the present analyses. This classification scheme is apparent in Appendix E, which identifies the specific PDI and non-PDI drugs taken by all participants as per the pharmacist review and as per self-report to the OT/CDRS just prior to their driving evaluations. The drug classifications only (i.e., used as analysis variables) are listed below:

- Antihypertensive diuretic
- Antihypertensive non-diuretic
- Anti-platelet/anticoagulant
- Anti-diabetic
- Neurologic
- Osteoporosis
- Gastric acid secretion reducer
- Cholesterol lowering
- Anti-spasmodics GU
- Non-steroidal anti-inflammatory drugs (NSAID)
- Antidepressants/antianxiety
- PDI eye preparations
- Sedating antihistamines
- Vitamins/minerals/supplements
- PDI other
- Non-PDI other

Dependent/criterion variables. Three broad criterion variables were selected for the primary analyses: *driving evaluation, brake response,* and *functional status.* For the planned analyses, a varying number of specific measures of interest were identified in each of these areas, each containing a specified number of data levels or categories. As noted earlier, these analyses were designed to test the ability of the regression model to sort study participants into categories of performance based on medication usage and other driver characteristics.

The measures selected for analysis under *driving evaluation* are identified below, with the outcomes categorized as indicated. All outcomes reflected scores assigned by the OT/CDRS, using the form referenced earlier (also see appendix D). A separate analysis was planned for each of the following measures:

- Overall rating of driving competence: four categories
  1 = Concerns about driving
  2 = Fair driver/ lacks numerous good driving habits
  3 = Adequate driver/few potential problems
  4 = Good driver/no concerns
- General driving errors: two categories
  1 = Safety is compromised: inconsistent performance; single error or pattern of errors
  2 = Safety is *not* compromised: consistent performance, only minor errors; skills are adequate (but a comment may be added as a qualifier)
- Controlled intersection driving errors: two categories *(same as above)*
- Uncontrolled intersection errors: two categories *(same as above)*
- Turns errors: two categories *(same as above)*
- Visual skills errors: two categories *(same as above)*
- Evaluator intervention: two categories
  1 = dual brake and/or steering intervention by evaluator required
  2 = no brake or steering intervention by evaluator required

For *brake response,* two behaviors were selected for analysis: the number of errors on the "alerted" trials—where the subject responded to the alerting stimulus instead of to the target stimulus—and the reaction time on the un-alerted trials. For the former measure, there were three alerted trials presented to each subject, so the range of possible scores (response categories) for number of errors was 0 to 3. These data were categorized as follows:

- Response errors/alerted trials: four categories
  1 = 0 errors
  2 = 1 error
  3 = 2 errors
  4 = 3 errors

For the latter measure, the raw brake reaction time (BRT), in milliseconds, was calculated as the mean of the three un-alerted trials presented to each subject; these means were then sorted into quartiles. The raw, un-alerted BRT means for the 44 field study participants, ranged from 0.653 s to 4.315 s. The categories selected for analysis are indicated below:

- BRT quartiles/unalerted trials: four categories
  1 = 0.653 s to 0.877 s
  2 = 0.877 s to 1.065 s
  3 = 1.065 s to 1.356 s
  4 = 1.356 s to 4.315 s

A Pilot Study to Test Multiple Medication Usage and Driving Functioning

For the remaining criterion variable, *functional status*, the measures selected for analysis included two measures of physical ability (leg strength/general mobility and head/neck flexibility); two measures of visual ability (static visual acuity, at high and low contrast); and four measures of cognitive ability (working memory, visual search with divided attention, visuospatial ability/visual closure, and visual information processing speed with divided attention). Categories of performance were assigned for each measure using cut points defined during the NHTSA research project, *Model Driver Screening and Evaluation Program*; also see Staplin, Gish, and Wagner (2003). These are indicated below:

- Head/neck flexibility: two categories – level of apparent deficit
  0 = no deficit (pass)
  1 = deficit present (fail)
- Leg strength/general mobility: three categories – level of apparent deficit
  1 = no deficit
  2 = mild deficit
  3 = serious deficit
- Acuity/high contrast: three categories *(same as above)*
- Acuity/low contrast: three3 categories *(same as above)*
- Working memory: three categories *(same as above)*
- Visuospatial ability/visual closure: three categories *(same as above)*
- Information processing speed, with divided attention: three categories *(same as above)*
- Visual search, with divided attention: three categories *(same as above)*

Preliminary runs using PROC LOGISTIC revealed additional problems associated with the selection of criterion variables as outlined above. Some of these variables have very few (one or two) individuals populating a given category level. This indicated a need both to reduce the overall number of outcomes examined in the analyses, and to further consolidate data into fewer categories for each of the remaining variables, to increase cell sizes.

These problems were addressed by selecting only four outcome measures – two *driving evaluation* measures and one each for *brake response* and *functional status* – for a revised analysis approach that could potentially allow a successful fit to the regression model. In addition, performance was recoded into only two categories for each measure, as follows.

- **Analysis 1.** This analysis of the overall OT/CDRS rating of driving competence seeks to predict which individuals received scores of 1 or 2 (fair driver, with numerous bad habits *or* OT has definite concerns) versus 3 or 4 (good driver, no concerns *or* adequate driver with only a few potential problems).
- **Analysis 2.** This analysis retains the "evaluator intervention" variable from the previous list, seeking to predict which study participants' behavior *did* versus *did not* elicit an intervention of *any kind* by the OT/CDRS.
- **Analysis 3.** This analysis of brake response time seeks to predict only which study participants scored in the top half (quartiles 1 *or* 2, as specified earlier) versus the bottom half (quartiles 3 *or* 4) of the BRT distribution, for the "unalerted" trials.

300 National Highway Traffic Safety Administration

- **Analysis 4.** This analysis focuses on the four cognitive measures (the last four items in the list above), seeking to predict which study participants scored in the "no deficit" *or* "mild deficit" ranges versus the "serious deficit" range for anyof these functional status indicators.

Secondary Analyses: Behavioral Variability Within Subjects

A secondary set of analyses explored differences in a measure of driver attention – moment-to-moment gaze direction – as a function of road and traffic conditions, for specified maneuvers, for independent driving versus the formal (OT/CDRS) driving evaluation carried out in this research, for a selected sub-sample of older drivers. An additional case study analysis contrasted speed choice by a single subject on identical roads, traversed alone (personal vehicle) and with the OT/CDRS. The following analyses used data obtained via the in-vehicle instrumentation package.

The first analysis required the two-camera (driver's face and forward road scene) video to be coded in terms of four elements: glance, infrastructure, traffic, and maneuver. These elements, in turn, were each defined in terms of a set of mutually exclusive attributes, as listed below. More extensive descriptions for coding attributes are provided in Appendix F.

GLANCE:
straight ahead through the windshield;
right only;
left only;
right+up (inside mirror);
down+ inside (dashboard, radio, etc.);
over shoulder (left or right).

INFRASTRUCTURE:
continuous, unbroken section of roadway;
stop-controlled intersection;
signalized intersection;
intersection with channelization for merge/yield— driver in turn lane;
school or pedestrian crossing;
at-grade rail crossing;
parking lot or garage.

TRAFFIC:
no threat of any conflicts with other traffic;
car following only—same or adjacent lane (rear-end crash potential);
opposing traffic only (head-on or angle crash potential);
car following and opposing traffic.

MANEUVER:
same path moving forward;
driver turns left;
driver turns right;
driver changes lanes (right or left);
driver overtakes/passes another vehicle;
backing/reverse movement;

driver's vehicle is stopped/no movement.

For each of the four elements above, one attribute was coded for every frame of video recorded in the independent drives and OT/CDRS driving evaluations, at 12 frames of video per second (12 Hz). In other words, subjects' data files included an entry for glance, infrastructure, traffic, and maneuver approximately every 1/8 of a second. The software tool used for this data coding task was Anvil (Kipp, 2001). The interface used for video data coding is displayed in Figure 9, showing each attribute value for the selected frame.

The coding of "behavior in context" from continuous, in-car video, as described above, provides data sufficient to address a large number of research questions relating to driver adaptation/compensation to varying traffic/demand conditions, in addition to providing heretofore scarce evidence of (older) drivers' actual (i.e., instead of self-reported) exposure patterns. Given the limited scope of this pilot investigation, two questions of particular interest to this research team were framed for the present analyses:

(1) *"Across all traffic, infrastructure, and maneuver attribute values excluding "car following only," "parking lot or garage," and "driver's vehicle stopped/no movement," respectively, how does drivers' glance behavior correlate between independent driving in their own vehicles and their driving evaluations with the OT/CDRS?"*

(2) *"For the specific scenario when an (older) driver is negotiating a signalized intersection – approaching and then continuing through without turning – what is the correlation in glance behavior between independent driving and driving with the OT/CDRS, under the same traffic (demand) conditions."*

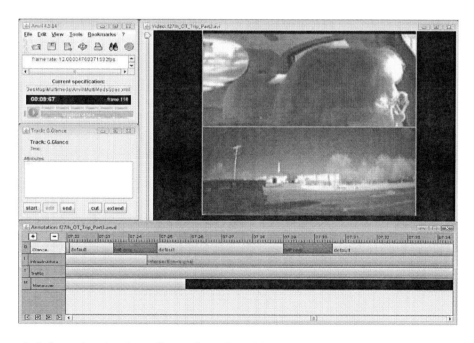

Figure 9. Software interface for coding attributes from driver face (top) and road camera (bottom) continuous video.

The former correlation was calculated using pooled data from the five drivers in the sub-sample, to offer an overall comparison between the two modes (independent driving versus driving evaluation). Virtually all aspects of road geometry, traffic operations, and driving maneuvers are included in this comparison. The latter correlation was calculated for only the selected video frames associated with codes denoting a "forward moving" maneuver, at a "signalized intersection," for matched traffic conditions.

In both cases, these correlations were based on the number of video frames where the included drivers were looking straight ahead, versus to the left, right, down/inside vehicle, up/right at the inside rearview mirror, or over their shoulder, for their independent drives versus their OT/CDRS driving evaluations, for just those frames where the driver was moving, on a public street or highway, and not in a car-following mode.

In the second, "case study" analysis, the correspondence between one subject's speed choice during independent travel compared to her OT/CDRS driving evaluation, for travel over identical sections of road, at roughly the same time of day, was examined. The date/time/place match between the two drives was based on GPS data, as were the speeds examined in this analysis.

It may be noted that the obtained match in driving locations for this subject was fortuitous; her independent driving while the on-board instrumentation package was installed was not scripted or directed in any way by the research team. Also, the reader should understand that this was a purely descriptive exercise, based on data analyzed for a single subject; its purpose was to explore the feasibility and utility of this approach for future investigations of within-subject variability in driving habits.

PILOT TEST RESULTS

Data Summary

Descriptive statistics reporting key sample characteristics follow. The composition of the study sample by age, gender, and location (residential community) is indicated in Table 12. As indicated, study participants ranged in age from 57 to 89, with a mean of 78.82 and median of 80. The sample was composed of 18 (41%) males and 26 (59%) females. Twenty-four, or 55% of the sample, were residents at the Cokesbury Village CCRC, while 20 (or 45%) were from the Erickson residential communities.

Table 12. Composition of study sample

Sample Characteristic	Cokesbury	Erickson	Overall
Number of Participants	24	20	44
Males/Females	12/12	6/14	18/26
Age Range	57-89	68-86	57-89
Mean Age	78.6	79.1	78.8
Median Age	80	82	80

An overview of the medication classes and subclasses used by study participants, in the aggregate, was presented earlier in Tables 10 and 11. A graphical summary of the number of classes of PDI and non-PDI drugs used by study participants according to their "brown bag" medication review with the visiting pharmacist review is presented in Figure 10; these same counts of PDI and non-PDI drugs according to study participants' self-reports on the day of their driving evaluations are displayed in Figure 11. As indicated, the number of medication (classes) that could potentially influence driving performance (or functional status) measures were fewer than the number identified in each individual's pharmacological inventory. For a comprehensive, person-level tabulation of the PDI and non-PDI drugs identified during the pharmacist reviews, and as taken on the day of each individual's driving evaluation, see Appendix E.

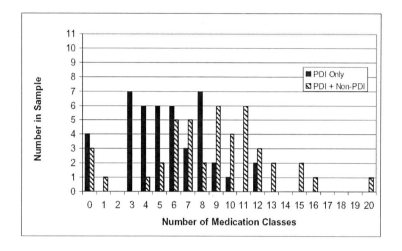

Figure 10. PDI and non-PDI medication usage by research sample: pharmacist review.

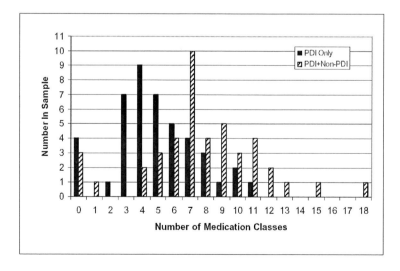

Figure 11. PDI and non-PDI medication usage by research sample: self-report before driving evaluation.

The correlation of study participants' ages with the number of PDI medications they reported on the day of their driving evaluations was calculated. The result was $r = 0.09$ (n.s.).

The request that study participants obtain letters/printouts listing their prescription medications from their pharmacists yielded very few responses; and those few could be incomplete, to the extent that individuals stated that they obtained medications from multiple sources. Thus, one clear-cut result in this work is the demonstrated superiority of the "brown bag" method to acquire information about the medication usage of (older) drivers. It is also important to note, however, that while a "brown bag" review may produce a complete inventory of the drugs in an individual's possession, some or many may be taken on an "as needed" basis, so studies attempting to relate the use of specific drugs or combinations of drugs to driving performance must query medication use at the time of testing.

The results for the driving performance measures obtained for this research sample are summarized in Table 13. Both the subjective (OT/CDRS ratings) and objective (un-alerted brake response time) data were categorized into four levels for analysis, as described earlier. Table 13 indicates the number and percent of study participants at each performance level, for the overall driving evaluation ratings. As shown, only 8 of 44 study participants were scored by the OT/CDRS at level 1 ("concerns about driving") or level 2 ("lacks numerous good driving habits"). This table also shows that the mean response time even for the slowest quartile of study participants, 1.87 sec, falls well within the "design driver" *perception-response time* of 2.5 sec used by the highway engineering community. However, while these trials are labeled "un-alerted," they represent data from an experiment where an evaluator was riding with the respondent, and so may not be compared directly with "surprise" conditions when a person driving independently, in traffic, must react to an unexpected object/threat in their path.

The results of the computer-based measures of functional abilities for the present research sample are displayed in Table 14. Forty study participants completed these measures; data are missing for four individuals due to equipment/software problems. Table 14 shows the number and percent of the sample for who *no* deficit, a *mild* deficit, or a *serious* deficit was indicated by the screening protocol, for each measure. Inspection of these results reveals that, as expected, only a minority of the research sample appeared to have a serious deficit on any given measure. An exception was shown for the "head/neck flexibility" measure, which has also been associated with an elevated failure rate in the Maryland pilot older driver study (Staplin et al., 2003). It is uncertain whether this reflects a methodological artifact or a genuine prevalence level of stiff/arthritic neck and upper torso conditions among this cohort.

Table 13. Data summary for subjective and objective driving performance measures

Measure	N	Performance level (number and percent of sample)			
		1 (worst)	2	3	4 (best)
OT/CDRS evaluation: overall rating	44	4	4	20	16
Brake response time: un-alerted trials	44	Performance level (mean RT by quartile, in seconds)			
		1 (slowest)	2	3	4 (fastest)
		1.87	1.20	0.94	0.75

A Pilot Study to Test Multiple Medication Usage and Driving Functioning

Table 14. Functional status of study participants, by screening measure

Measure	N	Functional Status (Number and Percent of Sample)		
		No deficit	Mild deficit	Serious deficit
Acuity/high contrast	40	38 (95%)	1 (2.5%)	1 (2.5%)
Acuity/low contrast	39	35 (90%)	3 (8%)	1 (2%)
Leg strength/mobility	40	34 (85%)	5 (13%)	1 (2%)
Head/neck mobility	40	17 (43%)	--	23 (5 8%)
Visuospatial ability/ visual closure	40	26 (65%)	8 (20%)	6 (15%)
Visual search/divided attention	40	10 (25%)	27 (68%)	3 (7%)
Working memory	40	27 (68%)	7 (17%)	6 (15%)
Information processing speed/divided attention	40	25 (63%)	6 (15%)	9 (22%)

In Table 15, additional detail is provided to show the number of study participants, average age of participants, and the average number of both the medication classes and PDI-medication classes—according to both the pharmacist review and as reported on the day of their driving evaluation—for all who scored in the "no deficit," "mild deficit," and "serious deficit" category on each functional test.

Table 15. Functional status by participant's age and medication use

Deficit Level	Number of Subjects	Average Age	Pharmacist Review: Average Number of MedicationClasses	Pharmacist Review: Average Number of PDI Medication Classes	Self-Report Before Driving Evaluation: Average Number of Medication Classes	Self-Report Before Driving Evaluation: Average Number of PDI Medication Classes
Measure: Acuity/high contrast						
No Deficit	38	78.4	8.79	5.48	7.74	4.87
Mild Deficit	1	85	8	5	8	5
Serious Deficit	1	81	9	4	7	4
Measure: Acuity/low contrast						
No Deficit	35	78.03	8.74	5.4	7.66	4.83
Mild Deficit	3	84.67	9	6.33	8.33	5.67
Serious Deficit	1	81	9	4	7	4
Measure: Leg strength/mobility						
No Deficit	34	78.3	9.09	5.59	7.94	4.97
Mild Deficit	5	82.6	5.8	3.2	5.2	3
Serious Deficit	1	69	13	10	13	10

Table 15. (Continued)

Deficit Level	Number of Subjects	Average Age	Pharmacist Review: Average Number of MedicationClasses	Pharmacist Review: Average Number of PDI Medication Classes	Self-Report Before Driving Evaluation: Average Number of Medication Classes	Self-Report Befor Driving Evaluation: Average Number of PDI Medication Classes
Measure: Head/neck mobility						
No Deficit	17	77.1	8.88	5.65	7.94	5.24
Serious Deficit	23	79.8	8.69	5.22	7.57	4.56
Measure: Visuospatial ability/visual closure						
No Deficit	26	79.7	7.65	4.66	7	4.31
Mild Deficit	8	76.3	9.75	6.63	8.25	5.88
Serious Deficit	6	77.3	12.33	7.0	10.17	5.83
Measure: Visual search/divided attention						
No Deficit	10	76.5	8.6	5.2	7.5	4.5
Mild Deficit	27	79.2	8.41	5.26	7.48	4.85
Serious Deficit	3	80.7	12.67	7.33	10.67	6.0
Measure: Working memory						
No Deficit	27	76.7	9.67	6.04	8.67	5.52
Mild Deficit	7	81.9	7.85	4.71	6.0	3.71
Serious Deficit	6	83.3	5.83	3.33	5.5	3.17
Measure: Visual information processing speed/divided attention						
No Deficit	25	78.9	8.36	5.04	4.6	7.32
Mild Deficit	6	79.2	9.83	5.83	5.5	8.83
Serious Deficit	9	77.6	9.22	6.11	5.11	8.11

These results indicate that poorer performance (greater deficit) was not always associated with increasing age, nor with increasing medication usage. These mixed findings are highlighted in the results for the measures of cognitive function, which are both the strongest crash predictors, and are those for which a relationship with medication usage might logically seem most likely. Specifically, the data for visuospatial ability and processing speed show no direct relationship with age, and only a weak relationship is evident for the visual search measure. The incidence of a serious deficit in working memory with increasing age is more pronounced, however. At the same time, there is a general trend toward greater deficits with increasing medication usage for three of four measures of cognitive ability; but for the memory measure there is an inverse relationship: those who manifested *greater* memory deficits were taking *fewer* drugs, overall, and fewer PDI drugs as well.

These results underscore the importance of (1) individual measures to determine functional (cognitive) status, rather than using chronological age as a proxy; and (2) looking beyond simply the number of drugs a person is taking when examining the potential associations between medication usage, age, and driving performance. A more detailed data summary for specific combinations of variables of interest follows. These include tabulations, presented graphically in Appendix G, of the *age x medication* profiles for study participants who are further classified according to (1) driving evaluation rating (four levels), (2) brake response time (four levels), and (3) evidence of cognitive deficit (3 levels), respectively.

Looking first at the age-by-drug profiles for performance, as scored by the OT/CDRS, only 4 participants "failed" the driving evaluation. The age range of these participants was 83 to 88, and the number of PDI medications ranged from 4 to 8. Moving to the color-coded profile for medication class by un-alerted brake response time quartile, the 11 participants who scored the poorest ranged in age from 76 to 89, with the majority (82%) 83 or older. The number of PDI medications for these 11 participants ranged from 0 to 8. Finally, the drug profile color- coded to denote levels of cognitive deficit (none, mild, or serious) shows subjects with serious cognitive deficits ranging in age from 68 to 88, and taking medications in 0 to 11 PDI drug classes. It appears that neither age nor number of PDI medications can adequately explain performance on these outcome measures.

One potential explanation for the small number of participants who failed the driving evaluation according to the OT/CDRS, compared to the number of participants with serious cognitive deficits, is that the demands of the test route were not high enough to elicit driving errors commensurate with the cognitive deficits suggested by the functional screening measures. It is interesting to note that the subset of failing older drivers (as scored by the OT/CDRS) is also the oldest. This may be explained by the fact that PDI medications are more impairing to driving performance for the oldest participants due to the way the aging liver metabolizes medications, and other physiological changes that occur with aging, i.e., reduced body mass and basal metabolic rate, reduced proportion of body water, increased proportion of body fat, decreased cardiac output, altered relative tissue perfusion, decreased plasma protein binding, reduced gastric acid production and gastric emptying time, and reduced gut motility and blood flow (Herrlinger and Klotz, 2001). Still, it should be noted that study participants who appear to have one or more serious cognitive deficits (denoted by red shading in the third graphic in Appendix G) include individuals in each decade from 68 to 88.

Part of the difficulty in detecting any pattern of changes in performance with changes in drug profiles is the strong overlap in the pharmacopeia of the research sample due to the inclusion criteria for the study. Participants were initially recruited on the basis of taking an ACE inhibitor to control hypertension, plus another PDI medication from one of three other classes (gastric acid secretion reducers, antidepressants, or cholesterol-lowering drugs). These criteria were subsequently relaxed to allow people taking any antihypertensive plus another PDI medication to participate. The result was that a large majority of study participants were taking antihypertensive medications (39 of the 44 were taking non-diuretic antihypertensive medications, and 23 were taking diuretic antihypertensive medications); and nearly as many (36 of 44) were taking cholesterol-lowering medications.

Despite this artifact of the selection strategy for study recruitment, the data relating age and medication class to driving performance, as summarized in the first graphic in Appendix G, may deserve a closer look – in particular, the entries for ACE Inhibitors. ACE Inhibitors (e.g., Lisinopril, Accupril, Altace) decrease the activity of angiotensin and as a result, blood vessels dilate and blood pressure is reduced. LeRoy and Morse (2005) found that drivers taking ACE inhibitors experienced a motor vehicle crash rate that was 23% greater

(OR=1.23) than that of drivers not taking these medications. Dizziness, drowsiness, excessive tiredness, weakness, and lightheadedness are potential side effects that could impair safe driving performance. In this context, it may be noteworthy that 75% of the sample who "failed" the OT evaluation in the present study were taking an ACE inhibitor, compared to 50% who received a rating of "fair," 35% who received a rating of "adequate," and 25% who received a rating of "good." A similar pattern was not observed in the graphic summarizing the (categorical) performance on the unalerted brake response time task, where 36% of both the best- performing and worst-performing participants were taking this medication. However, when considering the apparent level of cognitive deficit indicated by the included screening measures, 37% of those with a serious deficit and 36% of those with a mild deficit were taking ACE inhibitors, compared to only 14% of those without any apparent deficits. Thus, a pattern may be broadly discerned in this sample, whereby ACE inhibitors are associated with poorer outcomes on multiple safety surrogates.

At a still finer level, the combination of ACE inhibitors and thiazide diuretics appears potentially problematic. Side effects of thiazide diuretics include hypotension and dizziness. This combination may cause synergistic effects, increasing the risk of hypotension (abnormally low blood pressure) and leading to lightheaded, dizziness, and even fainting and seizures, if blood pressure becomes too low. The age-by-medication profiles depicted in Appendix G reveal that, of those "failing" the OT/CDRS driving evaluation, 25% (1 of 4) were taking this combination on the day of their evaluation, as were 25% (1 in 4) of those who scored "fair." This compares to 10% (2 of 20) of those scored as "adequate," and only 6% (1 in 16) of those scored as "good" on their driving evaluations. At the same time, 18% of those in the worst-performing quartile on the brake response time task were taking this combination, compared to 9% in the best-performing quartile. And, study participants without any apparent cognitive deficits were free of the ACE inhibitor/thiazide diuretic combination, while 14% of those with a mild deficit and 5% of those with a serious deficit were using these two drugs together.

These preliminary observations about possible driver-impairing effects of multiple medication usage are placed in context by scholarly reviews of the relationship between age and human drug metabolism (Herrlinger & Klotz, 2001; Schmucker, 2001; and Kinirons & O'Mahony, 2004). All of these authors conclude that although some measures of drug metabolism are diminished in the elderly, this population is characterized by significant inter-individual variability in drug metabolism, drug action, and adverse reactions. Certainly, the tentative results described above do not in any way diminish the importance of individual assessment of the ability to drive safely.

Logistic Regression

Four separate stepwise logistic regression analyses were performed using SAS, one for each of the following classification outcome variables:

- Cognitive status – seeking to predict which study participants scored in the "no deficit" *or* "mild deficit" ranges versus the "serious deficit" range for anyof the included functional ability measures in this domain.

A Pilot Study to Test Multiple Medication Usage and Driving Functioning 309

- OT intervention – seeking to predict which study participants' behavior *did* versus *did not* elicit an intervention by the OT/CDRS.
- Brake response time – seeking to predict which study participants scored in the top half (quartiles 1 *or* 2) versus the bottom half (quartiles 3 *or* 4) of the BRT distribution, for the "un-alerted" trials.
- Driver evaluation – seeking to predict which individuals received scores of 1 or 2 (fair driver, with numerous bad habits *or* OT has definite concerns) versus 3 or 4 (good driver, no concerns *or* adequate driver with only a few potential problems).

The analysis of effects statistics for each regression model appears below.

Analysis of effects for cognitive status *Analysis of effects for OT intervention*

Type 3 Analysis of Effects			
Effect	DF	Wald Chi-Square	Pr > ChiSq
Antidepressants_Anti	1	0.0042	0.9485
Antidiabetic	1	2.9847	0.0841
AntihypertensiveDiur	1	0.0092	0.9237
AntihypertensiveNonD	1	0.0381	0.8451
AntiPlatelet_Anticoa	1	0.0166	0.8976
Antispasmodics_GU	1	0.0468	0.8288
CholesterolLowering	1	0.0353	0.8509
GastricAcidSecretion	1	0.7668	0.3812
Neurologic	1	0.0130	0.9091
NSAIDs	1	0.0758	0.7831
Osteoporosis	1	0.1564	0.6925
PDIEyePreparations	1	0.2963	0.5862
PDIOther	1	1.7715	0.1832
SedatingAntihistamin	1	1.6977	0.1926

Type 3 Analysis of Effects			
Effect	DF	Wald Chi-Square	Pr > ChiSq
Antidepressants_Anti	1	0.0254	0.8733
Antidiabetic	1	0.0080	0.9288
AntihypertensiveDiur	1	0.0148	0.9032
AntihypertensiveNonD	1	0.0044	0.9469
AntiPlatelet_Anticoa	1	0.0093	0.9230
Antispasmodics_GU	1	0.0006	0.9806
CholesterolLowering	1	0.0005	0.9815
GastricAcidSecretion	1	0.0251	0.8742
Neurologic	1	0.0032	0.9551
NSAIDs	1	0.0161	0.8991
Osteoporosis	1	0.0170	0.8961
PDIEyePreparations	1	0.0071	0.9330
PDIOther	1	0.0116	0.9142
SedatingAntihistamin	1	0.0009	0.9762

Analysis of effects for brake response time *Analysis of effects for driver evaluation*

Type 3 Analysis of Effects			
Effect	DF	Wald Chi-Square	Pr > ChiSq
Antidepressants_Anti	1	0.0141	0.9055
Antidiabetic	1	1.0865	0.2973
AntihypertensiveDiur	1	1.1426	0.2851
AntihypertensiveNonD	1	0.0161	0.8991
AntiPlatelet_Anticoa	1	0.6569	0.4177
Antispasmodics_GU	1	0.0134	0.9079
CholesterolLowering	1	0.0175	0.8949
GastricAcidSecretion	1	0.1689	0.6811
Neurologic	1	0.0023	0.9616
NSAIDs	1	0.4581	0.4985
Osteoporosis	1	2.4712	0.1159
PDIEyePreparations	1	1.2059	0.2721
PDIOther	1	1.7511	0.1857
SedatingAntihistamin	1	0.2780	0.5980

Type 3 Analysis of Effects			
Effect	DF	Wald Chi-Square	Pr > ChiSq
Antidepressants_Anti	1	0.0586	0.8088
Antidiabetic	1	0.0176	0.8946
AntihypertensiveDiur	1	0.0086	0.9262
AntihypertensiveNonD	1	0.0052	0.9422
AntiPlatelet_Anticoa	1	0.0118	0.9134
Antispasmodics_GU	1	0.0525	0.8188
GastricAcidSecretion	1	0.0589	0.8082
Neurologic	1	0.0252	0.8739
NSAIDs	1	0.0211	0.8845
Osteoporosis	1	0.0125	0.9109
PDIEyePreparations	1	0.0025	0.9604
PDIOther	1	0.0191	0.8901

For each analysis, SAS used maximum likelihood estimates to order the predictors. The criterion for predictor entry into the model (SLENTRY) and predictor retention in the model (SLSTAY) were set close to 1 so that the full model could be obtained. Variables were entered in order from highest to lowest model effect size.

A significant Wald Chi-Square indicates that a predictor's regression coefficient is not equal to zero. The maximum likelihood estimates are compared to the proposed estimate (either 1 or 0 with a binary outcome, as in the present analyses) and are divided by the variance in the parameter estimate. The result is then compared to the normal distribution. The square of the difference is compared to the chi-square distribution, yielding an X^2 probability value as shown above. As indicated, *there are no significant effects among these analyses*.

With specific reference to the driver evaluation results, it may be noted that the predictor "Cholesterol Lowering" never reached the SLENTRY criterion for inclusion in the model, and the predictor "Sedating Antihistamine" was removed because it did not meet the SLSTAY criterion for retention in the model.

The absence of statistically significant drug effects for any of the outcome variables in these analyses may reflect several different factors. First, a larger sample is clearly needed to analyze the effects of classes of drugs - and especially specific drugs - on performance. Next, the consenting participants in this study may not be representative of older drivers. Based on unsolicited comments from rehabilitation services staff it is not only possible, but likely, that the "poorest" drivers would not volunteer for such a study. In addition, if drivers have been taking their medications for a long time, it is possible that they have learned ways to compensate for the effects that the drug has on their driving performance. Finally, the influence of other drugs – alcohol, in particular – is an unknown but possibly potent covariate that could explain individual differences in drug metabolism.

Table 16. Inter-rater reliability summary table

Rater	Glance Location	Frame Count	Percent
1	0	1578	77.9
1	1	61	3.0
1	2	63	3.1
1	3	300	14.8
1	4	0	0.0
1	5	24	1.2
2	0	1581	78.0
2	1	92	4.5
2	2	50	2.5
2	3	218	10.8
2	4	0	0.0
2	5	85	4.2
Correlation between raters: all locations, aggregate video			0.99
Correlation between raters: all locations except forward, aggregate video			0.93
Correlation between raters: frame by frame			0.77
Coefficient of determination (r-squared): frame by frame			0.60

Instrumented Vehicle Results and Case Study

The first analysis examining variability in driving behavior for a sub-sample of five study participants, comparing their independent driving to their driving during the evaluation with the OT/CDRS, measured the correlation in glance distribution across nearly all included traffic, infrastructure, and maneuver conditions. The second analysis examined the same correlation for a particular situation of interest: intersection negotiation.

Both of these analyses relied on the coding of driver behavior from video data recorded in the test vehicle and in participants' own cars. Specifically, the software tool (Anvil) was used to assign attribute values for glance location, infrastructure, traffic condition, and maneuver, for every frame of video, at 12 frames per second. Two video coders contributed to this task. To evaluate inter-rater reliability, glance location was scored independently, by both coders, in a test clip of slightly under 3 minutes. The results appear in Table 16.

As shown in this table, across all glance locations, for all video frames (i.e., in the aggregate), a very high correlation (0.99) was found. Because the driver was looking forward in most frames, and this was the easiest behavior to code, a separate correlation for glances away from the forward direction was also calculated; this was slightly lower but still impressive at 0.93. Of greatest interest was the consistency between raters on a frame-by-frame basis. This correlation fell to 0.77, due principally – based on a review of discrepant frames – to differences of a few frames in the perceived onset and offset of changes in glance direction by one coder versus another. These values, being in line with the reliability levels reported in a closely-related study on driver distraction using continuous video coded from a driver face camera (Stutts et al., 2003), were deemed satisfactory to support the planned analyses of behavioral variability in the independent drives versus driving evaluations.

Beginning with an examination of virtually all driving done by this sub-sample – excluding from video analysis only those frames where they were stopped, were following another vehicle, or were in a parking lot – there are modest differences in the proportion and distribution of glances away from the forward direction during independent driving versus the driving evaluations. With reference to Table 17, these study participants' behavior was marked by a substantial increase in the amount of time they were looking down/inside their vehicles, coupled with fewer glances to the inside rearview mirror (Right+Up location), during independent driving. Of course, traffic conditions were not identical; but the independent driving videos selected for this comparison were matched for road type and time of day/visibility condition with each individual's driving evaluation. Tentatively, then, this observed variability in driver behavior may be associated at least in part with the circumstances of the evaluation itself.

The correlation in overall glance distribution is almost perfect, due to the overwhelming percent of the time drivers are (appropriately) looking forward. Excluding the frames with a forward glance location, the correlation falls to 0.58; further, this change appears to be localized to a few specific differences in glance behavior. In particular, the differences associated with independent driving suggest a greater willingness to divide attention, engaging in secondary tasks and/or sampling information from inside the vehicle (e.g., radio controls) at the expense of sampling mirror information. These differences, while certainly not surprising, point to a degree of vigilance and self-monitoring to exclude distracting behavior during a formal driving evaluation, that individuals probably will not manifest in their everyday driving.

Table 17. Glance location for five participants during driving evaluations and independent driving, for all scenarios except parking lots, stopped vehicle, and car following

Glance Location	Driving Evaluation		Independent Driving	
	Count	Percent	Count	Percent
Forward	6113	84.93%	4845	82.54%
Right+Up	363	5.04%	206	3.5 1%
Right Only	288	4.00%	377	6.42%
Left Only	349	4.85%	219	3.73%
Down+Inside	26	0.36%	178	3.03%
Over shoulder	59	0.82%	45	0.77%
N =	7198		5870	
Correlation all 6 glance locations	0.998583			
Correlation excluding forward	0.5 80994			

Next, this comparative analysis of the present surrogate for attention (glance distribution) was performed for a much more restrictive set of conditions only when the driver approaches and continues straight through a signalized intersection as a lead or isolated vehicle, i.e., not in car following mode. This situation was selected for special examination because of the demands to actively and continuously search for potential conflicts with other road users while sampling signal status, other regulatory information, and formal and informal guidance cues in the environment; and because a considerable body of research has highlighted older drivers' errors leading to crashes at intersections as a preeminent safety concern. These results are presented in Table 18.

As shown in this table, the correlation for overall glance behavior remains very high, but when frames showing a forward glance are excluded the correlation falls to 0.24. This relatively weak correspondence may be explained by more glances down and inside the vehicle, coupled with fewer glances toward the inside rearview mirror and the complete elimination of over-the-shoulder glances during the independent drives. There was also a shift toward more "right only" and fewer "left only" glances during independent driving.

Again, it must be noted that while the video selected for this comparison was recorded during similar operating conditions, variability in traffic conditions and other factors during the driving evaluations versus the independent drives was inevitable. Such differences in, for example, the geometries of the particular intersections traversed by these study participants could account for the absence of over-the-shoulder glances. It is less obvious, however, why drivers continuing straight through the intersection would devote less attention searching to the left versus to the right during independent driving, given the nearly equal distribution of glances to the left and right at intersections during their driving evaluations. And the apparently greater willingness of study participants to devote attention to locations inside the vehicle during intersection negotiation – though still a small percentage of their overall glance distributions – highlights a difference between independent driving and (older) individuals' behavior during a driving evaluation that may have significant safety implications.

A Pilot Study to Test Multiple Medication Usage and Driving Functioning

Table 18. Glance location for five participants during driving evaluations and independent driving, for intersection negotiation only

Glance Location	Driving Evaluation		Independent Driving	
	Count	Percent	Count	Percent
Forward	644	79.3 1%	539	79.03%
Right+Up	55	6.77%	25	3.67%
Right Only	43	5.30%	76	11.14%
Left Only	37	4.56%	11	1.61%
Down+Inside	8	0.99%	31	4.55%
Over shoulder	25	3.08%	0	0.00%
N =	812		682	
Correlation all 6 glance locations	0.992106			
Correlation excludes forward	0.235991			

The comparative analysis with the closest congruence between independent driving and driving during the OT/CDRS evaluation was a "case study" carried out in the Hockessin, DE, vicinity for a selected research participant. Based on GPS data recorded with the in-vehicle instrumentation, the routes traversed by individual during the driving evaluation have been traced with a thin yellow line in Figure 12. Overlaid on the yellow line are thicker lines in red, blue, turquoise, and amber, which denote the routes this person traversed on four separate independent drives. With reference to this figure, some or all of each of these independent drives shares common road segments – presenting the same operational and infrastructure elements to drivers – with the driving evaluation route.

It is possible that this individual had other exposure during independent driving on route segments in common with the driving evaluation. However, there was a cell phone tower in the area that interfered with GPS reception, resulting in intermittent signal loss during independent driving. The available GPS recordings permitted location matches that are accurate to two significant digits for latitude and longitude coordinates, corresponding to a resolution of approximately 60 feet.

A database was created containing 318 records among the four independent drives, with coordinates that matched those on the driving evaluation route. For each location identified via matching coordinates, the driver's speed was examined. The number of matched locations where speed choice was higher and lower during independent driving, versus during the driving evaluation was tabulated. In addition, an average speed was calculated for all locations on each of the four independent drives where speed was higher, and where it was lower, than the same individual's speed on the same road segments during the driving evaluation. These results are presented in Table 19.

As indicated, this study participant drove faster at nearly all of the matched locations on the "red segment" during the driving evaluation, compared to independent driving, and at substantially more locations on the "blue segment" as well. In contrast, speed choice was higher during independent driving on the "turquoise segment," and even more so on the "amber segment." In fact, it is on the "amber segment" where the study participant's speed choice was higher during independent driving for the largest proportion of matched locations; and, this road segment has the lowest traffic volume – and so the driver's speed choice is least likely to be affected by other motorists – than on any of the other common road segments.

Table 19. Differential speed choice (mph) by one participant during the driving evaluation versus independent driving, on four common road segments

Common Road Segment	Higher Speed Choice During Driving Evaluation			Higher Speed Choice During Independent Driving		
	Mean speed: driving evaluation	Mean speed: independent driving	Matched locations in database	Mean speed: driving evaluation	Mean speed: independent driving	Matched locations in database
Red segment	38.3	30.8	86	26.8	27.8	2
Blue segment	40.7	32.6	87	26.7	36.9	50
Turquoise segment	29.4	24.6	22	23	25	40
Amber segment	22.7	20.2	8	23.2	31.1	22

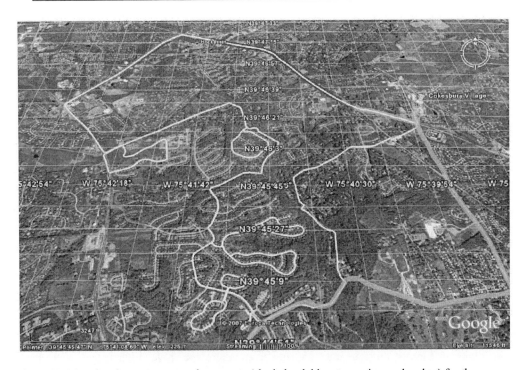

Figure 12. Map showing common road segments (shaded red, blue, turquoise, and amber) for the independent drives and the driving evaluation

RECENT REPORTS, STUDIES, AND NATIONAL SURVEYS ON POLYPHARMACY AND DRIVING

Overview and Objective

The purpose of this project task was to review all relevant technical literature published since the previous NHTSA report in this subject area.[1] This chapter contains summaries of recently published research on medication usage, injury data, and/or other relevant variables that could potentially impact the relationship between PDI medications and driving, that were posted in the SafetyLit database between October 2005 and October 2007. SafetyLit is a free service of the Center for Injury Prevention Policy and Practice at San Diego State University in collaboration with the World Health Organization. The weekly SafetyLit update provides abstracts of English language reports from researchers in 35 disciplines relevant to preventing unintentional injuries, violence, and self-harm. SafetyLit staff and volunteers regularly examine more than 2,600 scholarly journals from many nations, and also review conference proceedings and reports from government agencies and organizations. SafetyLit summaries are drawn from anthropology, economics, education, engineering specialties, ergonomics, law and law enforcement, medicine, physiology, psychology, public health, public safety, nursing, social work, traffic safety, and other fields.

Included in this chapter is an update on drug prevalence in fatal and non-fatal injury motor vehicle crashes. Studies are summarized providing new information about the effects of specific drugs/drug classes on driving, including an anti-seizure medication (topiramate) for migraine prevention and other therapies; acute and stable dosing of opioids; sedating and non-sedating antihistamines; antidepressants; short and long half-life sedative-hypnotics; an immediate-release versus extended-release anti-anxiety medication (benzodiazepine); a skeletal muscle relaxant (carisoprodol); and anti-diabetic medications. The chapter concludes with an examination of studies bearing on the risk of falling associated with chronic medical conditions versus the effects of the medications that treat these conditions.

Prevalence of Medications and Driving

Schwilke, Sampaoi dos Santos, and Logan (2006) reported on patterns of drug (illicit and therapeutic) and alcohol use in fatally injured drivers in Washington State between 2001 and 2002. These data were obtained for 370 drivers who died within 4 hours of a traffic crash. Driver culpability for the crash was not provided in the data that were analyzed; therefore drug use rates by crash-causing versus non-causing drivers could not be determined. The sample included 277 men ranging in age from 15 to 87 with a mean age of 38, and 93 women 16 to 91 with a mean age of 47.

Of the 370 cases tested, 150 blood samples were positive for alcohol. Of the 150 cases positive for alcohol, 63 (42%) were positive for one or more impairing drugs. For the most frequently identified drugs, the rate of drug and combined alcohol use included: cannabinoids (53%), cocaine (38%), methamphetamine (33%), diazepam (53%), and diphenhydramine (50%). Without considering alcohol, rates of drivers testing positive for drugs included the following: cannabinoids (12.7%), amphetamines (4.86), benzodiazepines (5.14%), cocaine/met (4.86%), diphenhydramine (2.7%), hydrocodone (1.89%), phenytoin (1.89%), morphine (1.62%), and amitriptyline (1.08%). The significance of the combined alcohol and drug use in this population is that the magnitude of impairing drug use by drivers may be underestimated because of the procedures used in DUI enforcement. Investigations of impairing agents in traffic stops typically end with a positive blood or alcohol result. These data suggest that individuals with impairing amounts of alcohol in their systems may more often have impairing drugs in their systems than is documented, which could have contributed to their driving impairment. The study authors note that if the patterns of drug and alcohol use in the sample population carry over into the general impaired driving population, as many as 40% of all individuals arrested for alcohol-related driving offenses could be at least partially under the influence of drugs.

The rate of benzodiazepines may be underestimated because clonazepam and lorazepam (two drugs with known effects on driving) are not detected by the autopsy blood test procedures, and would have gone undetected in the study population. The two most frequently detected benzodiazepines were diazepam (detected in 15 cases) and nordiazepam (detected in 7 cases). Midazolam was detected in 4 cases. The concentrations detected suggested therapeutic use. In these drivers, alcohol was detected in 54% of the diazepam-positive cases, 43% of the nordiazepam-positive cases, and 50% of the midazolam-positive cases.

Poly-drug use in this population was common, and often included a combination of illicit and prescription drugs. For the alcohol-free cases, 9.5% tested positive for two or more impairing drugs.

Kaplan, Kraner, and Paulozzi (2006) analyzed the prevalence alcohol and drug use in 458 drivers who were fatally injured in crashes between 2004 and 2005 in West Virginia. The West Virginia Office of the Chief Medical Examiner routinely screens all victims of motor vehicle crashes for evidence of impairment from alcohol, licit, and illicit drugs. This includes narcotics (e.g., heroin and opioid analgesics), marijuana, stimulants (e.g., cocaine and amphetamines), depressants (e.g., benzodiazepines and barbiturates), and other licit drugs (e.g., antidepressants and antihistamines). Up to three drugs may be listed in the database used for the analysis (Fatality Analysis Reporting System [FARS]), and if multiple drugs are found, they are recorded in the following order: narcotics, depressants, stimulants, marijuana, and other licit drugs. Drugs administered by emergency medical services are not included. Fifty percent of the drivers who were fatally injured had alcohol or drugs in their bodies, and 12.2% had both. Alcohol was detected in 33.8% of the deceased drivers. Detectable levels of at least one drug type were reported for 28.4% of the decedents, and two or more types of drugs in 9% of the deceased drivers. Opioid analgesics were present in 7.9%, depressants in 7.9%, stimulants in 4.4%, marijuana in 8.5%, and other licit drugs such as antidepressants and antihistamines in 9.4%. The three most common opioid analgesics were hydrocodone (2.8% of the fatally injured drivers testing positive for drugs), oxycodone (2.0%), and methadone (1.5%). The depressants were sedatives, including benzodiazepines (6.6%) and barbiturates (6.6%), and the muscle relaxant meprobamate/carisoprodol (0.6%). The most common benzodiazepines were diazepam and alprazolam. Cocaine was the most frequently identified stimulant (4.4%). A limitation of the research findings is that the FARS data do not describe the degree of intoxication, whether the drugs were used recreationally or therapeutically, or whether the user was an acute or stable user of a drug (e.g., level of familiarity). The database also does not assign driver fault, so some of the impaired drivers may not have been responsible for their crashes, and some impaired drivers who survived crashes but killed other road users are not included.

Kurzthaler et al. (2005) investigated the prevalence of benzodiazepines and alcohol (alone and together) in 1,611 non-fatally injured patients admitted to the emergency room at the University Hospital of Trauma Surgery in Innsbruck, Austria, between January 1 and December 31, 1995. In their sample, injuries were the result of a traffic crash for 269 patients. For the full sample of 1,611 patients, those 60 or younger tested positive for alcohol, as well as for benzodiazepines in combination with alcohol more often than patients over 60. All benzodiazepine concentrations were within the therapeutic range or lower. Almost all blood samples positive for benzodiazepines were traced to diazepam. Concentrating only on the sample of patients who were involved in traffic crashes, 7.1% tested positive for benzodiazepines; the mean diazepam plasma level was $87 + 64$ ng/L. This suggested that benzodiazepine use was associated with therapeutic use, rather than abuse of these drugs. In this same sample of 269 patients, 29.4% tested positive for alcohol; the mean blood alcohol concentration was $1.53 + 0.54$ g/l, which is above the legal limit in Austria at the time of the investigation (0.8 g/l). The percent of the traffic-crash sample testing positive for both alcohol and benzodiazepines was 1.9%.

Ch'ng et al. (2007) analyzed blood samples taken from 436 drivers injured in crashes in Victoria, Australia, and who were transported to a trauma center for care following the collision. The objective of the analysis was to examine the use of commonly abused drugs (amphetamines, benzodiazepines, opiates such as morphine and codeine) as well as cannabis and cocaine among drivers injured in motor vehicle crashes. Drivers who received opiates or benzodiazepines for treatment at the trauma center were eliminated from the analysis. The finding of particular interest to the present research is that benzodiazepines were found in 15.6% of the drivers across all age groups, but the use of benzodiazepines increased with age, and was highest among women drivers 65 and older. Four of the 13 women 65 and older (31%) tested positive for benzodiazepines.

Effects on Driving of Specific Drugs/Drug Classes

Topiramate (an anti-epileptic also used in migraine revention and other therapies)

Topiramate (Topamax) is a seizure disorder treatment that received additional FDA approval for prevention of migraine headaches in August 2004, and is being prescribed for off-label uses such as psychiatric disorders (e.g., schizophrenia and bi-polar disorder); eating disorders (e.g., bulimia, binge eating, obesity, and anorexia nervosa); as an adjunct therapy to treat weight gain associated with olanzapine, SSRIs, and other anti-psychotic medications; neuropathic pain; and alcohol and drug dependency (Gordon & Logan, 2006). Its potentially driver impairing side effects include sedation; dizziness; confusion; difficulty concentrating; shaky and unsteady body movements; rapid and repetitious involuntary eye movements; decreased visual acuity; hypoglycemia leading to loss of consciousness; and tingling or numbness in the arms and legs. The manufacturer states that patients should be warned about the potential side effects and advised not to drive or operate machinery until they have gained sufficient experience on topiramate to gauge whether it adversely affects their mental, motor, or visual performance.

318 National Highway Traffic Safety Administration

In forensic toxicology investigations of topiramate-positive drivers reported by Gordon and Logan (2006), psychomotor impairment was evident with blood concentrations within normal therapeutic range. As an example, a 31-year-old female was prescribed topiramate for an eating disorder. She drove off the highway and crashed into the median. Responding officers noted thick slurred speech, heavy eyelids and dilated pupils. She had a lack of coordination and could not stand unassisted and was arrested for DUI. Topiramate at therapeutic levels (8.1 mg/L) was identified in her blood as well as lorazepam at 0.01 mg/L. In the case of a 50-year-old female driver who was involved in a no-damage, non-injury collision, the driver was observed with severe lane drift, hitting curbs, and almost driving onto a sidewalk where children were playing. The only drug found in her blood was topiramate at a concentration of 14.2 mg/L. Gordon and Logan note that as anti-epileptic medications are increasingly used to treat psychiatric disorders, their prevalence in impaired driving cases has increased. Between 1998 and 2004, 68 suspected impaired drivers tested positive for topiramate in Washington State. The mean and median age of the drivers testing positive for the drug was 42. The majority (68%) of the cases were female. The median blood topiramate concentration was 6.4 mg/L (mean 8.4 mg/L, range 1-180 mg/L, sd 6.4). Alcohol was detected on only 5 of the 68 arrested drivers.

Opioids

New (Acute) Opioid Dosing. Verster, Veldhuijzen, and Volkerts (2006) compared driving performance, laboratory test performance, mood changes, and subjective measures of alertness for 18 healthy subjects who participated in a randomized, double-blind, placebo-controlled crossover study. Treatment sequences were randomized across the participants, and test days were separated by a wash-out period of seven days. Subjects were given the following medications/dosages: bromfenac 25 mg; bromfenac 50 mg; oxycodone/paracetamol 5/325 mg; oxycodone/paracetamol 10/650 mg; and placebo.

Bromfenac (Duract) is a non-steroidal anti-inflammatory drug that was indicated for short-term management of acute pain. Because it was pulled from the market during the data collection phase as a result of potentially serious side effects (liver damage), this summary will be limited to the results of the opioid drug (oxycodone) on subjects' performance. Oxycodone is an opioid agonist that is often prescribed in combination with paracetamol to reduce the opioid dosage while retaining the analgesic efficacy, to reduce opioid-related adverse effects. The recommended dosage is 5 mg oxycodone with 325 mg paracetamol.

Subjects were given a treatment dose or a placebo 30 minutes prior to a standardized breakfast. One hour after dosing, a standardized on-road driving test was given. The 100-km road test was conducted in a dual-controlled vehicle on a two-lane road. Subjects were instructed to maintain constant speed of 90 km/h (56 mph). Outcome variables included a measure of weaving (standard deviation of lateral positioning, or SDLP); and standard deviation of speed. The laboratory tests were given 2.5 hours after administration of the medications or the placebo, and included a Sternberg memory scanning test, a tracking task, and a divided attention task. Subjective assessments of their own driving performance following the drive test as well as the level of effort required to perform the test were obtained, in addition to subjective assessments of alertness level.

Drive test results showed no significant differences between the opioid treatments and the placebo; however, there was a significant difference in SDLP between the high dose (23 cm) and the low dose (20.5 cm) of the opioid medication. The difference between the high dose and the placebo (+1.9 cm) was not significant, and is less than that observed with blood alcohol concentrations of .05 grams per deciliter. There were also no significant differences between the opioid treatments and the placebo on any of the laboratory tests, although performance was worse under both opioid treatment conditions than the placebo condition.

Significant differences between the placebo and the opioid treatment were evident in the driving-related subjective assessments, the subjective assessment of alertness, and the mood change assessment. Level of mental effort invested in the driving task was assessed on a scale that ranged from "absolutely no effort" to "extreme effort," with consecutive sublevels including "almost no effort," a little effort," "some effort," "rather much effort," "considerable effort," "great effort," and "very great effort." Compared to the placebo, mental effort during driving was significantly elevated after the high dose of the opioid, but not after the low dose of the drug. Also, a significant dose-response relationship on mental effort was found for the opioid drug. The authors suggest that the lack of impairment on the drive test may have been related to the participants reporting increased effort during driving while under the influence of this drug. Alertness was assessed on a 21-point, equal-interval scale. Compared to the placebo, alertness was significantly decreased for both doses of the opioid, and there was also a significant dose-response relationship. Mood changes were assessed by the Addiction Research Center Inventory (ARCI_-49) Questionnaire. This questionnaire uses 49 yes/no questions that relate to five scales, differentiating between mood changes induced by psychoactive drugs. The five scales are: euphoria, dysphoria, sedation, intellectual efficacy and energy, and activation. After the drive test, sedation was significantly increased in the high-dose opioid condition, as was dysphoria.[2] There was a significant dose-response relationship for the opioid drugs on the dysphoria scores.

Stable Opioid Dosing. Byas-Smith, Chapman, Reed, and Cotsonis (2005) compared driving performance (on-road and closed course) and laboratory tests of attention and visual information processing for 50 normal volunteers with no pain, 11 opioid-free patients with chronic pain, and 21 patients who had chronic pain and were taking opiates. The most frequently used opioid analgesic was oxycodone. Of the 32 patients, only 2 used an opioid analgesic alone. Morphine equivalent daily opioid doses averaged 118 mg (median 40 mg).

Subjects participated in a community drive test in their own vehicles over 7 miles of urban residential driving and 4 miles of highway driving. The test administrator followed in another car and filmed the participant's car. The recorded videotape was used to identify driving errors (speeding, turning, stopping, and lane violations). The closed course consisted of five stations including a 50-yard straight course for driving forward; a 20-yard straight course for reverse driving; a 100-yard slalom course with frequent S-shaped turns; a circular-shaped course demanding constant turns; and parallel parking. The course was delimited with multiple, 3-foot tall, orange rubber cones. Test administrators positioned near the course recorded three measures: time to complete the station, number of touches of a cone by the automobile, and number of cones run over or knocked down.

Laboratory tests included the Test of Variables of Attention (TOVA) and the Digit Symbol Substitution Test (DSST).

Results of the community drive tests indicated no driving errors besides speeding for any groups; 90% of subjects in each group exceeded the speed limit by at least 5 mph, but none greater than 15 mph. There were no significant differences among groups on speeding. Results of the five stations of the obstacle course drive showed no significant group mean differences for total time, number of cones impacted or knocked down. There were also no group differences in accuracy of parking. To evaluate the effect of different doses of opioids on driving performance, the opioid group was divided into two subgroups: 16 patients taking more than 20 mg of morphine equivalent per day and those taking less than or equal to 20 mg per day. A comparison of these two subgroups found differences in only one analysis—patients in the higher dose group completed the circle course significantly faster than those in the lower dose group.

The laboratory tests showed no significant differences between groups on the TOVA. On the DSST, the healthy volunteers showed significantly higher scores, with no significant differences between the opioid and non-opioid patient groups. Group differences disappeared however, when age and years of education were controlled for.

The study authors state that these findings provide direct evidence that at least a subset of patients with chronic pain on a stable opioid analgesic regimen are capable of operating a motor vehicle safely during daytime, good-weather conditions. Given that there were no significant differences on the dependent measures between the opioid-treated patients with chronic pain, the opioid-free patients with chronic pain, and the healthy volunteers, Byas-Smith et al. (2005) indicate that an absolute prohibition against driving while taking opioid medications for pain control is contraindicated by the study findings.

Similar conclusions were drawn from a study of the effects of long-term treatment with controlled release oxycodone (CRO) using a computerized test battery (Gaertner, Radbruch, Giesecke, Gerbershagen, Petzke, Ostgathe, Elsner, & Sabatowski, 2006). The objective of the study was to demonstrate that patients treated with CRO did not perform significantly worse in the tests than the untreated controls. The test battery measured attention reaction, visual orientation, motor coordination, and vigilance. Performance of the patients treated with CRO was compared to that of the control sample, in addition to transformation of the control subjects' data equivalent to performance under the influence of .05 g/dL blood alcohol (from a prior study). The alcohol-impaired control data were used to define clinically significant impairment. Therefore, to show non-inferiority in test performance of opioid patients compared to controls, CRO patient performance would need to be significantly better that that of the control group with a blood alcohol concentration of .05. Performance of 30 patients suffering from non-cancer pain and treated with CRO for at least four weeks (and without a dose change in the prior 12 days) was compared to the performance of 90 controls, with three age-matched controls for each patient. Age ranged from 25 to 77. The average dosage of CRO was 76 mg/day (range 20 to 280 mg). The mean current pain intensity of the CRO patients was 4.8 on an 11-point scale where 0 = no pain and 11 = pain as severe as possible.

Combining the cognitive items of the battery, the CRO patients performed better than the age-independent control group with a blood alcohol level of .05, but the difference was not statistically significant. This result cannot demonstrate that CRO treatment is not un-impairing. The researchers also looked at the percentage of patients in the CRO and control group (not under the influence of alcohol) who passed the single tests in the test battery, acknowledging that this was a weaker statistical analysis, albeit one that is recommended by German legislation. In Germany, test batteries similar to the one used in the study are employed for "traffic delinquents" who are denied permission to drive if one or more of the tests is failed (i.e., a test result is below the 16th percentile of the age-independent reference range). The control group patients passed an average of 4.1 of the 5 tests, while the CRO patients performed only slightly worse, passing a mean of 4.0 tests. The difference in the

A Pilot Study to Test Multiple Medication Usage and Driving Functioning   321

percentage passing from the control group and the CRO group was not significant. The percentage of patients passing all 5 tests was 56% for the control group and 39% for the CRO group; this difference also was not significant. The daily oxycodone dosage correlated moderately (r=0.45, p-.01) with the number of wrong answers on the reaction time under pressure test. In addition, there was a moderate inverse relationship between dosage and the vigilance test score. The authors concluded that stable treatment with CRO in chronic non-cancer patients does not prohibit driving, however individual assessment is necessary.

Antihistamines

Tashiro et al. (2005) conducted a study to determine whether cellular phone use while driving further degrades the performance of drivers using antihistamines (both sedating and non-sedating). In a randomized, double-blind, placebo-controlled, three-way crossover study, healthy volunteers received fexofenadine HC1 120 mg (a non-sedating antihistamine), hydroxyzine HC1 30 mg (a non-benzodiazepine anoxiolytic/hypnotic, also used as a sedating antihistamine), and a placebo. Subjects were 18 male volunteers age 20 to 26. Brake reaction time while driving on a controlled course consisting of two straight lines 1.5 km in length connected by u-shaped turning roads at both ends, served as the dependent measure; 25 trials under each condition were performed. Subjective assessments of sedation (Stanford sleepiness scale and the line analog rating scale) were also provided. For each drug or placebo condition, the following four driving conditions were conducted: (1) driving only; (2) driving while answering simple arithmetic questions on the cellular phone; (3) driving while answering complex arithmetic questions on the phone; and (4) driving while engaged in conversation on the cellular phone, where the subject was asked to provide 1- to 2-minute answers on six to eight pre-determined topics.

Both assessment tests of subjective sleepiness showed that subjects given hydroxyzine were significantly less alert/more sedated than those who were administered fexofenadine or the placebo. There were no significant differences in subjective alertness/sleepiness between fexofenadine and the placebo groups.

Brake reaction time (BRT) showed significant differences as a result of drug administered and driving condition as follows. For the driving only condition, there were no significant differences in BRT as a function of the drug type (or placebo) given. For each of the three conditions where subjects used a cell phone, those driving under the influence of hydroxyzine had significantly slower BRTs that those taking either fexofenadine or the placebo: there were no significant differences in BRT for the fexofenadine and placebo groups.

The BRT of hydroxyzine vs. placebo was compared under the four driving conditions. Subjects who were administered the placebo and were engaged in discussions of simple calculations had slower BRTs than subjects administered hydroxyzine but were not using their cell phone at all. When the hydroxyzine subjects were engaged in discussions of simple calculations, their BRTs were slower than the BRTs of the placebo group engaged in discussions of simple calculations.

Similarly, subjects given the placebo and were engaged in discussions of complex calculations had slower BRTs than subjects given hydroxyzine and not talking on their cell

322National Highway Traffic Safety Administration

phone at all. BRTs of the placebo group performing complex calculations were not significantly different from BRTs of the hydroxyzine group completing the simple calculations.

Subjects given the placebo and who were engaged in general conversations on their cell phones had significantly slower BRTs than the hydroxyzine-treated subjects who were not using their cell phone, but significantly faster BRTs that the hydroxyzine-treated subjects who were engaged in general conversations on their cell phone.

Comparisons of BRT for fexofenadine versus placebo under the four driving conditions showed that for any driving condition where they were using their cell phones, placebo-treated subjects had slower BRTS than the fexofenadine-treated group who were not using cell phones. But no differences were shown as the result of the placebo versus the fexofenadine administration, when both groups were performing either of the three tasks while using their cell phones.

This study's findings are consistent with other research on the effects of fexofenadine (a non-sedating antihistamine) on driving performance, and furthers the state of the knowledge that fexofenadine does not impair driving performance even in the presence of divided attention tasks. Hydroxyzine, on the other hand (a sedating antihistamine) was associated with significantly greater sedation, and significantly slower BRTs when subjects were performing divided attention tasks. Thus, drivers given hydroxyzine will be slower at recognizing potential hazards or threats in the traffic situation ahead, and slower to apply their brake to stop or slow the vehicle as needed. Anything that divides their attention from the main task of driving (such as cell phone use) will exacerbate the risk of crashing. Although older drivers were not included in the sample, the negative effects of the sedating antihistamine on driving performance would likely be magnified, as would the combined effect of the antihistamine and the divided attention task.

Antidepressants

Brunnauer, Laux, Geiger, Soyka, and Moller (2006) evaluated the fitness to drive of 100 depressive inpatients on clinically relevant doses of various antidepressants (by antidepressant class). Inclusion criteria included antidepressant monotherapy, steady-state pharmacologic conditions (all patients were considered for discharge in at least three days), and possession of a valid driver's license. Mean age was 46.8 (sd = 13.6). Forty patients received tricyclic antidepressants (TCAs: amitriptyline, doxepin, maprotiline, or trimipramine), 25 received selective serotonin reuptake inhibitors (SSRIs: citalopram or paroxetine), 20 received a noradrenergic and specific serotonergic antidepressant (NaSSA: mirtazapine), and 15 received a serotonin-norepinephrine reuptake inhibitor (SNRI: venlafaxine). Subjects with a history of neurologic illness, substance abuse, or mental retardation were excluded. Fitness to drive was measured according to German guidelines for road and traffic safety using a computerized test battery that assesses the following domains: visual perception, selective attention, vigilance, and reactivity and stress tolerance. Sixteen percent of the depressive patients were considered unfit to drive (labeled as "severely impaired" and failing in more than 40% of test parameters) and 60% were considered "moderately impaired" (failed in less than 40% of test parameters) and in need of individual assessments of their ability to drive.

Only 24% of the patients passed the test according to German guidelines for driving (i.e., not more than 1 standard deviation below the mean of normative data in psychomotor domains). Looking at the global driving score, 10% of the patients taking TCAs passed the tests without impairments, as did 20% of those treated with venlafaxine, 28% treated with SSRIs, and 50% treated with mirtazapine. Comparisons between mirtazapine and each of the other antidepressants were statistically significant, indicating better performance with mirtazapine. On the psychomotor and visual perception tests, depressed patients taking TCAs were more impaired than those treated with SSRIs or mirtazapine. There were no significant differences in performance between patients treated with TCAs and venlafaxine. Subjects treated with mirtazapine showed significantly better performance on tests measuring reactivity and stress tolerance than those treated with TCSs, SSRIs, or venlafaxine. In the selective attention test, patients treated with SSRIs and mirtazapine performed significantly better than those treated with TCAs and venlafaxine.

It should be noted that all patients treated with mirtazapine were under steady-state pharmacologic conditions and received their doses in the evening (the night before testing). This is important because earlier studies on healthy subjects given mirtazapine as a daytime dose showed impairments in driving ability (Wingen, Bothmer, Langer et al., 2005; Rideout, Meadows, Johnsen, et al., 2003). In this study, depressive patients given mirtazapine in the evening performed better than patients in other groups, and greater percentages passed the driving test criteria for licensure. The findings indicate that antidepressant therapy affects fitness to drive differently in depressed patients, and physicians should be aware of this and conduct individual counseling for depressed patients wishing to drive.

Sedative-Hypnotics

Staner et al. (2005) investigated the driving abilities of patients diagnosed with primary insomnia, after repeated dosing of sedative hypnotic drugs. Single and repeated (7-day) doses of zolpidem (10 mg), zopiclone (7.5 mg), lormetazepam (1 mg) or a placebo were administered in a crossover design to 32 patients. Lormetazepam is a benzodiazepine not approved for sale in the United States or Canada, but is one of the most prescribed benzodiazepine hypnotics in France, where the study was conducted. Zolpidem (also known as "Ambien") is a strong hypnotic drug that has no significant muscle relaxant, anxiolytic, or anticonvulsant activity when administered at a clinically relevant dose, and zopiclone is an effective hypnotic that induces weaker myorelaxation than benzodiazepines. The average half-life of lormetazepam is 10 hours, compared to 5 hours for zopiclone, and 1.9 hours for zolpidem. Treatments were administered at bedtime from day 1 to day 7, and its effect was assessed at the beginning (day 2) and at the end (day 8) of each treatment period after a night spent in the sleep laboratory.

Driving simulator tests took place 9 to 11 hours post-dose. Driving simulation with EEG monitoring was conducted on a FAROS driving simulator with a roadway display video projection system that subtended a 120-degree visual field. It had no movement capabilities. Subjects "drove" for 60 minutes along the simulated highway during daytime; in light traffic; with occasional long, wide curves; and repetitive landscaping. The program calculated mean, median, and standard deviation of absolute speed, of deviation from the speed limit, of deviation from the ideal route, and the number of collisions (with other vehicles or crash barriers).

Results showed significantly poorer performance on the driving simulation measures of deviation of absolute speed and deviation from the speed limit for patients taking lormetazepam, compared to the placebo. Patients taking zopiclone had significantly more collisions than patients taking the placebo. Zolpidem had no effect on the driving performance measures. Both the lormetazepam and zopiclone had significant next-day effects (9 to 11 hours post dosages) on EEG correlates of vigilance level (benzodiazepine-like alterations in beta and alpha power), a phenomenon referred to as "pharmacological dissociation." Zolpidem did not alter next-day physiological EEG rhythms 9 to 11 hours post-dose. The authors suggest that the poor driving performance associated with lormetazepam and zopiclone was related to their prolonged CNS effects during the driving simulation test. The residual effects of the hypnotics increased with increases in their half-life. Zolpidem had the shortest half-life (1.9 hours), followed by zopiclone (5 hours) and by lormetazepam (10 hours).

Anti-Anxiety Medications

Leufkens, Vermeeren, Smink, van Ruitenbeek, and Ramaekers (2007) compared the effects of extended-release (XR) and immediate-release (IR) alprazolam on the on-road driving performance of 18 healthy volunteers age 20 to 45. Citing Isbister, O'Regan, Sibbritt, and White (2004) and others, Leufkens et al. state that alprazolam (e.g., Xanax) is the most frequently used benzodiazepine for the treatment of panic disorder and anxiety. Alprazolam IR has a half-life ranging from 10 to 18 hours, and a peak blood plasma concentration is reached within 0.7 to 1.8 hours after ingestion. Patients report side effects including drowsiness, dizziness, and reduced alertness. Alprazolam XR was developed to reduce the adverse side effects associated with alprazolam IR. Its peak plasma concentrations are approximately half those of alprazolam IR and they occur between 5 and 12 hours after ingestion.

As a requirement for participation in the study, subjects were prohibited from using any other prescription medications and drugs of abuse throughout the study duration and for 1 week prior to their participation in the study. They also had to refrain from alcohol and caffeine use 24 hours before testing, were not allowed to smoke during testing, and were not allowed to consume food 3 hours prior to arrival for testing. Treatments were single oral doses of alprazolam 1 mg IR, alprazolam 1 mg XR, and placebo. The study was a double-blind, placebo-controlled, three-way crossover design. Study medication was supplied at 9 a.m. on each test day, with a minimum period between testing days of 7 days. Before the first treatment, subjects received comprehensive training on the driving task. The standardized driving task was administered between 4 and 5 hours post-dose, at the time blood plasma concentrations of the XR formulation were expected to be at the maximum.

The driving test lasted one hour and was conducted in an instrumented vehicle over a 100 km (61 mi) highway while operating at a constant speed of 95 km/h (58 mph) and maintaining a steady lateral position between the lane lines of the right (slower) lane. Subjects were accompanied by a licensed driving instructor in a vehicle with dual controls. The standard deviation of lateral position (SDLP) was the primary outcome measure, and is a measure of road tracking error or "weaving."

Ten driving tests (7 under the influence of alprazolam IR and 3 under the influence of alprazolam XR) were terminated prematurely because the driving instructor judged the subject to be too drowsy to continue safely. SDLP scores were calculated from the data collected until termination of each ride. There was a significant treatment effect, with both drug formulations significantly increasing SDLP. The mean SDLP after alprazolam XR was significantly lower as compared to alprazolam IR. The IR formulation produced a mean increase in SDLP of 8.2 cm and the XR formulation produced a mean increase of 3.9 cm. However, the impairment was still severe with the XR formulation, equivalent to a blood alcohol level that is above .05 g/dL (the legal limit in many countries). It is concluded that the impairing effects of alprazolam XR 1 mg on driving performance were less than those of the IR equivalent dose, but still of sufficient magnitude to increase the risk of becoming involved in a crash.

The authors note that a study limitation is that the effects were assessed after a single dose. Alprazolam-induced impairment may become less severe after chronic administration, as tolerance to the sedating effects may develop after repeated use. However, they also note that tolerance to the impairing effects of benzodiazepines is never complete.

Skeletal Muscle Relaxants

Carisoprodol (Soma, Vanadom), an often abused drug, is a muscle-relaxing medication with CNS depressant side effects that is generally prescribed for managing acute lower back pain (Bramness, Skurtveit, Morland, & Engeland , 2007). The study objective of Bramness et al. was to determine if dispensing a prescription for carisoprodol was associated with an increase in motor vehicle crash risk by using population-based prescription, crash, and population registry databases in Norway. The pharmacy database (NorPD) covers the entire Norwegian population (4.6 million inhabitants). Exposure to carisoprodol was studied in community-dwelling patients age 18 to 69 who filled a prescription for carisoprodol, but did not fill a prescription for other impairing drugs during the study period. The other impairing drugs included natural opium alkaloids, benzodiazepine anxiolytics, and hypnotics. The Norwegian Road Accident Registry (NRAR) provides information about motor vehicle crashes involving personal injury. Drivers age 18 to 69 involved in crashes during the study period were extracted for analysis. A third database (Norwegian Central Population Registry) was used to obtain demographic information on crash-involved patients. Data from the three databases were linked using the unique 11-digit identifier assigned to all individuals living in Norway.

Crash incidence among the exposed patients was compared to crash incidence among unexposed patients by calculation of a standardized incidence ratio (SIR). SIRs above one (1.0) indicate increased crash risk with personal injury as a driver. The SIR for a 7-day exposure period, across all age groups (n=66) was 3.7, and dropped to 2.4 for a 14-day exposure. The SIR for older males (age 55 to 69, n=2) was 1.5 and for older females (n = 6) was 4.1 after a 7-day exposure. The study authors indicate that their study findings are not surprising, based on the earlier studies that showed that carisoprodol may produce

326   National Highway Traffic Safety Administration

psychomotor impairment, that it may impair driving performance, and that it is issued to patients with a warning against driving motor vehicles. They note that physicians should be made aware of the potential driving problems connected with the use of carisoprodol, and should inform their patients of the risk.

Anti-Diabetic Medications

Hypoglycemia is a common side effect of some anti-diabetic medications that can result in cognitive-motor slowing and loss of consciousness. Hemmelgarn, Levesque, and Suissa (2006) conducted a case-control study using linked insurance databases in Quebec to assess whether the use of anti-diabetic drugs (specifically insulin, sulfonylureas, and biguanides) by older drivers increases their crash risk. The only biguanide in Canada at the time the study was conducted was metformin. Cases included 5,579 drivers age 67 to 84, who had been in an at-fault injurious motor vehicle crash, and controls included 13,300 older drivers who were not crash involved. Anti-diabetic drug exposure was assessed for the year preceding the date of the motor vehicle crash for cases and a randomly selected date during the follow up for the controls. Anti-diabetic drug exposure was also assessed during the 30 days prior to the index date to reflect current exposure. Exclusion criteria for cases and controls were: residence in a long-term care setting during the study period; hospitalization in the 60-days that preceded the index date; and hospital admission in the year before the index date lasting 30 days or more. Exposure was defined as the dispensing of at least one prescription for an anti-diabetic agent. A reference group of cases and controls was defined as those not using any anti-diabetic agents in the year preceding the index date.

A rate ratio of injurious motor vehicle crash for all anti-diabetic drugs was estimated using logistic regression. Rate ratios were adjusted for potentially confounding effects of age (within 1 year), sex, previous motor vehicle crash, and place of residence (rural or urban). The use of central nervous system (CNS) agents and the chronic disease score (excluding diabetes) were also evaluated as possible confounders using a change-in-estimate method. Rate ratios were adjusted for these factors only if the resulting estimate changed by more than 10%. Use of CNS agents was defined as receipt of a prescription for any of the following medications within 60 days preceding the index date: benzodiazepines and other sedatives/hypnotics; analgesics; antidepressants; tranquilizers/anti-psychotics; lithium; and centrally acting muscle relaxants. The chronic disease score was based on patterns of selected medication use in the preceding year, and includes medications used to treat chronic conditions such as heart disease, hypertension, and respiratory disease.

The adjusted risk of injurious motor vehicle crashes for current users of any insulin was 1.3 relative to non-users, with the use of insulin alone higher at 1.4. The adjusted rate ratio for the combined use of insulin and oral agents was 1.0, indicating no increased crash risk.

Use of oral hypoglycemics only (no insulin) was associated with no increased risk, with an adjusted rate ratio of 1.0 for use of sulfonylureas only and metformin only. However, the combined use of sulfonylureas and metformin (without insulin) was associated with an adjusted rate ratio of 1.3. Among individuals using oral agents, the risk of an injurious crash was greatest for those managed with high doses of combined therapy using sulfonylurea and metformin, for an adjusted rate ratio of 1.4. The rate ratios for current exposure to anti-diabetic agents were slightly higher than the ratios for any use in the year preceding the index date.

In summary, among drivers ages 67 to 84, the use of insulin alone or a combination of sulfonylurea and metformin, especially at high doses, is associated with an increase in the rate of involvement in injurious motor vehicle crashes of 30 to 40%. The authors note that metformin alone does not usually cause hypoglycemia, however it does when combined with a sulfonylurea. The use of insulin is associated with hypoglycemia. Use of insulin as well as the combined use of metformin and sulfonylurea in high doses is also associated with retinopathy and neuropathy (complications of more advanced diabetes). The authors recommend that for individuals treated with insulin alone or high doses of combined oral therapy, efforts to reduce their risk of injury due to motor vehicle crashes may include assessment of vision and peripheral neuropathy, and measurement of blood glucose levels prior to driving.

ILLNESS VERSUS MEDICATIONS AND THE RISK OF FALLS

This section addresses a recurring theme in assessing the behavioral consequences of medication usage among (older) people, i.e., gauging the risk associated with prescription and OTC drugs versus the medical conditions treated by the medications. It is included because the same medications that mediate falls risk—specifically with respect to cardiovascular adverse drug reactions—may also mediate motor vehicle crash risk.

Lee, Kwok, Leung, and Woo (2006) found that chronic medical conditions were often more important than medications in causing falls in high-functioning community-dwelling older people. They reviewed demographic data, falls history in the previous 12 months, medical diagnoses, current medications, and self-rated health for 4,000 ambulatory community-dwelling men and women over age 65 in an urban community in Hong Kong. The purpose of the investigation was to determine whether medical illnesses or the medications used to treat them were the cause falls in the older population. This study is included in this research update, because vehicle crash involvement in the elderly has been significantly associated with a history of falling in the past two years (see Staplin, Lococo, Stewart, & Decina, 1999), and as falling and crashing are two adverse mobility outcomes, they may share the same underlying causes.

In this sample, 19.7% of subjects reported at least one fall, and 5.9% reported two or more falls. After adjusting for age and gender, medications associated with any falls included: aspirin, diabetic drugs, nitrates, NSAIDS, and paracetamol. Medications associated with recurrent falls included: calcium channel blockers, diabetic drugs, nitrates, NSAIDS, aspirin, and statins. Psychotropic drugs including benzodiazepines, antidepressants, and antipsychotics were not significantly associated with any falls or recurrent falls.

Multivariate models were applied to determine the association between each medication and falls history (any falls) with adjustment to significant non-drug factors. Being female, having heart disease, and having shorter stride length were highly associated with falling. Eye disease was moderately associated with falls in the nitrates model. Lower body musculoskeletal pain, previous stroke, and eye disease were slightly associated with falls in all medication models. *The only medication that was significantly associated with any falls was nitrate* (OR=1.489, p<.027). Multivariate models were also run for recurrent falls. Again, being female and having a shorter stride length were strongly associated with recurrent falls. Eye disease was moderately associated, and heart disease and lower musculoskeletal pain showed a slight association. *Among medications, only anti-diabetics showed a significant association with recurrent falls*(OR=2.9, p=.001). Because the study cohort contained a large proportion of diabetic patients not on drug treatment (25.7%), direct comparisons between diabetics with anti-diabetic medication and those without this medication could be made. The study indicated that anti-diabetic medications were related to recurrent falls, but being diabetic was not. Thus, more advanced diabetes or hypoglycemics side effects of drugs could be the cause of falls among older diabetics.

Van der Velde, van den Meiracker, Pols, Stricker, and van der Cammen (2007) conducted the first prospective cohort study of geriatric patients to investigate the effects of withdrawal of all fall-risk-increasing drugs (FRIDs) on tilt-table test abnormalities. The tilt-table test evaluates how blood pressure is regulated in response to simple stresses. At times, the nerves that control blood pressure may not operate properly and may cause a reaction that causes the blood pressure to drop.[3] This reaction may produce a fainting spell or symptoms such as severe lightheadedness. Tilt-table testing can determine the likelihood that a patient is susceptible to this type of reaction. In the tilt-table test, patients lie down on a table and their baseline blood pressure and EEG are taken for 10 minutes. Then, the table is tilted head-up to 30 degrees, and blood pressure and EEG are taken again for 5 minutes in this tilted position. The table is then tilted head-up to 60 degrees, and measurements are taken for 45 minutes in this position. The table is then lowered to the flat position and a dose of isuprel is given, simulating the amount of adrenaline the body would produce when walking up a staircase. The table is then tilted to the 60-degree position and blood pressure and EEG are again taken for 15 minutes. If this portion of the test can be completed, the table is returned to the flat position, the dose of isuprel is increased, and the table is again tilted to 60 degrees for a third and final time.

Certain drugs increase the risk of falls in older people. These include psychotropic drugs such as antipsychotics, antidepressants, and sedatives, as well as cardiovascular drugs such as diuretics, type Ia antiarrhythmics, and digoxin (Leipzig, Cumming, & Tinetti, 1999). Cardiovascular adverse drug reactions include syncope (fainting or a sudden loss of consciousness) and falling, and are thought to result from carotid sinus hypersensitivity (CSH), vasovagal collapse (VVC), as well as orthostatic hypotension (OH). Explanations of these cardiovascular abnormalities follow. The carotid sinus is the point where the common carotid artery, located in the neck, divides into its two main branches. The carotid sinus can be oversensitive to manual stimulation, which is known as "carotid sinus hypersensitivity." Manual stimulation can cause large changes in heart rate and/or blood pressure. Symptoms can be produced by turning the head, wearing garments with tight-fitting collars, or manual stimulation of the neck as when shaving or taking a pulse in the neck. Orthostatic hypotension consists of symptoms of dizziness, faintness, or lightheadedness which appear only upon standing, and are caused by low blood pressure. Vasovagal collapse (also known as vasovagal syncope and neurocardiogenic syncope) is a fainting spell that often occurs when upright, although it can occur while sitting. Often, there are no precipitating circumstances, and it is most likely to occur in situations such as: during a large meal in a warm restaurant; when watching a production in a hot theater; when flying; or after prolonged standing.[4] The majority of the fall-risk-increasing drugs are known to induce OH, VVC, and/or CSH, which may be causal factors in drug-induced falls (and by extension, to drug-related crashes, as falls and crashes have been associated). The study was conducted to determine whether the removal of FRIDs resulted in a reduction of falls, and in improvement in tilt-table test outcome (indicating normalization of cardiovascular abnormalities resulting from the drugs).

Study participants were 211 new, consecutive outpatients at a geriatric outpatient clinic, 65 and older, with a mini-mental status exam score of 21 points or higher and able to walk 10 m without a walking aid. Falls history was considered positive if at least one fall occurred in the previous year; 135 subjects had a positive fall history. All subjects underwent tilt-table testing at baseline. First, carotid sinus massage was performed. CSH was defined as a fall in blood pressure greater than 50 mmHg or asystole (a state of no cardiac electrical activity) of 3 seconds or more. OH was measured for the first 5 minutes of head-up tilt after 10 minutes of quiet resting. OH was defined as a 20-mmHg fall in systolic blood pressure or a 10-mmHg fall in diastolic blood pressure. To provoke VVC, head-up tilt was continued until collapse occurred or 30 minutes of head-up tilt was reached. VVC was defined as a fall in blood pressure greater than 50 mmHg or asystole of 3 seconds or more.

Following tilt-table testing, all potential FRIDs were considered for withdrawal in the subgroup of fallers. FRIDs were able to be discontinued for 65 patients and dosages reduced for 6 patients. The subgroups of drugs withdrawn included psychotropics (sedatives, antidepressants, and neuroleptics), cardiovascular (antihypertensives, nitrates, antiarrhythmics, nicotinic acid, and timolol eye drops), and others (analgesics, antivertigo preparations, hypoglycemics, and urinary antispasmodics). Sedatives and antihypertensives were the largest two groups of drugs withdrawn. At a mean follow-up period of 6.7 months, tilt-table testing was repeated. Findings indicated that although overall FRID withdrawal was favorable for normalizing tilt-test-table results, it was significant only for OH. For the subgroup of patients who had cardiovascular FRIDs withdrawn, there was a significant reduction in OH and in CSH. This indicates that a substantial subgroup of geriatric patients experiences drug-induced cardiovascular adverse events, which are reversible after withdrawal of these drugs. For VCC, cardiovascular FRID withdrawal appeared favorable, but it was not statistically significant.

The association between cardiovascular improvements and nonoccurrence of falls during follow-up was also significant. Given the significant association between normalization of tilt-table test outcomes and nonoccurrence of falls, Van der Velde et al. (2007) comment that it is likely that part of the reduction in falls after FRID withdrawal in this cohort of geriatric patients was due to improvement in OH and in CSH. In this study, FRID-related falls were mediated through cardiovascular side effects.

FEASIBILITY OF ANALYSES USING LARGE ADMINISTRATIVE DATABASES

Overview of Candidate Databases

This project task examined the feasibility of collecting and analyzing data from a National database and from at least two other large, administrative databases to improve our understanding of the associations between multiple medication use among older adults and motor vehicle crashes. These future analyses would support case-control studies by identifying the relative frequencies of various combinations of medications used by those with and without motor vehicle crash involvements in a given period of time.

The National databases chosen for review were the Medicaid Analytic eXtract (MAX) files; the Medicare Current Beneficiary Survey (MCBS) and associated Access to Care files, and the Cost and Use files; and the Veteran's Health Administration (VHA) Pharmacy Benefits Management (PBM) database. Requests for information about other national databases were also made to the Agency for Healthcare Research and Quality) regarding its research program called the Centers for Education and Research on Therapeutics and associated databases, and specifically to the HMO Research Network.

The General Practice Research Database in the United Kingdom was also reviewed in this task; with 3 million active patient records and 35 million patient-years of data, it is the world's largest source of primary care data from a single country. It also appears to be the most comprehensive database included in this review, in terms of the data elements it contains. However, the GPRD is very costly to access; and, it is unclear that analysis outcomes using this resource would generalize to U.S. experience, given the cultural and infrastructure differences between the two countries.

Additional, large administrative claims databases – including Kaiser Permanente and Independence Blue Cross – were identified as potential candidates but were judged less desirable according to criteria detailed in this chapter, and were excluded from further, in-depth review. However, a proprietary research database (Ingenix LabRx) using United Healthcare data, operating under the parent company UnitedHealth Group, was selected for detailed review.

Nine database administrators were contacted in this task. Based on responses from each to a questionnaire, and follow-up telephone calls, the leading candidates for future NHTSA data mining activities appear to be (1) the VHA/PBM database; and (2) the Ingenix LabRx database. The VHA/PBM, which appears to be a good choice overall, requires a caveat: a VHA collaborator on the research team is mandatory in the type of work envisioned by NHTSA. Because of the close scrutiny of all data entered in insurance claims among contributing organizations, the Ingenix LabRx database may offer the most accurate and reliable data among the present alternatives.

This chapter describes pertinent characteristics of each administrative claims database identified as a potential candidate for NHTSA research purposes and discusses its strengths and weaknesses, to provide a rationale for the included recommendations. An overview of the most salient features of each database reviewed herein is provided in Appendix H. Appendix I presents a set of questions sent to administrative claims database administrators to obtain the information needed for the detailed review of their appropriateness for NHTSA investigations of medication usage and driving safety.

Detailed Review of Administrative Databases

A "straw man" in evaluating the strengths and weaknesses of each candidate database is to consider what an ideal database would be to support future NHTSA research on this topic. The ideal database would contain patient-level information on multiple millions of people[5]

A Pilot Study to Test Multiple Medication Usage and Driving Functioning

who have been continuously enrolled in the insurance program for at least 6 months and preferably for one year or more. This database would contain linked medical, hospital, and pharmaceutical data for each eligible person, and, ideally, would be the *only* provider of service for each eligible person. All prescriptions obtained would be through the insurance provider, so that a complete record of drug utilization would be captured in the claims database. Data fields would include:

- Dates of inpatient *and* outpatient hospital and doctor services;
- Diagnosis codes to document the reason for the healthcare visit, including E-codes with 4 digits to indicate external causes of injury for all injury diagnoses (so claims resulting from a motor vehicle cash may be identified, and the injured person may be identified as either the driver or a passenger);
- Patient demographics, including date of birth/age, gender, and ZIP code of residence;
- Pharmacy data including:
  - Drug dispensed (NDC);
  - Therapeutic drug class (decoded);
  - Active ingredient;
  - Quantity and date dispensed;
  - Drug strength;
  - Days supply;
  - Dollar amounts;
  - New fill/refill/partial indicator; and
  - Medical condition for which drug prescribed.

Not surprisingly, the present review, conducted in 2006, failed to identify such an ideal database. Details describing the following candidates for future analyses complete this chapter:

- Medicaid Analytic eXtract Database;
- Medicare Current Beneficiary Survey;
- VHA Pharmacy Benefits Management Database;
- General Practice Research Database (United Kingdom);
- Nationwide Inpatient Sample/Healthcare Cost and Utilization Project;
- Kaiser Permanente;
- Independence Blue Cross;
- Ingenix LabRx (United Healthcare) Database;
- The Centers for Education and Research on Therapeutics; and
- HMO Research Network.

Medicaid Analytic eXtract Database

Information describing MAX data was obtained from the following two Web sites: www.cms.hhs.gov/MedicaidDataSourcesGenInfo/07_MAXGeneralInformation.asp#TopOfPage and www.cms.hhs.gov/MSIS. A contact with the Centers for Medicare and Medicaid

332 National Highway Traffic Safety Administration

Services provided additional information about the feasibility of use of the MAX data by NHTSA.

The MAX data – formerly known as State Medicaid Research Files – are a set of person-level data files on Medicaid eligibility, service utilization, and payments. The MAX data are extracted from the Medicaid Statistical Information System. The MAX development process combines MSIS initial claims, interim claims, voids, and adjustments for a given service into this final action event. Unlike fiscal-based MSIS quarterly files, MAX files are annual calendar year files.

MAX data are derived from MSIS, and because it is necessary to allow for the delay between service delivery dates and claims adjudication dates, the availability of MAX data for a particular time period lags behind that of the MSIS data. Since the MAX data contain individually identifiable data, they are protected under the Privacy Act. They are available for approved research activities only through a Data Use Agreement (DUA) with the Centers for Medicare & Medicaid Services. Note that only approved academic research projects and certain government agencies are entitled to a DUA to obtain MAX data.

Prior to Federal fiscal year 1999, the Medical Statistical Information System (MSIS) was a voluntary program and those States participating in the MSIS project provided data tapes from their claims processing systems to the Centers for Medicare & Medicaid Services in lieu of the hard-copy statistical 2082 tables. Beginning in 1999, the program became mandatory for all States.

MAX 2002, 2001, 2000, and 1999 data are available for all States and the District of Columbia. Data for all States and DC for 2003 became available in late 2006, and data for all States and DC for 2004 should be available in 2007.

There are 5 MAX data sets: (1) a Person Summary file; (2) an Inpatient Hospital file; (3) a Long-Term Care file; (4) a Prescription Drug file; and (5) an Other Services file. The Person Summary File contains one record for each person enrolled in Medicaid for at least one day during the reporting year. The file includes the enrollee's demographic data as well as annual and monthly Medicaid enrollment data. It also contains information regarding the person's eligibility for Medicare (known as crossover claims or dual eligibility). Finally, it includes an annual summary of Medicaid utilization and expenditures for each enrollee by major Medicaid types of service. The four paid claims files contain information from adjudicated medical service related claims and capitation payments. Four types of claims files representing inpatient, long term care, prescription drugs and non-institutional services are submitted by the States. These are claims that have completed the State's payment processing cycle for which the State has determined it has a liability to reimburse the provider from Title XIX funds. Claims records contain information on the types of services provided, providers of services, service dates, reimbursement amounts, types of reimbursement, and selected demographic variables. The Other Services file contains information on outpatient services, excluding pharmacy services (pharmacy charges are included in the pharmacy database).

Data validation reports provide a wide array of basic statistics on data elements from each State and file type. Data anomaly reports are available that document data inconsistencies (which can't be fixed) and work-around solutions. They also describe situations where data are valid, but unexpected results occur because of broken time series, newly covered services, etc.

Medicaid data limitations include those related to eligibility, services, payments, completeness, timeliness, and the lack of provider characteristics. In terms of eligibility, there is minimal information on other insurance coverage, there is no beneficiary name or address, income data are unavailable, and eligibility is not continuous for all enrollees—therefore there is eligibility "churning." The concept of churning eligibility means that eligibility for Medicaid is determined monthly, based on a categorical relationship to Medicaid entitlement (e.g., age, disabled, poverty adult or child, etc.), income and assets. Because circumstances change from month to month people may be enrolled in Medicaid intermittently—on and off the program. The services limitations include the following: services are included only during times of eligibility, only Medicaid-covered services are present (and coverage varies by State), services are incomplete for duals (only the residual after Medicare payment), and services are incomplete for people in prepaid plans. Payment limitations include: missing payments (due to aggregate adjustments, end-of-year settlements, and disproportionate share hospital), incomplete for third-party payments, and drug payment amounts are prior to rebates.

The database contact for the current project task provided some specific information about the feasibility of the MAX databases for future NHTSA analyses of medications and motor vehicle crashes. First, it was stated that the databases include data that are necessary to meet reporting requirements or to get medical claims paid. Therefore, some of the data that would be necessary for future NHTSA work may not be present. For example, although the agency manuals state that cause of injury codes and diagnoses should be coded, diagnoses and injury codes are often not required for payment, and researchers have found that cause of injury (E-codes)are dramatically underreported in Medicare and Medicaid data.

In a study population utilizing 5% of the Medicare-aged sample from 1997 to 1999, approximately 75% of the Medicare claims reporting an injury diagnosis (800-995) were *not* E-coded (Bishop et al., 2002). E-coding in the MAX database varies by State, by injury severity, and by site of fracture. Western and northern regions of the country report more E-codes than Midwestern and southern regions. The more severe the injury, the more likely that E-coding will be present. Strains and sprains are less likely to be E-coded than fractures. As an example, back sprains were associated with E-coding in 12% of the cases, compared to fractures of the femoral neck, which were associated with E-coding in 45% of the cases. Bishop et al. (2002) conducted a logistic regression on a 5% sample of aged fee-for-service Medicare beneficiaries in the year 1999. For the 48,636 fracture episodes, E-codes were present in 40% of the cases. Bishop et al. (2002) reported that E-codes are more frequently reported in fracture episodes for older elders; the odds ratio for an E-code for people age 75 to 84 was 1.06, compared to 1.13 for people 85 and older. In addition, the probability that a fracture episode for a rural beneficiary includes an E-code is 10% greater than that for an urban beneficiary. Fractures treated outside of a hospital are less likely to have an E-code (16% of the claims were E-coded), compared to fractures treated during an inpatient stay in the first week of an episode (57% of the claims were E-coded) and fractures treated in an emergency room without a hospital stay (54% of the claims were E-coded). Although the odds of E-codes in episodes with hospital care are low in States that require cause of injury in hospital discharge data, odds are even lower in States with no E-code requirement for hospital discharge.

A further concern with the use of CMS Medicaid data is how E-codes are reported. In a memo commenting on motorcycle accidental E-codes in the Medicaid eXtract Analytic files for the year 2000, it was reported that *when* E-codes were reported, they were often reported using only the 3-digit code (Benedict & Brinker, 2005). To identify vehicle type, a 4-digit E-

334 National Highway Traffic Safety Administration

code must be reported. This would be problematic in future NHTSA research, because not only is vehicle type important (trains vs. automobiles versus trucks vs. motorcycles), occupant type (driver versus passenger) is important. The 4th digit must be present in an E-code to identify the injured person. Only drivers would be of interest in studies of vehicle crashes and medication use.

Another caveat to the use of the data is that prior to January 2006, coverage for prescription drugs under Medicare was nonexistent (except for limited coverage of drugs related to End-Stage Renal Disease and transplantation), so there is no pharmacy data for Medicare-only patients up to this date. Prescription drug data are available for Medicaid recipients (including dual Medicaid-Medicare enrollees), however. In 2002, the Medicaid database contained data for approximately 7 million individuals 65 and older. Prescription drug information is not available for inpatient hospital stays; because inpatient hospitalbills aggregate the drugs into one cost center (no names are available). The outpatient medications are listed individually by NDC code, but the NDC code does not provide the therapeutic drug class. If that was required, a separate filter would need to be applied. Existing license agreements prevent CMS from sharing data that includes therapeutic use codes with third parties. Alternatively, the Food and Drug Administration maintains a free filter for therapeutic drug classification.

The lag between claims incurred for pharmacy claims and entry into the database should theoretically take no more than 45 days. But States vary in their compliance to these regulations, and there is no penalty for failure to comply with reporting requirements.

In order to gain access to the database, first the files required for research must be identified among the five available: Inpatient hospitalizations; Long term care; Prescription drug; other ambulatory services; and the Person file (includes Medicaid eligibility information). Then, the States of interest and years of interest would need to be identified. Access is governed by the Privacy Act/HIPAA. Requests for these files must include a study protocol along with a Data Use Agreement. The use of the files must then meet approval by the Privacy Board. CMS does no custom programming or data extraction. A CMS processing fee may apply.

Based on the "churning eligibility," the fact that E-codes are generally reported only for the most serious injuries (and many of those including only 3 digits), and the incomplete data resulting from dual eligibility, it doesn't appear that the MAX databases are the most robust among those evaluated in this task for the type of data-mining efforts of interest to NHTSA. CMS initiatives begun in 1998 may improve Medicare E-coding. A suggestion provided by an analyst at CMS[6] was to consider the possibility of linking the Medicaid research files to a State motor vehicle crash file and to an auto insurance crash file, with the most promising common variables being a Social Security number in each database and at least one other demographic, such as year of birth. The Medicaid research files contain an SSN and an individually assigned Medicaid identifier for each enrollee, but they do not contain driver license numbers or addresses. It would be important to obtain the State of residence of the individual being linked, and not the State where the crash occurred and is being reported from. It would be important to match the individual with the Medicaid research file from the State of residence. A fair number of motor vehicle crashes occur when people are driving out-of-State. An auto insurance database might provide a third linkage, providing a driver's license number and an address, and personal demographics.

Medicare Current Beneficiary Survey (MCBS)

Much of the information presented about the Medicare Current Beneficiary Survey CMS database was obtained from the CMS Web site[7], which presents detail on the interview population, as well as the two major files produced by MCBS: the Cost and Use File and the Access to Care File. A request for information was also sent to the director of the Enterprise Databases Group (Office of Information and Systems) at the Centers for Medicare and Medicaid Services, and to the Research Data Assistance Center at the University of Minnesota.

MCBS interview data are linked to Medicare claims and other administrative data to enhance their analytic power. The survey and claims data together constitute a more complete utilization data set for the MCBS sample than is available from either source. The final file consists of survey, administrative, and claims data. All personal identifying information is removed.

The MCBS is a continuous, multipurpose survey of a representative national sample of the Medicare population, conducted by the Office of Strategic Planning of the Centers for Medicare & Medicaid Services. The central goals of MCBS are to determine expenditures and sources of payment for all services used by Medicare beneficiaries, including co-payments, deductibles, and non-covered services; to ascertain all types of health insurance coverage and relate coverage to sources of payment; and to trace processes over time, such as changes in health status, spending down to Medicaid eligibility, and the impacts of program changes.

MCBS contains a variety of data on each sampled person, including topical supplements; combining survey and administrative data. Beneficiaries sampled from Medicare enrollment files (or appropriate proxies) are interviewed in person three times a year using computer-assisted personal interviewing (CAPI). The first round of interviewing was conducted from September through December 1991, and the survey has been continuously in the field since then. The data are designed to support both cross-sectional and longitudinal analyses. Interviews at 4-month intervals are designed to yield longitudinal series of data on the use of health services, medical care expenditures, health insurance coverage, sources of payment (public and private, including out-of-pocket payments), health status and functioning, and a variety of demographic and behavioral information, such as income, assets, living arrangements, family supports, and access to medical care.

The MCBS contact for this database review task advised that the MCBS would not be a feasible data set for future NHTSA research on older drivers, medications, and crashes, because it does not contain any prescribing information, other than self-reported prescription drugs. There are no pharmacy or prescription claims data; only self-reported medication use. So there is no way to determine if a survey respondent was taking a prescription drug on the date of service for a Medicare claim. In addition, the Medicare claims data include E-code data, but it is unreliable (i.e., it is only available when an E-code is required for billing purposes). None of the MCBS survey questions relate to motor vehicle crashes. Finally, information in the database relating to Medicare HMO utilization and other insurers and payers outside of Medicare is based on self-reported information and imputation.

Veteran's Health Administration Pharmacy Benefits Management Database

Three research studies using the VHA PBM database deserve mention in this chapter, as certain variables, procedures, anomalies, and limitations revealed therein speak to the feasibility of using the database to associate medication use and motor vehicle crashes (a specific type of adverse event).

In the first study, French, Campbell, Spehar, and Angaran (2005) linked outpatient prescription data with clinical data to develop a risk adjusted binary model that associates benzodiazepine use with the risk for a healthcare encounter for an injury. They used 3 years of outpatient benzodiazepine prescription data (totaling 133,872 outpatient prescriptions) for 13,745 patients for a VA medical center (James A. Haley VA Hospital in Tampa, FL). The PMB database contains information on the strength of the drug, prescribed daily amount, fill date, quantity supplied, and a unique patient identifier. The daily milligrams consumed was computed as the product of the prescribed daily amount (number of pills) and strength (mg) and then converted from daily milligrams consumed to daily oral dosing equivalents or valium equivalents. Using the patient identifier, the pharmacy data were combined with VHA healthcare utilization data extracted from the centralized VHA National Patient Care Database. This database includes patient demographics, injuries, and diagnoses. Dates of the injuries were unavailable in the database; the researchers used the date of the associated healthcare encounter (inpatient admission and outpatient clinic visit). Primary and secondary diagnoses using the ICD-9-CM codes 800-999 for injuries and poisonings in both inpatient and outpatient datasets were examined. Only those encounters associated with an injury code while receiving benzodiazepines were used in the analyses and only the first injury episode of care while using benzodiazepines was used, to avoid analytical problems with multiple episodes for one patient. Certain injuries were excluded, as they were unlikely to result from benzodiazepine use. These included complications devices, implants, grafts, and complications of surgical procedures or medical care. These were identified using the Agency for Healthcare Research and Quality Clinical Classification Software (CCS) that aggregates the injury ICD-9-CM codes into homogenous diagnosis groups. Thus, CCS categories 237 and 238 for the two types of complications were removed. Also, because of coding anomalies, CCS category 227 (spinal cord injuries) were removed. Anomalies resulted with this code because almost all spinal cord injury patients were being treated for follow-up care, as opposed to being treated for the original spinal cord injury.

Controlling for co-morbidities (secondary diagnoses that did not relate to the principal diagnosis, screened through a diagnosis related group) and demographic factors (age and marital status), French et al. (2005) found that increases in dose and duration were associated with an increased risk for an injury-related episode of care. Increasing the dose by 1 U (valium equivalent) may increase the risk of injury on average by 6% and a 1-U increase in duration (one additional week on the drug) may increase the risk by 4%. The authors note a limitation to the study is that the sample was overwhelmingly male, and thus generalizability of the results to females is questionable. Also, the mechanisms of injury (E-codes) could not be ascertained for all injuries under study because of the lack of E-coding for most of the healthcare injury encounters. Preliminary analyses found that less than 50% of injury discharges in the VHA system have an E-code. However, this compares to national studies of civilian injury hospitalizations where E-coding was present for 60% of the discharges (Shinoda-Tagawa & Clark, 2003).

In the second study, French, Chirikos, et al. (2005) evaluated the concomitant use of benzodiazepines and other drugs on the likelihood of an injury-related healthcare episode. They used the VHA data from the pharmacy benefit management system for the James A. Haley VA Hospital, as described earlier. Drug combinations were limited to those defined by Micromedex software likely to result in major interactions. Pair-wise combinations of a benzodiazepine and one of the other medications were then constrained to just those being used within the 30-day period prior to the date of the healthcare encounter for the injury. There were a total of 54,591 prescriptions involving the concomitant use of benzodiazepines and other drugs for 6,223 unique patients. Results indicated that 12.7% of the patients with concomitant use of benzodiazepines and other drugs had an injury or adverse event, as compared with 4.3% of the patients taking benzodiazepines who did not have concomitant drug use. The most common combinations were benzodiazepines with a muscle relaxant (17% of the concomitant prescriptions) and opioids (79% of the concomitant prescriptions).

More recently, French, Campbell, et al. (2006) used data from the national VHA ambulatory event database to identify which specific medications (within recognized major problematic drug categories that increase risk of falling) were prescribed to veterans before their outpatient treatment for a fall. The database includes data from all 21 Veterans Integrated Service Networks for approximately 5.1 million unique patients with approximately 72 million outpatient encounters. The study population was all VHA patients age 65+ who had a fall-related outpatient encounter (as indicated by a diagnostic E-code) during the year 2004 and who received one or more outpatient medications during the study period. Using unique encrypted patient identifiers, the encounter data were merged with outpatient pharmacy data from the VHA decision support system (DSS) for the same year. The DSS pharmacy data contains information on the drug, fill date, and quantity supplied for each patient. It does not include medications filled outside of the VHA system, or information on nonprescription drugs, or drug samples acquired independently by the patient. The authors note, however, that many veterans have an incentive to use the VHA for their medications because of the low VHA co-payment. The researchers identified patients with a fall-coded encounter and exact age and sex matched comparison subjects from a pool of over 180,000 outpatient nonspecific chest pain patients, because nonspecific chest pain is one of the most common reasons for outpatient visits and an important symptom in cardiovascular disease, and to analyze differences in particular medications between this patient group and the group that fell. Fall related injuries due to slips, trips, or falls unrelated to transportation were identified by E-codes E860-E888). Records were included in the analysis if a fall E-code appeared in any of the 10 diagnosis fields (1 primary diagnosis and 9 secondary diagnosis fields).

The drugs of interest were in three major drug categories: central nervous system (CNS), cardiovascular system (CVS), and musculoskeletal system (MSS). The most comprehensive and evidence-based published list of specific problematic fall-related medications is the Canadian Safety Council's Risk Assessment tool, which is divided into classes with generic and trade names. The data from the DSS outpatient prescription file only contain information about drugs on the VHA formulary, therefore, drugs from the Canadian fall risk assessment tool and the Beers Criteria list were reclassified using the U.S. national drug code. Linking of outpatient medications and outpatient encounters was temporarily constrained, and included only those medications actively prescribed up to the time of the encounter. There were 20,551 patients with fall-coded encounters and 20,551 exact age- and sex-matched comparisons. Of the patients selected for the study, 95% were male. There was no significant difference in the number of patients who used fall-related medications in the nonspecific chest pain group and fall-coded group. More patients with nonspecific chest pain received CVS medications and more patients with fall-coded encounters received CNS medications. There were no statistically significant differences in the overall MSS category between the two groups, but more patients in the nonspecific chest pain group than in the fall-coded group used (prescription) non-steroidal anti-inflammary drugs. Within the CNS category, significantly more fall-coded patients used opioid analgesics and narcotics, hypnotics, anti-Parkinson agents, and the psychotropic drug classes of cholinesterase inhibitors, anticonvulsants and barbiturates, antidepressants (including SSRIs, tricyclic antidepressants, and others), antipsychotics (including both atypical antipsychotics and typical neuroleptics) and benzodiazepines. There were no differences between groups in the use of antihistamines and antinauseants.

One limitation to French, Campbell, et al. (2006) study (other than the population being limited to veterans and mostly males) is that some veterans can receive care under the Medicare program from non-VHA providers and facilities, and that these data were not captured in the analyses. The authors state that future research at the Patient Safety Center in Tampa, Florida, will link available Medicare data from the U.S. Department of Veterans Affairs Medicare data sets so that this health care utilization is captured.

French, Campbell, et al. (2006) note that this is the first national study of veterans that examined their outpatient use of particular drugs temporally linked with a fall-coded health encounter. This study is of particular interest to the current topic of examining multiple drug use and vehicle crashes. In the past NHTSA study of polypharmacy, classes of drugs were identified as being potentially driver impairing and were linked to increased crash risk in older drivers using a non-proprietary database. The list of drug classes and specific medications developed in that project (available at www.drivinghealth.com/ PDIdrugindex.html) could be used by NHTSA in future research with the VHA PBM database. French, Campbell, et al. (2006) state that no U.S. medication safety studies have been based on National outpatient medication data linking information about outpatient prescriptions, including dosing and timing, to health care utilization associated with injuries. They state that, *"The data available through the VHA system allows one to study the association between a particular drug and an injury or adverse event by identifying a population at risk and then linking outpatient medications with healthcare utilization in that population."* They further state that in their opinion, there is no other comparable National drug safety research capability that includes a National electronic medical record and data on health care utilization across as many care settings in the United States.

French, Campbell, et al. (2006) indicated that comprehensive National outpatient medication usage data at the patient level are currently not available for researchers from the Medicare program. The new Medicare Part D outpatient medication benefit was implemented in January 2006. Because of the large number of private Medicare prescription drug plans with nonstandard formularies, they state that it is not clear how, when, or if any of the outpatient medication data in the Part D benefit will be available to researchers. They further state that countries with national health care systems (Canada, Australia, Finland, Sweden, and the United Kingdom) and large managed health care systems in the United State currently have the ability to link data in such a way.

A Pilot Study to Test Multiple Medication Usage and Driving Functioning 339

Contact with the program manager of Outcomes Research at the VA Center for Medication Safety revealed that there are 8 million veterans nationwide who use the VA for health care. Of this group, over 5.1 million get their prescriptions from inside of the VA system. Some of these patients who are 65 and older may use outside systems to obtain their medications, but it is rare, based on the fact that the co-pay for VA medications is so low (only $8 per prescription). There are cases where a VA patient may go to a non-VA facility for health care, as in the case of an acute condition, where an ambulance takes the patient to the closest hospital that may be non-VA. It is sometimes possible to link with the Medicare database, but the Medicare database is two years behind in claims, whereas the VA system is current to within three months. But, the patients always return to VA centers for follow-up, so their information will be picked up at their next regular visit. Although the VA population includes physically and cognitively disabled people who would not be drivers, a "fair number" of the veterans are drivers. Motor vehicle crashes are coded in the VA database. While drivers and passengers are not separately identified, the database contains ICD-9-CM E-codes, so presumably the 4th digit identifying the injured person as a passenger or driver is present. The VA PMB database includes data for both inpatient and outpatient health care visits. It is a nomenclature-based database, so exact drug names, rather than drug codes are included. The exact drug names can be easily matched to the NDC codes, however.

A potential drawback to the use of this database is that it has been historically proprietary, and can only be used by non-VA researchers if a collaborative agreement is made with an investigator within the VA. Alternatively, the data has been made available if a VA employee is on staff with the researchers. The VA doesn't provide a data file to anyone other than a VA collaborator. This is due to HIPAA requirements, as well as the need for internal knowledge of the VA database and its coding to ensure the accuracy of the results." In order for the VA to release data, NHTSA and its researchers would need to identify the kind of information needed and provide an analysis plan, and then the VA IRB would review the request. They would only provide the data to the VA principal investigator or a research member who is affiliated with the VA. Costs for data range from $8,000 to $150,000. The cost for data and data cleaning for a study population of 40,000 (the magnitude of the French, Campbell et al., 2006 study) would run approximately $30,000. This covers the costs of pulling ICD-9 codes and medicines. If data analysis were required by VA staff, the salary of programmers and statisticians would need to be covered. This would increase the cost by an additional $25,000 to $75,000. Requests would need IRB approval from both the researchers and the VA IRB. In summary, it appears that this database contains all the necessary elements to perform analyses of interest to NHTSA. The only drawback is the inability to obtain an extracted dataset for independent work, if a non-VA researcher is proposed.

General Practice Research Database

The General Practice Research Database is operated by the GPRD Division of the Medicines & Healthcare products Regulatory Agency in London. The GPRD is considered by many as the "gold standard" of longitudinal anonymised patient databases from primary care, and its usage has resulted in over 400 clinical reviews and papers.[8] With over 3 million current patient records (8.9 million total) and over 35 million patient years of data from over

340   National Highway Traffic Safety Administration

350 practices, it is the world's largest source of longitudinal primary care data covering the full cross-section of the population in the UK. GPRD contains comprehensive data from real life clinical practice on diagnoses, prescribing, ADRs, co-prescription, co-morbidity, dosage details, off-label prescription, and patient age, sex and other demographic details. The data are anonymised and collected directly from records held on general practitioners' surgery computers.

Information obtained from the GPRD Web site is presented below, supplemented by comments from the head of GPRD/GPRD Group.

There are several ways to access Full Feature GPRD (FF-GPRD), either as datasets, through commissioned research and reports or through secure on-line access. Unlike flat files, the database is pre-structured and ready to query online, minimizing the need for IT support. This is cost-effective because it saves time and resources compared to building and periodically updating datasets. Included as part of the online access licenses are software packages and tools for constructing queries, and results can be exported for further analysis to most statistical spreadsheet packages. The GPRD Division has an experienced research team who assists customers with queries, advises on study design and carries out additional commissioned research projects. Best practice guidance is issued as new methodologies are developed, allowing customers to make the most of the system and the data. These services complement the comprehensive training included with all online access packages. Additionally, online access customers are supported by the Helpdesk to help resolve any IT-related issues.

As some GPRD customers may not have the resources to have continued access to FF-GPRD via the on-line services, datasets for single study analysis may be provided. Datasets are built from the FF-GPRD but are static representation of the data. Datasets are usually supplied, following ISAC approval on a CD-ROM. Charges are based on the number of patients and the data element required.

A direct contact with GPRD provided additional information about the feasibility of using this database for future studies of medications and crashes. While the clinical data (medical, basic hospital care, and pharmaceutical care) are within one database called the GPRD, what NHTSA studies would require is external linkage via the National Health Service 10-digit ID to National Hospital Episodes data for patents who are hospitalized and to other more regional datasets for patients who attend the emergency room but are discharged without being admitted to a hospital bed. The GPRD is a generalizable, "5.5% of the UK population based dataset." Patients 65 and older make up approximately 17% of the sample.

In the United Kingdom, the general practitioner is the gatekeeper to all care, and as such, stores not only primary care information, but essentially all details of care. Linkage of medical, hospital, and pharmaceutical data is via a unique patient identifier (the NHS 10-digit unique ID). Diagnoses are coded using the ICD10 (ICD9 for earlier data) and READ. Four-digit coding is used with up to 12 ICD codes allowed after the primary code. Codes V40.n to V48.n are available to distinguish car related events and the driver (.0, .5, or .9) and equivalent codes for lorries, buses, etc. Codes identify when a patient is a passenger or the driver. Procedures are coded using the OPCS4; and pharmaceutical claims are coded using the British National Formulary, ATC code, and UK-wide Multilex. ICD9 E-codes (coded by coding clerks) are present in the database. The percentage of injury discharges with an E-code could be made available to us at a later date, if required. Dates of motor vehicle crashes are unknown; the data of first admission for care relating to a crash would be used as the data of the crash, for analyses. The database includes socioeconomic class and regional markers (rather than zip codes). Privacy rules would allow the release of patient age; date of birth would be released by year only. Also, patient gender is available for release.

The database contains information that would allow the identification of what prescriptions were filled or refilled within a specified window of time, in proximity to a motor vehicle crash. Prescriptions are based on a 28-day cycle. There may be some level of misclassification, because some prescriptions might not be picked up; but, the sequence of prescribing for chronic drugs will indicate, for the most patients, this will not be an issue. Dates are associated to the date that the prescription was written, not filled. For acute drugs, this is known to be an accurate marker, and for chronic drugs, the sequence of refills is the key. All drug coding is done to the names of individual drugs (using generic names). The following information about drugs is also available: medical condition for which the drug was prescribed (from the linked consultation ID file of therapy and diagnosis); drug name, active ingredient, and NDC code; quantity provided; strength; decoded therapeutic class; and day's supply.

The database contains all information for a patient, regardless of what physician and what pharmacy was used (the database is NHS total care). Variables are not available (nor are they necessary) to indicate whether a patient has other coverage; there is a small volume of private care in the United Kingdom, but this would not significantly bias the research that could be undertaken. Because of the NHS and the fact that there is no charge for those over age 65 and those with chronic conditions, together with the relatively low charge for others, 99% of the drugs used are obtained through the NHS system. Only over-the-counter (essentially, the very safe drugs) are obtained outside of the NHS.

Data are available to the GPRD approximately one year after a claim is made (i.e., the lag time is one year). Continuity of eligibility is tracked via the patient roster file, as NHS care is cradle to grave for essentially 99.9% of the U.K. population.

The cost of having selected fields extracted from the database and anonymized could not be provided by the database contact, without further detail about the studies (e.g., the protocol). The GPRD Web site provides the following range of costs for the listed services.[9]

- Online access   £30,000 to £325,000 per year.
- Datasets   £8,000 to £65,000.
- Commissioned studies   £30,000 to £250,000.

The procedure to obtain the data would be to submit a protocol, and then have it undergo approval by the relevant Scientific and Ethical committees. The GPRD team would advise on the procedures necessary. A linking agreement would also be required from a committee called PIAG. There would be no barriers to the release of the data to NHTSA; however, it would need to be under legal agreement and the study must be published.

The completeness of the GPRD recommends it for future NHTSA data-mining activities. However, it may be cost-prohibitive. Also problematic are the substantial differences in the availability of/access to public transportation facilities; geometric and operational characteristics of streets and highways; licensing policies/practices; and gasoline costs (and therefore miles driven per capita) that differ between the two countries, and that may call into question the generalizability of U.K. analysis outcomes to the United States.

Nationwide Inpatient Sample/Healthcare Cost and Utilization Project

Information about the NIS was obtained from the NIS Web site,[10] i.e., there was no direct contact with a database administrator, other than an e-mail inquiry to User Support. According to the NIS Web site, NIS is the largest all-payer inpatient care database in the United States. It contains data from approximately 8 million hospital stays each year. NIS 2003 contains all discharge data from 994 hospitals located in 37 States, approximating a 20% stratified sample of U.S. community hospitals. The sampling frame for the NIS 2003 is a sample of hospitals that comprises approximately 90% of all hospital discharges in the United States.

NIS is the only national hospital database with charge information on all patients, regardless of payer, including people covered by Medicare, Medicaid, private insurance, and the uninsured. NIS's large sample size enables analyses of rare conditions, such as congenital anomalies; uncommon treatments, such as organ transplantation; and special patient populations, such as children. NIS data are available from 1988 to 2003, allowing analysis of trends over time. The number of States in the NIS has grown from 8 in the first year to 37 currently.

For most States, NIS includes hospital identifiers that permit linkages to the American Hospital Association's database and county identifiers that permit linkages to the Area Resource File. The NIS contains clinical and resource use information included in a typical discharge abstract, with safeguards to protect the privacy of individual patients, physicians, and hospitals (as required by data sources). The NIS can be weighted to produce national estimates. The NIS excludes data elements that could directly or indirectly identify individuals. Purchase of the files is open to all users who sign a Data Use Agreement (PDF file, 55 KB; HTML). Users must agree to use the database for research and statistical purposes only and to make no attempts to identify individuals.

Identities of institutions are available only in States where data sources already make that information public or agree to its release. For these institutions and for research purposes only, linkage is possible to data from the Annual Survey of the American Hospital Association.

An e-mail contact was made to HCUP User Support to determine whether medication use and injury codes were included in the datasets. HCUP User Support replied that HCUP data include ICD-9-CM external cause of injury codes (E-codes) and previous studies have found the E-code data fairly complete and reliable (Barrett, Steiner, & Coben, 2004). Barrett et al. (2004) found that across 33 States that provided inpatient data to HCUP, E-code completeness on injury records averaged 87.2%. For inpatient data, motor vehicle traffic accounted for 18.2% of all unintentional injuries. Across the nine States that provided emergent department data to HCUP, E-code completeness on injury records averaged 92.5%. In these nine States, motor vehicle traffic accounted for an average of 12.1% of the unintentional injuries.

Although E-code data are complete and reliable, HCUP does not include complete or reliable pharmacy data, nor can HCUP data be linked to pharmaceutical data. Thus, it would not be possible to determine what prescriptions were filled or refilled within a specified window of time. Since it would not be possible to identify medication use for patients hospitalized with injuries resulting from motor vehicle crashes, the NIS database would not be feasible for future NHTSA data-mining activities.

Kaiser Permanente

The database contact stated that Kaiser does not sell or distribute data; it would not download data and provide it to NHTSA or its researchers. Further, it only does research in-house, and only when it is of value to its members. In order to engage in research on medications and crashes among the older population of members, Kaiser would first need to find a collaborative researcher in-house with an interest in the topic. It would then require the use of its own investigator, statisticians, and programmers to complete the work, according to a research plan that NHTSA would provide, under a formal contract to ensure that its research costs were covered.

Kaiser Permanente has 8.3 million members distributed throughout 8 regions nationally, the largest of which is the Northern California region with 3.3 million members. In the Northern California region there are 600,000 members age 65+. There are presently 80 databases that can all be linked through each member's 7-digit membership number. Many months into the future, a new database—HealthConnect—will be installed, which contains most of the fields presently existing in the 80 databases; the new database will then need to be verified before it can be used. The present databases contain inpatient, outpatient, and emergency room medical data. The kinds of data that are included in the databases are diagnoses, radiology, pharmacy data, clinical laboratory data, and pathology. It is unknown whether etiology data (the reason for the visit) are present in any of the databases. The database contact did not know whether motor vehicle crashes were coded, although they could be obtained through chart review, and future encoding. If E-codes are not presently included in the databases, the cost for chart review would likely be prohibitive.

Based on the fact that Kaiser cannot provide a data set to NHTSA or its researchers, and the high likelihood that E-codes for motor vehicle crashes are not presently part of the databases, the use of the Kaiser databases for future NHTSA research is not recommended.

Independence Blue Cross

A contact at Independence Blue Cross provided several reasons that the Independence Blue Cross (IBX) database would not be feasible for use in future NHTSA research. First, IBX outsources all drug claims for payment; this means that there is no mechanism to link pharmacy data with claims data relating to injuries. Second, it's questionable whether coding for injuries goes beyond coding for diagnoses. It is very likely that there are no E-codes present in the database. Finally, the IBX legal department expressed concern regarding patient privacy, and advised that a separate authorization would need to be sent to all patients to obtain their permission (to comply with HIPAA), even though our description of the future work specified that any files obtained would be anonymized.

Ingenix LabRx Database (United Healthcare Data)

Ingenix LabRx is a proprietary research database that incorporates de-identified medical and pharmacy claims, lab results, and enrollment data on more than 35 million lives spanning

4.5 years (a National managed care population). Of particular interest is that the database has more than 21 million continuously enrolled covered lives for 12 months. A database contact indicated that it would be feasible to use the LabRx database in future NHTSA data mining research, as this type of work is performed quite frequently using LabRx.

LabRx is a database linking five datasets: administrative data, pharmacy claims data, physician and facility claims data, lab test results data, and consumer elements. It contains 35 million people with *both* medical and pharmacy benefits between May 2000 and December 2005. There are 55 million lives covered in the United Health Care Group, interacting with 450,000 physicians and 5,000 health care institutions. Of the 35 million lives included in LabRx, 61% have at least one pharmacy claim. Only 5.5% of this population (1,943,152) is 65 or older. However, although the number of lives covered drops significantly as age approaches 65, this will change dramatically in the coming years, because United recently acquired Pacific Care (a Medicare and Supplemental carrier) and Ovations (the largest Medicare provider in the Nation).

Within the population of 35 million lives, approximately 33 million are covered by commercial insurance, 1 million by Medicaid, 700,000 by Medicare, and 4,000 by other or unknown payers. It contains approximately 14 million covered lives per year, and is updated monthly. The data are blinded to protect patient privacy, yet the database supports patient-linked longitudinal analyses.

The data elements included within each of the five data sets are listed below.

Administrative Data: Member Identifier; Plan; Gender; Age; Dates of Eligibility.

Pharmacy Claims Data: Member Identifier; Prescribing Physician; Drug Dispensed (NDC); Therapeutic Drug Class; Quantity and Date Dispensed; Drug Strength; Days Supply; Dollar Amounts.

Physician and Facility Claims Data: Member Identifier; Physician or Facility Identifier; Procedures (CPT-4, revenue codes, ICD-9); Diagnosis (ICD-9-CM, DRG); Admission and Discharge Dates; Date and Place of Service; Dollar Amounts.

Lab Test Results Data: Member Identifier; Lab Test Name; Result.

Consumer Elements: Member Identifier; Income; Net Worth; Education; Race and Ethnicity; Life Stage; Life Style Indicators.

A ballpark cost estimate of providing a data file to NHTSA that includes 40,000 patients with two years of data is $50,000.

The database contact in this task indicated that E-codes are indeed captured, and it is much more common for them to be coded using 4 digits rather than 3. A "quick and dirty" run of the database (excluding the recent additions from Ovations and Pacific Care) identified 126 members age 65+ with 4-digit E-codes in the range of E8130 to E8139 (motor vehicle traffic accident involving collision with other vehicle). It was noted, however, that this older population group is increasing in the database as a result of bringing more Medicare Part D members into the plans that supply Ingenix with data. In summary, the Ingenix LabRx database appears to have the necessary elements for use in future NHTSA studies on medications and crash risk.

The Centers for Education and Research on Therapeutics

The Centers for Education and Research on Therapeutics is a research program administered by the Agency for Healthcare Research and Quality, in consultation with the Food and Drug Administration, within the U.S. Department of Health and Human Services. The mission of the CERTs is to conduct research and provide education that will advance the optimal use of drugs, medical devices, and biological products.[11] There are seven CERTs centers, each with the following emphasis:

- Duke University Medical Center (therapies for disorders of the heart and blood vessels);
- HMO Research Network (drug use, safety and effectiveness studies in HMO populations);
- University of Alabama at Birmingham (therapies for musculoskeletal disorders);
- University of Arizona Health Sciences Center (reduction in drug interactions that result in harm to women);
- University of North Carolina at Chapel Hill (therapies for children);
- University of Pennsylvania School of Medicine (therapies for infection and antibiotic drug resistance); and
- Vanderbilt University Medical Center (prescription drug use in a Medicaid population).

An e-mail request was sent to the director of pharmaceutical studies at the Agency for Healthcare Research and Quality regarding the feasibility of using CERT databases for future NHTSA research. At the time this chapter was developed as a project interim report in 2006, no contacts had been received. In parallel with requests made at the administrative level within CERTs, a request was made to a particular CERTs center, the HMO Research Network. A summary of the results of this contact follows.

HMO Research Network
The CERTs HMO Research Network comprises the investigators, information resources, delivery systems, and the following health maintenance organizations that are committed to public domain research (www.certs.hhs.gov/centers/hmo.html):

- Harvard Pilgrim Health Care, Boston, MA;
- Meyers Primary Care Institute/Fallon Community Health Plan, Worcester, MA;
- Group Health Cooperative of Puget Sound, Seattle, WA;
- HealthPartners Research Foundation, Minneapolis, MN;
- Kaiser Permanente Georgia, Atlanta, GA;
- Kaiser Permanente Northern California, Oakland, CA;
- Kaiser Permanente Northwest, Portland, OR;

- Kaiser Permanente Colorado, Denver, CO;
- Kaiser Permanente Hawaii, Honolulu, HI;
- Kaiser Permanente Southern California, Pasadena, CA;
- Lovelace Clinic Foundation, Albuquerque, NM;
- Henry Ford Health System – Health Alliance Plan, Detroit, MI;
- Scott and White Health System, Temple, TX; and
- Marshfield Clinic Research Foundation, Marshfield, WI.

The HMO Research Network focus is on use, safety, and effectiveness studies of therapeutics using health plans for defined populations. Key projects include patient interventions to increase adherence to beta blocker therapy after heart attack; working with the FDA to develop new methods for rapid discovery of adverse drug reactions; and assessing medication errors in ambulatory cancer care.

The principal investigator of the HMO Research Network served as the contact for our request. He indicated that the center has considered research like this over the years, and concluded that health plan records were probably unable to satisfactorily identify the operators of vehicles involved in motor vehicle accidents. The studies of which he is aware use motor vehicle registry data to identify the individuals of interest, and then they link this information to health plans' data on drug exposures and other conditions. He stated that he didn't know of any reason the health plan records would have improved in this regard. So, the participation of the HMO Research Network would require developing a linkage agreement with relevant motor vehicle registries. He also indicated that the HMO CERT often collaborates with external investigators, but doesn't work as a data vendor.

Based on the information provided by the HMO CERT, this database is not recommended for future data mining activities by NHTSA.

Discussion and Recommendations

This research has contributed evidence that can help guide continuing investigations into the relationship between (multiple) medication usage and driving safety. Such studies will provide the knowledge base upon which to develop and implement new programs to inform key health care providers,[12] and consumers themselves, about specific drugs and combinations of drugs that place (older) adults at greatest risk when they drive. The proliferation of poly-pharmacy among older people who remain frequent, active drivers—including not only a wide range of potentially driver-impairing (PDI) medications, but also drugs on the Beers list of inappropriate medications for older adults—only underscores the need for such educational countermeasures. To that end, this pilot study has provided an update on the prevalence of prescription medications in the older population, and the effects on driving of specific drugs/drug classes. In addition, its results point to what appear to be relatively stronger, and weaker, strategies for carrying out future work in this vital area of research.

The literature review in this project updated the information presented in *Identifying Strategies to Study Drug Usage and Driving Functioning Among Older Drivers* (Lococo & Staplin, 2006). Relevant reports were identified by monitoring summaries of recently published research on medication usage, injury data, and other variables bearing on the relationship between PDI medications and driving, that were posted in the SafetyLit database between October 2005 and October 2007. This service regularly examines more than 2,600 scholarly journals from fields including education, engineering specialties, ergonomics, law and law enforcement, medicine, physiology, psychology, public health, public safety, nursing, social work, and traffic safety. This chapter presents a number of new findings identified in this manner. Specifically, new information is reported about the effects on driving of an anti-seizure medication (topiramate); acute and stable dosing of opioids; sedating and non-sedating antihistamines; antidepressants; short and long half-life sedative-hypnotics; an immediate-release versus extended-release anti-anxiety medication (benzodiazepine); a skeletal muscle relaxant (carisoprodol); and anti-diabetic medications.

The current review of the technical literature also provided insight into the risk associated with chronic medical conditions versus the effects of the medications that treat these conditions. This question was examined in the context of studies bearing on the risk of falls; there is evidence that the same medications that mediate falls risk, may also mediate motor vehicle crash risk. What emerges in this review is that some geriatric patients experience an increased risk of falling due to cardiovascular adverse effects of sedatives, antihypertensives, and other medications, and that when these fall-risk-increasing-drugs are withdrawn there is a resulting, persistent benefit a significant reduction in the occurrence of falls (Van der Velde et al., 2007). At the same time, researchers have found that chronic medical conditions were often more important than medications in causing falls in high-functioning community-dwelling older people (Lee et al., 2006).

At least two recommendations are warranted by these results. First, an ever-expanding volume of work in this area makes it fruitful for NHTSA to sponsor future, periodic updates to remain current with new research. Also there are likely to be safety benefits for many older people from an individualized medication review by their pharmacist, with physician follow-up, that may lead to the withdrawal of selected medications, for selected conditions, and/or their replacement with alternative prescriptions without known PDI (or fall-risk-increasing) effects.

Next, the efficacy of data-mining using large, patient-level administrative databases was highlighted in this project. Ideally, such a database would contain linked medical, hospital, and pharmaceutical data for each eligible person, and, ideally, would be the *only* provider of services. All prescriptions obtained would be through the insurance provider, so that a complete record of drug utilization would be captured in the claims database. Data fields would include dates of inpatient *and* outpatient hospital and doctor services; diagnosis codes to document the reason for the healthcare visit, including E-codes with 4 digits to indicate external causes of injury for *all* diagnoses (so claims resulting from a motor vehicle cash may be identified, and the injured person may be identified as either the driver or a passenger); patient demographics, including date of birth/age, gender, and zip code of residence; and comprehensive pharmacy data.

While this ideal database does not presently exist, several promising candidates for future NHTSA investigations were identified. One such candidate is the Ingenix LabRx database (United Healthcare). Four-digit E-codes are captured in this database, including codes in the range of E8130 to E8139 (motor vehicle accident involving collision with other vehicle); and, the number of older people in the database is increasing as a result of bringing more Medicare

Part D members into the plans that supply Ingenix with data. The estimated cost of providing a file to NHTSA that includes 40,000 patients with two years of relevant data is $50,000.

Another candidate that may be recommended is the Veteran's Health Administration Pharmacy Benefits Management Database. According to French, Campbell et al. (2006), the data available through the VHA system allows one to study the association between a particular drug and an injury or adverse event by identifying a population at risk and then linking outpatient medications with healthcare utilization in that population. There are 8 million veterans nationwide who use the VA for health care. Of this group, over 5.1 million get their prescriptions from inside of the VA system. Many are over the age of 65. Motor vehicle crashes are coded in the VA database. While drivers and passengers are not separately identified, the database contains ICD-9-CM E-codes; the 4th digit identifies the injured person as a passenger or driver. This database is a nomenclature-based database, so exact drug names, rather than drug codes are included; the exact drug names can be easily matched to NDC codes, however. One potential drawback is that the VHA/PMB has been historically proprietary, and can only be used by non-VA researchers if a collaborative agreement were made with an investigator within the VA. For the VA to release data for a traffic safety study as presently contemplated, NHTSA and its researchers would need to identify the needed information and provide an analysis plan to the VA IRB, which would review the request. They would only provide the data to the VA principal investigator or a research member who is affiliated with the VA. If the request is approved, the cost for data and data cleaning—but not the actual data mining analyses—for a study population of 40,000 would cost approximately $30,000.

The data mining exercise undertaken in this research consisted of a set of exploratory analyses in a proprietary database that is the property of NHTSA, the PharMetrics Patient-Level Database developed through a prior contract (LeRoy & Morse, 2005). The main objectives were to refine our understanding about the exposure of seniors to PDI prescription medications, and to prioritize specific combinations of these drugs for subsequent field study. This database consists of cases and controls—individuals with and without motor vehicle crash involvement—who have been continuously enrolled for 6 months or more in prescription medication insurance plans. It includes E-codes identifying causes of injury, plus entries for patient demographics, number of medications dispensed, combinations of medications, and disease prevalence. A subset of 22,574 cases (versus 100,557 controls) was considered in the present analyses.

The range of driver ages encompassed in this exercise included 16-49, then 5-year cohorts through age 74, and 75+. The number of PDI drugs taken by individuals in the study population ranged from zero to 16. These analyses revealed that the rate of use of multiple PDI medications by crash-involved drivers climbs steadily with age, until leveling off at the 65- to 69-year-old cohort. It was also interesting to note that from one-third to one-half of crash-involved drivers in each cohort older than 50 were taking no PDI medications at all.

In the context of the present project, the key findings of this data mining exercise were a set of 2-PDI drug combinations to serve as inclusion criteria in the subsequent field study. Based on the prevalence of specific combinations of medications among drivers 65 and older in the PharMetrics database, a primary focus on medications to lower blood pressure (hypotensives) was recommended. Specifically, it was recommended that the pilot study should attempt to examine the effects on driving performance of this drug class in combination with one or more other classes of PDI medications – lipotropics, beta blockers, calcium channel blockers, NSAIDS, SSRIs, and gastric acid secretion reducers.

The field study conducted in this project included 44 generally healthy individuals recruited from residential communities in Delaware and Maryland, ranging in age from 57 to 89, who drove an average of 50 miles and/or three days each week. Data collected for this sample included medication usage—via one-on-one medication reviews with a visiting pharmacist—plus functional status information using a computer-based battery of measures validated as significant at-fault crash predictors in previous NHTSA research (see Staplin, Gish, & Wagner, 2003). Next, driving performance measures were collected, including an on-road evaluation by an occupational therapist/certified driver rehabilitation specialist (OT/CDRS) and brake response time measures, using an instrumented vehicle. For a subsample of 5 individuals, video, GPS and speed recordings in their own, private cars were also carried out to examine the variability in selected behaviors—surrogates of driver attention/distraction, plus speed choice—during independent driving versus drives with the OT, under comparable conditions.

Considerable difficulties were encountered in recruiting the research sample, with eventual success realized principally due to the generous support of management and staff at the participating residential communities. Attempts to relate observed differences in functional (cognitive) status, driving evaluation outcomes, and brake response time to medication usage, via stepwise logistic regression, were similarly challenging, and ultimately unproductive due to the small sample size relative to the number of drugs and drug classes used as predictors in the linear model. None of the differences in outcome measures, even when coded only as binary (e.g., pass/fail) variables, were significantly predicted by any particular drug combination represented in the study sample. In retrospect, this result might have been anticipated, given that all sample members were selected according to common and fairly narrow entry requirements.

A descriptive summary of these data indicated that the small subset (4) of drivers who "failed" the OT evaluation also were among the oldest. This may be explained by the fact that PDI medications are more impairing to driving performance with increasing age, due to a wide range of (age-related) physiological changes and changes in how these drugs are metabolized (see Herrlinger & Klotz, 2001). The descriptive data summary also suggested that ACE inhibitors, generally, and ACE inhibitor/thiazide diuretic combinations, in particular, may be deserving of special attention in future research; but this must be regarded as a tentative conclusion given the research limitations noted above.

The analyses of behavioral variability during independent driving versus a formal driving evaluation, based on instrumented vehicle data, were more revealing. A case study with an 82-year-old showed that, while speed choice was often lower when driving independently than during the driving evaluation, on those specific road segments that were common to both sets of drives and which had the lowest traffic volumes – and therefore the fewest constraints on drivers' speed choice – this sample member was more likely to drive *faster* on her own than when observed by the OT.

Analysis of continuous driver face and external road view video recordings compared glance direction – an indicator of driver attention – for both types of driving, and found that for five sample members, in the aggregate, there was more time spent looking down and inside the vehicle and less looking toward the inside rearview mirror when driving independently. And, this trend was more pronounced during intersection negotiation, even when the driver was notin car-following mode – in other words, when active scanning of the road environment is critical. The apparently greater willingness of study participants to devote attention to locations inside the vehicle during intersection negotiation – though still a small percentage of their overall glance distributions – highlights a difference between independent driving and (older) peoples' behavior during a driving evaluation that may have significant safety implications.

The field study results indicate that small-sample empirical investigations are not likely to be the most practical route to a better understanding of (multiple) medications and driving impairment. Not only will the prevalence of PDI drugs in any population-based sample work against successfully modeling the predictor-criterion relationships of greatest interest, but—based on experience in this project—sample recruitment will be daunting without a high level of support and assistance from others who are already familiar to and trusted by the prospective research participants.

Two other research methods explored in this pilot project may be much more strongly recommended. First, data mining in large administrative claims databases with patient-level information holds a clear promise for pinpointing the most problematic drugs and combinations of drugs to target in future information and education interventions; specific candidate databases are highlighted in this chapter. Also of potentially great value are new studies utilizing miniature in-car instrumentation, integrating affordable off-the-shelf technology to unobtrusively monitor the behavior of (consenting) drivers. Measures of behavioral variability as a function of driving context, as well as normative exposure data long sought as the denominator by traffic safety analysts, may realistically be expected to result from such investigations.

APPENDIX A. SAMPLE PARTICIPANT RECRUITMENT MATERIAL

IRB approval #06-0248, Univ. of North Carolina, Chapel Hill, Office for Human Research Protection

Do you Drive Several Times a Week? Join a First-of-its-kind Research Study!

This is an opportunity to support the National Highway Traffic Safety Administration develop educational materials for older drivers who are taking prescription medications for high blood pressure, high cholesterol, heart conditions, diabetes, and many other common medical conditions.

Men and women who hold a valid license and routinely drive 3 or more days per week are asked to join a research study. Other eligibility requirements are:

1) You have been taking a prescription medication for high blood pressure for three months or longer. Of special interest are the 'ACE Inhibitor' type drugs. Some common brand names for these medications are: *Prinivil, Zestril, Altace, Zestoretic, Prinzide, Vaseretic, Vasotec, Accupril, Lotensin,* and *Monopril.*

2) You are also taking a prescription medication for *any* of the following conditions: *depression, thyroid deficiency, gastric acid reflux, high cholesterol, chronic pain or inflammation.*
3) You have NOT been involved in more than 2 crashes serious enough to be reported, in the past 5 years.
4) You do NOT have epilepsy or another seizure disorder that can cause you to lose consciousness.

Approximately three hours of your time will be needed, over a period of 1 or 2 months. You will receive a free consultation with a pharmacist about the medications you are taking. You will also receive a professional driving evaluation by a Certified Driving Rehabilitation Specialist, at no charge. And, you may be asked to drive according to your normal habits for a week with instruments in your car that record how and where you drive.

All data from this study will be absolutely confidential. Only group statistics – no individuals – will be included in the study results. Your license will not be affected in any way.

A $100 payment is offered for research participants who qualify. If interested, please contact Loren Staplin at 1-866-650-5380 (toll free number).

By joining this research study you will help others drive more safely.

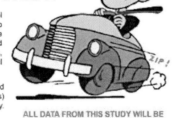

APPENDIX B. REASONS FOR NOT PARTICIPATING SURVEY

Did you Receive the Flyer Asking You to Join the Medications-and-driving Study?

You may recall that flyers were distributed earlier this year, asking for older persons who are active drivers to join a study sponsored by the National Highway Traffic Safety Administration. We want to thank those residents who agreed to participate, and learn why others decided not to join this research effort. Please read the following statements and *check all that apply* to you.

"I did not participate in this study because:

__ I did not qualify for the study based on the medications I am taking."

__ I do not drive enough to qualify for the study."

__ I was out of town."

__ I was too busy; I did not want to commit to the time required for study participation (3 hours)."

__ I did not feel the incentive payment ($100) offered for study participation was enough."

__ I did not want to reveal my medication usage or medication history."

__ I did not want to drive with a stranger (for the driving evaluation part of the study)."

__ I did not want to drive an unfamiliar car (for the driving evaluation part of the study)."

__ I did not want instrumentation that would record my driving behavior to be installed in my car."

__ I did not trust that the results of my driving evaluation would remain confidential."

__ I was worried that the results of my driving evaluation would be reported to the DMV."

__ of reasons other than those listed above." (Please explain below.)

_____

_____

_____

_____

We appreciate your anonymous feedback. Please return this sheet to _____.

APPENDIX C. SAMPLE MEDICATION REVIEW FORM

Client Name: Xxxxxx Xxxxx **Age:** 82
Address: Xxxxxxxxxx
Phone: xxx-xxx-xxxx
Date of Visit: July 27, 2007
Referral: UNC Driving Study
Source of Information: patient

CC/HPI: This is a medication review that is part of a driving study.

PMH: XX is an 82 yr old woman who notes that she is being treated for high cholesterol, h/o stroke in 1999/2000 and high blood pressure. She notes she is very active in various activities such as working out about 3-4 times a day.

Medical Provider: Dr. X

Pharmacy/Insurance: Mail order via Express Script

Allergies: Nosebleeds with aspirin

Medications:

Plavix	Stoke Prevention (anticoagulant)	75mg	1 tablet once daily	Dr. X
Fosinopril	High Blood Pressure (ACE inhibitor)	10mg	1 tablet once Daily	Dr. X
Simvastatin	High Cholesterol (HMG coA reductase inhibitor)	10mg	1 tablet once daily in the evening	Dr. X
Glucosamine/ Chondrotin	Arthritis	750mg/600mg	1 tablet once daily	Dr. X
B complex	Health Maintenance		1 tablet once daily	Dr. X
Calcium and Vitamin D	Bone Health	600/200	1 tablet twice daily	Dr. X
Tylenol	Arthritis (analgesic)		As needed	

Review of Systems: unremarkable except for a nosebleed last week which she attributes to the dry environment.

Recommendations:

1) Medication management: pt appears to be appropriately managing her medications and monitors for effectiveness by having her weight and blood pressure checked at the health club. Her medication regimen is appropriate for her history and there are no clinically significant interactions occurring.

Follow-up:

Will be followed up by Xxxx Xxxxx, OT for driving evaluation.

Work-up done by:

Xxxxx Xxxxx, PharmD, CGP, BCPP

APPENDIX D. SAMPLE ON-ROAD DRIVING EVALUATION FORM

Identifier: (m/f, birth year, first & last initial)_____

Date _____ Time _____ Evaluator _____

Valid License: YES/verified   Road Conditions: _____

What medications have you taken in the last 12 hours? _____

National Highway Traffic Safety Administration

_____

_____

What is your past medical history? _____

_____

_____

_____

Substance use history _____

_____

Driving History/Record/Restrictions? _____

_____

Behind the Wheel Driving Performance:

Key: ✔ = performs consistently and independently, very minor errors do not compromise safety

* = performed task/skill adequately but comment is added as a qualifier

– = single error or performs inconsistently, 25-75% of available opportunities, pattern of errors may indicate that safety is compromised

X = requires physical or verbal instructor intervention to manage hazards or prevent crash, performs less than 25% of available opportunities

Vehicle Entry
_____ manages key to open and close the door
_____ properly positions self in the driver's seat
_____ secures any mobility aides
_____ adjust seat
_____ adjusts mirrors
_____ fastens seatbelt
_____ accommodates and adjusts to vehicle; understands the usual placement of the turn signal, can manage the column shift, looks for symbols for P, R, N, D)

Comments: _____

_____

Initiating Driving/Starting Procedures
_____ turns key to start
_____ depresses brake prior to shifting gears
_____ shifts to proper gear
_____ checks mirrors
_____ checks blind spots
_____ signals intent
_____ applies accelerator/brake as appropriate

A Pilot Study to Test Multiple Medication Usage and Driving Functioning   355

_____ demonstrates intact "practical" brake reflexes
Comments: _____

_____

General Driving
_____accelerates gradually
_____brakes smoothly
_____maintains consistent speed appropriate to area and road conditions
_____on roadways that do not have lane markings, keeps right position in preparation for/potential of oncoming vehicles
_____on roadways that have lane markings, maintains lane position, does not drive on or cross lane lines left, does not hit or near curb or right lane markings
_____ in travel lane, maintains central path of travel, alters path in response to obstacles (bicyclers, pedestrians, potholes, speed bumps, other vehicles etc.)
_____anticipates other vehicles and hazards
_____signals intent for lateral maneuvers in sufficient time frame
_____performs lane changes at an appropriate place
_____cancels signal after lane changes
_____yields right of way
_____demonstrates awareness of posted speeds and looks for signs
_____ maintains appropriate space cushion for speed of travel
_____ alters speed of travel for potential hazards (fast moving side vehicles, pedestrians, bicyclers, speed bumps, potholes/road debris etc.)
_____regularly uses rearview and side view mirrors to note traffic to the rear and sides
_____checks blind spots via mirrors and head checks for merges and lane changes
_____completes organized process for lane changes (look, signal, headcheck, move, recheck traffic)
Comments: _____

_____

Controlled Intersections (traffic light or stop sign, with/without specified turn lanes)
_____anticipates traffic lights/stop sign
_____positions vehicle in appropriate lane
_____respects pedestrian crosswalk
_____comes to a complete stop as req'd-stops at/before the stop line or stop sign
_____checks for oncoming traffic from right, left, and straight ahead
_____correctly manages amber light
_____observes "no turn on red"
_____proceeds when safe and indicated
_____understands right of way issues at 2, 3, 4, way stop intersections and yields right of way as required
Comments: _____

_____

Uncontrolled Intersections

_____despite lack of intersection control, recognizes the need to slow and search for traffic and potential hazards

_____ anticipates other vehicles/pedestrians

_____ yields right of way

_____ proceeds when indicated

Comments: _____

_____

Turns (those with/without a designated turn lane or specific turn signal)

_____chooses and makes the turn from the appropriate lane

_____signals intent

_____yields to oncoming traffic

_____checks blind spot prior to turning

_____coordinates speed through the turn, accelerates out of the turn

_____coordinates upper extremities for steering

_____allows recovery of steering wheel

_____corrects for over steering wheel as needed

_____maintains lane position through turn

_____understands time and space requirements for unprotected left turns (judges traffic for appropriate amount of space and drives at speed necessary to safely move across and turn in with traffic)

_____understands time and space requirements for unprotected right turns (judges traffic for appropriate amount of space and drives at speed necessary to safely turn in with traffic)

Comments: _____

_____

Visual Skills

_____recognizes color of traffic light

_____notes and responds to arrow signals

_____reads speedometer or understands the relative placement of the arrow/needle to the speed

_____reads large regulatory signs-speed limit, no turn on red, construction etc.

_____recognizes that the road bends or curves and moves smoothly through them

_____recognizes and avoids road dividers, islands or curbs

_____has 20-30 second forward scan allowing for anticipation of road issues

_____uses ground scan to note lane markings, arrows, directions for parking lots, cues from other cars etc.

_____uses mirrors, completes head check for blind spots

_____anticipates areas of limited space or the need to change lanes

_____follows lane markings

_____observes warning signs as demonstrated by an appropriate adaptive response or comment

_____notes and obeys stop signs or other traffic controls

Comments: _____

Lot Parking
_____approaches the parking space in the appropriate lane
_____checks for traffic in the rear
_____signals intent
_____stops in appropriate spot
_____places foot on brake prior to changing gears
_____checks rear window, mirrors, front bumpers etc. when backing up
_____maneuvers vehicle into designated space) selects gears, steers in correct direction)
_____accurately judges distances to curb and other vehicles
_____avoids obstacles
_____centers the car in the parking space
Comments: _____

OverallComments/notes:_____
_____
_____

General Rating:
Good driver/no concerns
Adequate driver/few potential problem/driving habits
Fair Driver/lacks numerous good driving habits
Concerns about driving
Instructor intervened for:
_____ braking   Other: _____
_____ steering   _____
_____ speed   _____
_____ lane position   _____

How familiar are you with the major roads on which you traveled during your driving evaluation today? (please circle a number on the scale below)

very unfamiliar = 1 2 3 4 5 6 7 = very familiar

In your normal driving habits, how often do you drive on the major roads on which you traveled during your driving evaluation today? (please circle a number on the scale below)

very rarely = 1 2 3 4 5 6 7 = very often
When is it convenient for the research team to add the equipment into your vehicle?
_____
What type of car will you be driving? _____
What number can you be reached to coordinate this installation? _____

SUGGESTIONS:

_____ M.S.,OTR/L, CDRS
_____ DATE

APPENDIX E. COMBINED MEDICATION CLASSES FOR ANALYSIS

Medication Classes Per Pharmacist Review. (1=PDI Drug Class, 2= Non-PDI Drug Class)

Subject ID/Drugs	DriverID / Age
Antihypertensive Non Diuretic	Alpha Adrenergic Blocker
	Beta Blocker
	ACE Inhibitor
	Calcium Channel Blocker
	Combo Calcium Channel Blocker / ACE Inhibitor
	Angiotensin Receptor Antagonist
Antihypertensive Diuretics	Loop Diuretic
	Potassium Sparing Diuretic
	Thiazide Diuretic
	Combination Diuretic
Anti-Platelet/ Anticoagulant	OTC Antiplatelet
	Anticoagulant / Coumadin Type
	Antiplatelet
Antidiabetic	Sulfonylurea
	Biguanide
	Alpha Glucosidase Inhibitor
	Thiazolidine
	Dipeptidyl peptidase 4
Neurologic	Antipsychotic
	Anti Mania
	Anti Convulsant
	Cholinesterase Inhibitor
	Dopamine Agonist
Osteoporosis	Calcitonin Hormone
	Bisphosphonate
	Selective Estrogen Receptive Modulator
Gastric Acid Secretion Reducer	OTC Antacid
	OTC H2 Blocker
	Proton Pump Inhibitor
Cholesterol Lowering	HMG CoA Reductase Inhibitor
	Antilipemic
Anti-spasmodics GU	Antispasmodics GU
NSAID	NSAID
Antidepressants-Antianxiety	Benzodiazepine Anti Anxiety Non BZD
	SNRI
	SSRI
PDI Eye Preparations	Glaucoma Drops
	Steroid Eye Drops
	Immuno-modulator / Dry Eyes
Sedating Antihistamine	OTC Analgesic Antihistamine
	OTC Antihistamine / Sedating
	Nasal Spray / Antihistamine
Vitamins/ minerals/ supplements	Potassium Supplement
	OTC Vitamin/ Mineral
	OTC Herbal
	OTC / Fish Oil Supplement
	OTC / Joint Supplement
	OTC / Eye Supplement
PDI-Other	Antiarrhythmic
	Aromatase Inhibitor
	CNS Stimulant / ADHD
	Thyroid Supplement
	Narcotic Analgesic
	Opiate Agonist
	Antibiotic
	Nasal Spray / Steroid
	Corticosteroid
	Beta Adrenergic Agents Inhaled Steroid
	Phospho-diesterase 5 Enzyme Inhibitor
	Hormone Replacement Topical Cream
	Topical Antibiotic
	Alpha Reductase Inhibitor
Non-PDI Other	Antihistamines Non Sedating
	Nasal Spray Anticholinergic
	OTC Analgesic
	OTC Topical Analgesic
	OTC Cough Drops
	OTC Laxative
	OTC Eye Tears
	OTC Saline Nasal Spray
	OTC Antiflatulent
	OTC Antifungal Topical
	Count - All
	PDI Count
	Non-PDI Count

Medication Classes Taken on the Day of the OT Evaluation (1=PDI Drug Class, 2= Non-PDI Drug Class)

Subject ID	DriverID →	f526n	f42bit	f38mw	f38bb	f38ctg	f38ad	f36alh	f35dw	m34kgs	m32fij	f371vj	m31fp	f31ss	m31mm	f31mm	f30aw	f29cm	f28sgj	f28esh	m27gm	m27fl	f27fh	m27rc	f26hb	f26jc	m36crq	f25nti	f25gs	m24wi	f24ph	m24js	f23wm	f23cih	f22cih	f22xh	f22sp	f22pv	m21ef	m20lru	m19pib	m19lmg	m18let	Count
	Age →	57	65	68	69	69	60	71	72	73	75	76	76	76	76	77	78	79	79	80	80	80	80	81	81	82	82	82	83	83	84	64	85	85	85	85	86	87	87	88	68	89	
Antihypertensive Non Diuretic	Alpha 1 Adrenergic Blocker									1												1																	1	1	1	1		5
	Beta Blocker			1	1				1								1						1								1								1		1	1	1	10
	ACE Inhibitor	1	1	1	1										1	1	1	1							1				1					1				1	1	1	1			16
	Calcium Channel Blocker			1		1	1			1					1		1					1					1				1				1				1	1				11
	Combo Calcium Channel Blocker ACE Inhibitor						1																																					1
	Angiotensin II Receptor Antagonist		1									1		1							1	1		1	1				1	1				1	1		1	1					14
Antihypertensive Diuretics	Loop Diuretics		1			1										1																												4
	Potassium Sparing Diuretic															1																												1
	Thiazide Diuretic				1					1			1		1		1		1		1	1	1			1				1			1	1	1									14
	Combination Diuretic				1			1	1																			1																1
Anti-platelet/ Anticoagulant	OTC Antiplatelet		2		2	2		2	2	2	2		2	2		2			2	2	2	2	2	2	2		2	2			2	2	2	2	2	2	2	2	2	2	2	2	2	30
	Anticoagulant / Coumadin Type		1							1					1	1								1						1	1		1											7
	Antiplatelet																								1			1	1			1												4
Antidiabetic	Sulfonylurea	1			1														1									1							1						1	1		6
	Biguanide	1																																	1									2
	Alpha Glucosidase Inhibitor					1																																						1
	Thiazolidine			1	1																								1	1														4
	Dipeptidyl peptidase 4																													2														1
Neurologic	Antipsychotic											1																																1
	Anti Mania				1																																		1					2
	Anti Convulsant			1											1																													1
	Cholinesterase Inhibitor																			1																								1
	Dopamine Agonist				1																																							1
Osteoporosis	Calcitonin Hormone															2																					2							2
	Bisphosphonate		2	2												2					2	2			2													2	2					8
	Selective Estrogen Receptive Modulator									2							2	2																										3
Gastric Acid Secretion Reducer	OTC Antacid																							1													1							2
	OTC H2 Blocker																																											
	Proton Pump Inhibitor			1							1			1		1		1	1		1	1		1	1		1				1			1				1						14
Cholesterol Lowering	HMG Coa Reductase Inhibitor	1		1	1	1	1	1	1	1	1	1	1		1		1	1	1		1			1	1		1	1	1	1	1	1	1	1			1	1	1	1	1	1	34
	Antilipemic		1	1	1	1	1	1		1	1		1			1				1					1						1			1				1						10
Anti-spasmodics GU	Antispasmodics GU				1													1												1	1	1									1			5
NSAID	NSAID					1							1		1				1	1					1																			7
Antidepressants/ Antianxiety	Anti-Anxiety Non BZD														1																													1
	SNRI		1		1																																							2
	SSRI																															1												1
PDI Eye Preparations	Glaucoma Drops							1		1			1																															3
	Immunomodulator / Dry Eye				1																																							1
Sedating Antihistamina	OTC Analgesic Antihistamine																																					1						1
	OTC Antihistamine / Sedating																																				1							1
	Nasal Spray / Antihistamine									1									1																									2
Vitamins/ minerals/ supplements	Potassium Supplement					2													2																									2
	OTC Vitamin/ Mineral	2		2	2	2	2	2	2	2		2		2	2	2	2	2	2	2	2	2	2	2	2	2	2		2	2	2	2		2	2	2	2	2	2		2	2		37
	OTC / Herbal									2						2																												2
	OTC / Fish Oil Supplement		2							2		2		2	2															2									2					7
	OTC / Joint Supplement			2						2		2	2	2		2				2							2											2	2				11
	OTC / Eye Supplement									2				2													2											2					4
PDI-Other	Hormone Repl. Topical Cream													1																													1
	Topical Antibiotic													1		1																							1					2
	Corticosteroid Inhaled Steroid / Asthma															1																												1
	Nasal Spray Steroid								1									1																					1					2
	Antibiotic																																											1
	Opiate Agonist								1																																			1
	Aromatase Inhibitor															1																												1
	CNS Stimulant																																											
	Thyroid Supplement			1	1									1			1		1	1										1												1		7
	Antiarrhthmic																																									1		1
Non-PDI Other	5 Alpha Reductase Inhibitor																				2																							1
	OTC Antiflatulant														2																													1
	OTC Eye Tears			2																									2			2					2		2		2			8
	OTC Laxitive			2																																								
	OTC Analgesic								2																			2								2								3
	Antihistamines Non Sedating					2												2																										
	Count - All	5	8	7	15	10	10	8	9	10	8	11	9	11	18	9	7	9	9	11	6	4	8	7	8	6	5	1	7	5	12	7	9	19	5	7	8	12	7	7	4	11	7	
	PDI Count	4	0	3	11	10	6	7	7	4	5	0	9	5	10	8	3	8	7	4	7	4	2	5	4	4	3	0	5	3	9	5	6	0	8	3	4	5	6	3	4	8	5	
	Non-PDI Count	1	6	4	4	3	4	1	2	6	1	5	0	6	8	3	4	1	2	5	4	2	2	3	3	4	2	2	1	2	2	3	1	0	2	3	3	6	4	3	1	3	2	

Appendix F. Anvil Coding Manual

Nodes	
G Group	...
I Group	...
T Group	
M Group	...

Generated by Anvil on Tue Nov 13 15:14:20 EST 2007

Annotation G. Glance

Where is the driver looking now? The default is looking **straight-ahead** (through the windshield). Code elements as:

Attributes
ValueSet (6 tokens) GlanceStatus ---

Attribute Values

GlanceStatus

default	Straight ahead through the windshield
right+up	Right and up glance (e.g., rearview mirror); includes sharp eye cuts without a head turn, as well as head turns toward the inside rearview mirror
right only	Rightward only glance; includes sharp eye cuts to the right without a head turn, as well as head turns toward the right
left only	Leftward only glance; includes sharp eye glances to the left without a head turn, as well as head turns toward the left
down+inside	downward glance or apparent glance inside vehicle.
over shoulder	driver performs direct head check over shoulder (left or right)

Annotation I. Infrastructure

What are the significant aspects of the infrastructure? Default condition is driver traveling on continuous, unbroken section of roadway. Code elements as:

Attributes
ValueSet (7tokens) InfrastructureStatus ---

Attribute Values

InfrastructureStatus

default	continuous, unbroken section of roadway
intersection+stop	Intersections with stop signs. Begin at stop bar; end at other side of intersection intersection with Merge locations at
intersections with merge/yield	channelization and yield signs or merges at highway interchanges. Begin at stop bar in adjacent through lane; end at solid lane marking after turn/merge
intersection+signal	Intersections with traffic signals. Begin at stop bar; end on other side of intersection.
school/ped	School crossing or other mid-block pedestrian crossing crossing
railroad crossing	At-grade railroad crossing. Begin at stop line (if present) or just before tracks; end after tracks. Do not include area marked with advanced RRX signs or markings
parking lot	Parking lot or garage

Annotation T. Traffic

What is the level of attentional demand associated with other traffic? The default is no traffic in scene OR traffic in scene but far away or separated by a physical barrier. Code as follows:

Attributes

ValueSet (4 tokens)	TrafficStatus	---

Attribute Values

TrafficStatus

Default	No traffic in scene OR traffic in scene but is not an immediate threat (e.g., too distant or is separated by a physical barrier) OR is on an intersecting path removed from driver's current position.
Car following ONLY	Driver is following another vehicle (same lane or adjacent lane); potential for rear-end crash if not attending. NOTE: A leading vehicle is an immediate threat if it is within 4 seconds from the driver, which corresponds to an image size of 1/8 inch (3.2 mm) wide or larger.
Opposing traffic ONLY	Potential for head-on crash (but no car following/rear-end crash potential). NOTE: opposing approaching vehicles are an immediate threat as soon as they become visible in the driving scene (e.g., at a 5 sec preview distance), unless they are separated by a physical barrier.
Car following AND opposing traffic	Potential for rear-end crash and head-on crash.

Annotation M. Maneuver

What is the driver's maneuver? The default is same path moving forward Code elements as:

Attributes
    ValueSet (7 tokens)   ManeuverStatus   ---

Attribute Values

ManeuverStatus

Default	Same path moving forward
Left Turn	Driver turns left
Right Turn	Driver turns right
Lane Change	Driver changes lanes, either to the left or to the right
Overtaking/Passing	Driver overtakes/passes another vehicle
Backing	Driver performs a backing/reverse maneuver
Stopped	No vehicle movement

APPENDIX G. MEDICATION USE IN THE 12-HOUR PERIOD PRIOR TO THE OT EVALUATION, BY (1) OVERALL DRIVING EVALUATION SCORE, (2) UNALERTED BRAKE RESPONSE TIME QUARTILE, AND 3) LEVEL OF COGNITIVE DEFICIT

Medication use in the 12-hour period prior to the ot evaluation, by overall driving evaluation score.

Color coded according to OT Evaluation "Overall Score." Green = good driver/no concerns; blue = adequate driver/few potential problem/driving habits; yellow = fair driver/lacks numerous good driving habits; red = concerns about driving. 1=PDI Drug Class; 2=Non-PDI Drug Class

MEDICATION USE IN THE 12-HOUR PERIOD PRIOR TO THE OT EVALUATION, BY OVERALL DRIVING EVALUATION SCORE.

Color coded according to OT Evaluation "Overall Score." Green = good driver/no concerns; blue = adequate driver/few potential problem/driving habits; yellow = fair driver/lacks numerous good driving habits; red = concerns about driving.

MEDICATION USE IN THE 12-HOUR PERIOD PRIOR TO THE OT EVALUATION, BY UNALERTED BRAKE REACTION TIME QUARTILE.
Color Coded According to Unalerted BRT: Red = slowest > 1356; Yellow=>1065 and <=1356; Blue = >877 and <=1065; Green = fastest <=877 1=PDI Drug Class; 2=Non-PDI Drug Class

MEDICATION USE IN THE 12-HOUR PERIOD PRIOR TO THE OT EVALUATION, BY LEVEL OF COGNITIVE DEFICIT.

Green = no deficits in any measure of cognitive function; Yellow = at least 1 mild deficit but no serious deficits; Red = 1 or more serious deficits. White = no measures of cognitive function collected. 1=PDI Drug Class; 2=Non-PDI Drug Class

APPENDIX H. FEATURES OF EACH DATABASE IDENTIFIED AS A POTENTIAL CANDIDATE FOR NHTSA RESEARCH PURPOSES

Database	N of Database	E –Codes	Pharmacy data	Demographic Data	Special Consideration
Medicaid Analytic eXtract (MAX) Database	~ 7 million individuals age 65+	• Present for ~ 25% of claims reporting injury diagnoses, but more likely to be present for higher severity episodes (present in 45-55% of the claims). • Often contain only 3 digits (i.e., 4th digit to identify the injured person as a passenger or the driver is missing).	• For outpatient services only. • NDC code; requires a filter to obtain therapeutic drug class. • Prescribed date • Fill date • New or refill • Days supply • Other First Data Bank Proprietary data (Access restricted to license holders): NDC format, drug class, multi source code, HICL, therapeutic class-general, therapeutic class- specific, American hospital formulary code, Smart key, Medispan code, over-the-counter indicator	• Date of Birth • Age Group • Sex • Race/Ethnicity • State • County of Residence • Zip Code of Residence	Data Limitations: • Churning eligibility (people are enrolled in Medicaid intermittently). • Minimal info on other insurance coverage. • Income data are unavailable. • Only Medicaid-covered services are present. • Services are incomplete for people with dual eligibility (only the residual after Medicare payment), and for people in pre-paid plans. • CMS does no custom programming or data extraction (i.e., CMS will provide the full file). • Feasibility of database for future NHTSA work very limited.
Medicare Current Beneficiary Survey (MCBS)	Sample size of 12,000 individuals ranging in age from 0 to 85+, with the 85+ sample overrepresented by a factor of 1.5.	• Unreliable; only available when required for billing purposes. • Unlikely to have 4th digit	• No pharmacy or prescription claims data; only self-reported medication use.	• SSN • Age • Gender • Race/Ethnicity • Income • Marital Status • Living Arrangements	• Impossible to determine what medications the sample was taking on the date of a claim for hospital services, because there are no pharmacy or prescription claims data; only self-reported medication use.

(Continued)

Database	N of Database	E –Codes	Pharmacy data	Demographic Data	Special Consideration
				(lives alone, with spouse, with children, with others). • Schooling • Metropolitan Area resident	• Database not feasible for future NHTSA research.
Veteran's Health Administration (VHA) Pharmacy Benefits Management (PBM) Database	~ 8 million veterans Nationwide use the VA for healthcare, and 5.1 million of them get their prescriptions from inside of the VA system	• Available for approximately 50% of the injury discharges.	• Outpatient pharmacy data currently only viable for research • NDC Code • Station product name or description • VA product name • VA drug class • Regional formulary indicator • National formulary indicator • Fill date • Prescription number • Quantity dispensed • Dispensing unit • Dosing instructions • Days supply • New fill/refill/partial indicator • Mail or pickup window indicator • Medication counseling acceptance indicator • Purchase price	• SSN • Scrambled SSN • Date of Birth • Age • Gender • Low-income identifier (means test) • Zip Code	• Use of data requires a collaborative agreement with a VA investigator. • Cost for data and data cleaning for a study population would average $30,000, not including data analysis services by VA, if needed. Data analysis would increase the cost by $25,000 to $75,000. • Database feasible for future NHTSA research.

(Continued)

Database	N of Database	E–Codes	Pharmacy data	Demographic Data	Special Consideration
General Practice Research Database [United Kingdom]	• 3 million current patient records (8.9 million total patient records). • 17% of the sample is patients age 65+	Codes V40.n to V48.n are available to distinguish car-related events; codes identify whether the patient was the driver or a passenger. Percentage of injury discharges with E-codes could be made available at a later date, if required (it is presently unknown).	• Drug name • Medical condition for which drug prescribed • Active ingredient • NDC code • Quantity provided • Strength • Decoded therapeutic class • Days supply • Date prescription written	• Socioeconomic class • Regional markers (rather than zip code) • Age • Date of birth (year only would be released) • Gender	• The cost of a dataset ranges from $14,000 to $120,000. • Database feasible for future NHTSA research, although not an American population.
Nationwide Inpatient Sample (NIS)/Healthcare Cost and Utilization Project (HCUP)	• Data from 8 million hospital stays each year, from 1988-2004. • Contains discharge-level records, not patient-level records	• E-code completeness on injury records averaged 87% across 33 States. MVCs accounted for 18% of all unintentional injuries	• HCUP contains no pharmacy data, nor can it be linked to pharmaceutical data	• Age • Gender • Median household income for patient's zip code • Race	• Database not feasible for future NHTSA research as it contains no pharmacy data, nor can it be linked to pharmacy data.
Kaiser Permanente	• 8.3 million members Nationally Northern CA region (largest region): 3.3 million members with 600,000 members age 65+	• Availability of E-code data unknown	• 80 databases can be linked, providing pharmacy data, diagnoses, radiology, clinical laboratory data, and pathology data.	• Available but specific variables not identified in this task	• Database not feasible for future NHTSA research as Kaiser will not provide data; they only do in-house research on topics of interest to their staff and members. • Also, if etiology data are not coded, chart reviews to pull out MVCs would be cost-prohibitive.

(Continued)

Database	N of Database	E –Codes	Pharmacy data	Demographic Data	Special Consideration
Independence Blue Cross	Not provided	Not provided	Not provided	Not provided	Database not feasible for future NHTSA research for several reasons: • IBX outsources all drug claims for payment • It is unlikely that e-codes are available • Concern in IBX legal dept. regarding patient privacy • No in-house interest at IBX for collaboration on this topic
Ingenix LabRx® (United Healthcare) Database	• 35 million patients, 61% of which have at least 1 pharmacy claim, 5.5% of which are age 65+ • Number of older patients should increase in the coming years with acquisition of Pacific Care and Ovations	• Available, most often with 4-digit codes than with 3-digit codes. • Percentage of injury claims with E-codes not presently known, however, preliminary data run identified 126 members age 65+ with 4-digit E-codes in the range of E8130 to E8139.	• Drug Dispensed (NDC) • Therapeutic Drug Class • Quantity and Date Dispensed • Drug Strength • Days Supply • Dollar Amounts	• Gender • Age • Income • Net Worth • Education • Race & Ethnicity • Life Stage • Life Style Indicators	• Approximate cost to provide a data file to NHTSA that includes 40,000 patients with 2 years of data, is $50,000. • Database feasible for future NHTSA research.
HMO Research Network1 of 7 Centers for Education and Research on	Not provided	The center has considered research such as that proposed in the current project, and has concluded that the health plan records included in this Network were	Not provided	Not provided	In addition to the limitation of this database resulting from lack of complete E-code data, HMO CERT often collaborates with external investigators but doesn't work as a data vendor. • Database not feasible for future NHTSA research

Database	N of Database	E –Codes	Pharmacy data	Demographic Data	Special Consideration
Therape-utics/ CERTS		probably unable to satisfactorily identify the operators of vehicles involved in motor vehicle crashes. Participation of the Network would require developing a linkage agreement with relevant motor vehicle registries.			•

APPENDIX I. QUESTIONS FOR INSURANCE CLAIMS DATABASE ADMINISTRATORS

A research activity under NHTSA Task Order NTS-01-5-05194, Contract DTNH22-02-D-85121 *"A Pilot Study to Test Multiple Medication Usage and Driving Functioning"*

- Do you have linked medical, hospital, and pharmaceutical data? If yes....
  - How are they linked?
  - Are the ID codes patient-specific (i.e., are family members clearly separated)?
  - Are the claims in one database?
  - What coding systems are used for diagnosis, procedures, and pharmaceutical claims?
  - How many digits are used in the medical claims coding (e.g. 4th digit or 5th digit ICD9-CM)?
  - What is the time lag for the various types of claims?
  - How are claims reversals handled?
  - How is continuity of eligibility tracked?
- Are ICD9-CM "E" codes —codes assigned by trauma registrars and medical record coders in hospitals and doctors' offices to identify the causes of external injury— present in the database to indicate the reason a patient received emergency room or other medical service, and incurred the medical claim?
- What percent of *injury* discharges following inpatient service have an E-code (of any type)? (One study of the VHA system reported that less than 50% of injury discharges were E-coded, and it referenced recently published national studies of civilian injury hospitalizations where E-coding was present for 60% of the discharges).
- What percent of services for treatment of *injuries* during outpatient visits are E-coded?
- Do E-codes that are associated with a motor vehicle crash (motor vehicle traffic accident codes E810 to E819) have the 4th digit to identify the injured person (e.g., 0 for driver of a motor vehicle other than a motorcycle vs. 1 for *passenger* in a motor vehicle other than a motorcycle)?
- Is there a data checking process to ensure accuracy of E-code assignment and entry into the database for driver vs. passenger? (Because the influence of medication is only relevant to the *driver* in a crash, and misdesignation of driver vs. non-driver could influence the results of the analyses).
- Is the date of the motor vehicle crash available in the database? If no, can the date of an emergency room visit or hospital or medical service associated with the diagnosis code of motor vehicle crash be obtained?
- Are claims for both inpatient and outpatient visits available in the database?
  - If yes, is there a designation for the place of service?
- How many patients are in the database?
- What percentage of the patients are age 65 or older?
- Is zip code of patient residence available (as a surrogate for urban vs. rural residence) and able to be released (HIPAA)?

A Pilot Study to Test Multiple Medication Usage and Driving Functioning

- Would patient age and/or date of birth be able to be released (HIPAA)?
  - If not, would patient age be available for release?
  - If age is not available, are strata indicators available for the patients?
- Would patient gender be able to be released (HIPAA)?
- Would it be possible to determine what prescriptions were filled or refilled within a specified window of time (in proximity to the motor vehicle crash occurrence).
- How are the drugs coded (e.g., NDC?). How are the drug classes coded? Is it possible to identify the drug as well as its therapeutic class without using proprietary software?
- Associated with each prescription drug, is the following information available:
  - Medical condition for which the drug was prescribed?
  - Major drug class, drug name, active ingredient, NDC code?
  - Date the prescription was filled?
  - Quantity provided?
  - Strength of medication?
  - Decoded therapeutic class?
  - Days Supply
  - Are claims reversals backed out with the corresponding claim, so as to not have 3 claims for one fill?
- Does the database contain all claim information for a patient, regardless of what physician he/she saw and what pharmacy he/she used to obtain prescriptions (i.e., is the database the central "clearing house" for patients with plan coverage? Is there a way to track prescriptions obtained by mail order or Internet (e.g., drugstore.com)
- Is it possible to determine the duration of treatment for the various drugs prescribed, so that de novo exposure and prolonged exposure vs. crash risk can be assessed? (New users of a drug may initially be at higher risk of a crash, whereas long-time users may have lower risks because they are better acquainted with the adverse effects of the medicine).
- Is there a variable indicating that the patient has other coverage?
- Are data complete for the over-65 patients, that is, if they have crossover claims from Medicare, Medicaid, Veteran's Administration, other commercial insurances are they available in the database?
  - If not, do databases need to be linked somehow, for the data to be all inclusive? If linking is required, is this do-able (by the database administrator, as the data will be anonymized by the time it reaches the researchers)?
- How long are records available for use (in longitudinal studies) before being archived? (NHTSA would need at least 90-180 days before an index event date plus a buffer period. Additional time will be needed to determine "effectively" de novo exposure).
- Are there any known irregularities, inconsistencies, or omissions in the database, with respect to any of the aforementioned variables? If yes, which variables, and what are the coding anomalies?
- What would be the cost of having selected data fields including, but not limited to, those referenced above extracted from the database, anonymized, and delivered to NHTSA?

- What procedures are required to submit a request for data?
- Are there any known barriers to the release of these data to NHTSA?

REFERENCES

Administration on Aging. (2004). *"A Profile of Older Americans."* http://www.aarp. org/research/ reference/statistics/aresearch-import-519.html

Allard, J., Hébert, R., Rioux, M., Asselin, J. & Voyer, L. (2001). "Efficacy of a Clinical Medication Review on the Number of Potentially Inappropriate Prescriptions Prescribed for Community-Dwelling Elderly People." *Canadian Medical Association Journal, 164(9)*, 1291-1296.

Bramness, J. G., Skurtveit, S., Morland, J. & Engeland, A. (2007). "The Risk of Traffic Accidents After Prescriptions of Carisoprodol." *Accident Analysis and Prevention, 39*, pp. 1050-1055.

Barrett, M., Steiner, C. & Coben, J. (2004). *Healthcare Cost and Utilization Project (HCUP) E Code Evaluation Report*. HCUP Methods Series Report # 2004-06 Online. U.S. Agency for Healthcare Research and Quality. Available at http://www.hcupus.ahrq .gov/reports/methods.jsp.

Benedict, B. & Brinker, C. (2005). *Comments on Medicaid Inpatient Stays and Ambulatory Final Paid Claims with Motorcycle Accidental E-Codes*. CMS/ORDI Memo dated May 12, 2005.

Bishop, C., Gilden, D., Hakim, R., Blom, J., Kubisiak, J. & Garnick, D. (2002). *Opportunity Missed: Undercounting Causes of Injury for the Elderly*. Presented at the Annual Meeting of the American Public Health Association, Philadelphia, Pa. November 11, 2002.

Brunnauer, A., Laux, G., Geiger, E., Soyka, M. & Möller, H.J. (2006). "Antidepressants and Driving Ability: Results from a Clinical Study." *Journal of Clinical Psychiatry, 67(11)*, 1776-1781.

Byas-Smith, M. G., Chapman, S. L., Reed, B. & Cotsonis, G. (2005). "The Effect of Opioids on Driving and Psychomotor Performance in Patients with Chronic Pain." *Clinical Journal of Pain, 21(4)*, 345-352.

Carr, D. B. (2004). "Commentary: The Role of the Emergency Physician in Older Driver Safety." *Annals of Emergency Medicine, 43(6)*, 747-748.

Ch'ng, C. W., Fitzgerald, M., Gerostamoulos, J., Cameron, P., Bui, D., Drummer, O.H., Potter, J. & Odell, M. (2007). "Drug Use in Motor Vehicle Drivers Presenting to an Australian, Adult Major Trauma Centre." *Emergency Medicine Australasia; 19(4)*, 359-365.

De Vries, F., de Vries, C., Cooper, C., Leufkins, B. & van Staa, T-P. (2006). "Reanalysis of Two Studies With Contrasting Results on the Association Between Statin Use and Fracture Risk: the General Practice Research Database." *International Journal of Epidemiology, 35*, 1301-1308.

French, D. D., Campbell, R., Spehar, A. & Angaran, D.M. (2005). "Benzodiazepines and injury: a risk adjusted model." *Pharmacoepidemiology and Drug Safety, 14(1)*, 17-24.

French, D. D., Campbell, R., Spehar, A., Cunningham, F., Bulat, T. & Luther, S. L. (2006). "Drugs and Falls in community-Dwelling Older People: A National Veteran's Study." *Clinical Therapies, 28(4)*, pp. 619-630.

French, D. D., Chirikos, T. N., Sephar, A., Campbell, R., Means, H. & Bulat, T. (2005). "Effect of Concomitant Use of Benzodiazepines and Other Drugs on the Risk of Injury in a Veterans Population." *Drug Safety, 28(12)*, 1141-1150.

Gaertner, J., Radbruch, L., Giesecke, T., Gerbershagen, H., Petzke, F., Ostgathe, C., Elsner, F. & Sabatowski, R. (2006). "Assessing Cognition and Psychomotor Function Under Long-Term Treatment With Controlled Release Oxycodone in Non-Cancer Pain Patients. *Acta Anaesthesiologica Scandinavica 2006; 50(6)*, pp. 664-672.

Gordon, A. M. & Logan, B.K. (2006). "Topiramate-Positive Death-Investigation and Impaired-Driving Cases in Washington State." *Jour. of Analytical Toxicology, 30(8)*, 599-602.

Gurwitz, J. H. (2004). "Polypharmacy: A New Paradigm or Quality Drug Therapy in the Elderly?" *Archives of Internal Medicine, 164*, 18, 1957-1959.

Gurwitz, J. H., Field, T. S., Harrold, L. R., Rothschild, J., Debellis, K., Seger, A. C., Cadoret, C., Fish, L. S., Garber, L., Kelleher, M. & Bates, D. W. (2003). "Incidence and Preventability of Adverse Drug Events Among Older Persons in the Ambulatory Setting. *" Journal of the American Medical Association, 289(9)*, 1107-1116.

Gurwitz, J. H., Soumerai, S. B. & Avorn, J. (1990). "Improving Medication Prescribing and Utilization in the Nursing Home." *Journal of the American Geriatrics Society, 8(5)*, pp. 542-552.

Hemmelgarn, B., Levesque, L. E. & Suissa, S. (2006). "Anti-Diabetic Drug Use and the Risk of Motor Vehicle Crash in the Elderly." *Canadian Journal of Clinical Pharmacology,* Vol. *13(1)*, Winter 2006. e112-e120.

Herrlinger, C. & Klotz, U. (2001). "Drug Metabolism and Drug Interactions in the Elderly." *Best Practice & Research Clinical Gastroenterology*, 15, 897-918.

Insurance Institute for Highway Safety (2003). *"Fatality Facts 2003: Older People."* http://www.highwaysafety.org/safety_facts/fatality_facts/olderpeople.htm.

Isbister, G. K., O'Regan, L., Sibbroitt, D. & Whyte, I. M. (2004). "Alprazolam Is Relatively More Toxic Than Other Benzodiazepines in Overdose." *British Journal of Clinical Pharmacology, 58*, pp. 88-95.

Kaplan, J., Kraner, J. & Paulozzi, L. (2006). "Alcohol and Other Drug Use Among Victims of Motor-Vehicle Crashes—West Virginia, 2004-2005." *Morbidity Mortal Weekly Report, 55(48)*, pp. 1296-6. Centers for Disease Control and Prevention, Atlanta, GA.

Kinirons, M. T. & O'Mahony, M.S. (2004). "Drug Metabolism and Aging." *Br. J. Clin. Pharmacol, 57*, 540-544.

Kipp, M. (2001) "Anvil - A Generic Annotation Tool for Multimodal Dialogue". In: *Proceedings of the 7th European Conference on Speech Communication and Technology* (Eurospeech), pp. 1367-1370. http://www.anvil-software.de/

Kurzthaler, I., Wambacher, M., Golser, K., Sperner, G., Sperner-Unterweger, B., Haidekker, A., Pavlic, M., Kemmler, G. & Fleischhacker, W. (2005). "Alcohol and/or Benzodiazepines Use: Different Accidents—Different Impacts?" *Human Psychopharmacology, Clinical and Experimental*, 20, pp. 583-589.

Lee, J., Kwok, T., Leung, P. & Woo, J. (2006). "*Medical Illnesses Are More Important Than Medications as Risk Factors of Falls in Older Community Dwellers?* A Cross-Sectional

Study." *Age and Aging,* Advance Access published online on February 23, 2006, at http://ageing.oxfordjournals.org/cgi/content/abstract/afj056v1?ct.

LeRoy, A., & Morse, L. (2005). *Exploratory Study of the Relationship Between Multiple Medications and Vehicle Crashes: Analysis of Databases.* Final Report (draft), NHTSA Contract No. DTNH22-02-C-05075. Washington, DC: National Highway Safety Administration.

Leufkens, T., Vermeeren, A., Smink, B., van Ruitenbeek, P. & Ramaekers, J. (2007). "Cognitive, Psychomotor, and Actual Driving Performance in Healthy Volunteers After Immediate and Extended Release Formulations of Alprazolam 1 mg." *Psychopharmacology, 191,* 951-959.

Lococo, K., & Staplin, L. (2006). *Identifying Strategies to Study Drug Usage and Driving Functioning Among Older Drivers.* Report No. DOT HS 810 558. Washington, DC: National Highway Safety Administration.

Meier, C. R., Schlienger, R. G., Kraenzlin, M. E., Schlegel, B. & Jick, H. (2000). "HMG-CoA Reductase Inhibitors and the Risk of Fractures." *Journal of the American Medical Association, 283,* 3205-3210.

Ridout, F., Meadows, R., Johnsen, S. et al. (2003). "A Placebo-Controlled Investigation Into the Effects of Paroxetine and Mirtzapine on Measures Related to Car Driving Performance. " *Human Psychopharmacology, 18,* 261-269.

Schmucker, D. L. (2001). "Liver Function and Phase I Drug Metabolism in the Elderly: A Paradox." *Drugs Aging 18,* 837-851.

Schwilke, E., Sampaio dos Santos, & Logan, B. (2006). "Changing Patterns of Drug and Alcohol Use in Fatally Injured Drivers in Washington State." *Journal of Forensic Sciences, 51(5),* 1191-1198.

Shinoda-Tagawa, T. & Clark, D.E. (2003). "Trends in hospitalizations after injury: are older women replacing young men." *Injury Prevention, 9,* 214-219.

Staner, L., Ertlé, S., Boeijinga, P., Rinaudo, G., Arnal, M., Muzet, A. & Luthringer, R. (2005). "Next-Day Residual Effects of Hypnotics in DSM-IV Primary Insomnia: A Driving Simulator Study With Simultaneous Electroencephalogram Monitoring." *Psychopharmacology, 181,* 790-798.

Staplin, L., Gish, K. & Wagner, E. (2003). "MaryPODS revisited: Updated Crash Analysis and Implications for Screening Program Implementation," *Journal of Safety Research, 34(4),* 389-397.

Staplin, L., Lococo, K., Stewart, J. & Decina, L. (1999). Safe Mobility for Older People Notebook. Publication No. DOT HS 808 853. Washington, DC: National Highway Safety Administration.. Available at www.nhtsa.dot.gov/people/injury/olddrive/safe/

Stuck, A. E., Beers, M. H., Steiner, A., Aronow, H. U., Rubenstein, L. Z. & Beck, J. C. (1994). "Inappropriate Medication Use in Community-Residing Older People." *Archives of Internal Medicine, 154(19),* pp 2195-2200.

Stutts, J., Feaganes, J., Rodgman, E., Hamlett, C., Meadows, T., Reinfurt, D., Gish, K., Mercadante, M. & Staplin, L. (2003). *Distractions in Everyday Driving: Causes and Consequences.* Washington, DC: AAA Foundation for Traffic Safety.

Tashiro, M., Horikawa, E., Mochizuki, H., Sakurada, Y., Kato, M., Inokuchi, T., Ridout, F., Hindmarch, I. & Yanai, K. (2005). "Effects of Fexofenadine and Hydroxyzine on Brake Reaction Time During Car-Driving With Cellular Phone Use." *Human Psychopharmacology, Clinical and Experimental, 20,* pp. 501-509.

Transportation Research Board. (1988). *Transportation in an Aging Society, Special Report 218, Volumes 1 and 2*. Washington, DC.

Van der Velde, N., van den Meiracker, A. H., Pols, A. A. P., Stricker, B. H. & van der Cammen, T. J. M. (2007). "Withdrawal of Fall-Risk-Increasing Drugs in Older People: Effect on Tilt-Table Test Outcomes." *Journal of the American Geriatrics Society, 55*, 734-739.

Van Staa, T-P., Wegman, S., de Vries, F. Leufkens, B., & Cooper, C. (2001). "Use of Statins and Risk of Fractures." *Journal of the American Medical Association, 285*, 1850-1855.

Verster, J. C., Veldhujzen, D. S. & Volkerts, E. R. (2006). "Effects of an Opioid (Oxycodone/Paracetamol) and an NSAID (Bromfenac) on Driving Ability, Memory Functioning, Psychomotor Performance, Pupil Size, and Mood." *Clinical Journal of Pain, 22(5)*, 499-504.

Walsh, J. M., de Gier, J. J., Christopherson, A. S. & Verstraete, A. G. (2004). "Drugs and Driving." *Traffic Injury Prevention, 5*, 241-253.

Wilkinson, C. & Moskowitz, H. (2001). *Polypharmacy and Older Drivers: Literature Review*. Unpublished Manuscript, Southern California Research Institute, Los Angeles, CA.

Wingen, M., Bothmer, J., Langer, S., et al. (2005). "Actual Driving Performance and Psychomotor Function in Healthy Subjects after Acute and Subchronic Treatment with Escitalopram, Mirtazapine, and Placebo: A Crossover Trial." *Journal of Clinical Psychiatry, 66*, pp. 436-443.

End Notes

[1] Literature Review, Lococo, K.H., and Staplin, L. "Polypharmacy and Older Drivers: Identifying Strategies to Study Drug Usage and Driving Functioning Among Older Drivers." Contract DTNH22-02-D-85121, Report DOT HS 810681. Washington, DC: National Highway Traffic Safety Administration. Available on the Web at http://www.nhtsa.gov/staticfiles/DOT/NHTSA/Traffic%20Injury%20Control/Articles/Associated%20Files/Polyphar macy.pdf.

[2] Characterized as a state of feeling unwell or unhappy, *Merriam-Webster Medical Dictionary*, 2007-2008. See http://medical.merriam-webster.com/medical/dysphoria.

[3] The tilt-table test procedure was obtained from information provided on Columbia University Medical Center's Web page at http://hora.cpmc.columbia.edu/dept/syncope/tiltfaq.html

[4] PatientPlus Web site at: http://www.patient.co.uk/showdoc/40001942/ and http://www.syncope.co.uk/neurocardiogenic_vasovagal_syncope_causes_of_fainting.htm

[5] Based on the PharMetrics analysis reported by Leroy et al. (2004), it may be anticipated that 15-20% of all patients enrolled in the database will be 65+; but, only 5-8% of *crash-involved* patients will be in this older cohort.

[6] Beth Benedict, CMS/ORDI.

[7] http://www.cms.hhs.gov/apps/mcbs/default.asp

[8] See http://www.gprd.com/whygprd

[9] In June 2006, 1 British pound = 1.8517 dollars

[10] http://www.hcup-us.ahrq.gov/nisoverview.jsp

[11] Visit www.certs.hhs.gov

[12] For example: NHTSA's "Pharmacist Education—Medication Impaired Driving" has produced an ACPE-approved curriculum to foster increased interaction with older consumers about drugs and driving safety.

INDEX

A

abuse, 2, 10, 317, 324
accelerator, 292, 354
accuracy, 12, 262, 320, 339, 372
acid, 8, 29, 83, 84, 85, 86, 88, 89, 90, 266, 283, 284, 297, 307, 349, 351
acidosis, 35
acute renal failure, 205
adaptation, 301
adaptations, 7
adjustment, 327
administrators, 319, 330
adverse event, 9, 10, 329, 336, 337, 338, 348
agencies, 315, 332
agonist, 83, 84, 86, 88, 89, 90, 318
alcohol use, 36, 315
alcoholism, 3
alertness, 318, 319, 321, 324
alkaloids, 325
allergy, 203, 205
alters, 355
Alzheimer disease, 270
American population, vii, 1, 5, 6, 272, 369
amphetamines, 315, 316, 317
analgesic, 28, 31, 318, 319, 320, 353
anaphylactic shock, 203
angina, 281
anorexia, 9, 317
anorexia nervosa, 317
anthropology, 315
anti-asthma, 21, 28
antibiotic, 345
anticholinergic, 8
anticholinergic effect, 8
anticoagulant, 297, 353
Anticoagulants, 35, 86, 90, 269
anticonvulsant, 21, 323
antidepressant, 270, 322, 323
antidepressant medication, 270
Antidepressants, 29, 31, 269, 271, 282, 322, 374

Antigout, 269
antihistamines, 1, 5, 10, 28, 33, 266, 297, 315, 316, 321, 338, 347
Antihistamines, 269, 296, 321
antihypertensive agents, 271
antihypertensive drugs, 9
anti-inflammatory drugs, 281, 297
Antineiplastics, 270
Antiplatelets, 270
Antiseizure, 269
antispasmodics, 329
anxiety, 21, 26, 29, 31, 33, 35, 36, 38, 203, 266, 270, 271, 315, 324, 347
apnea, 37
appointments, 285
arithmetic, 321
arthritis, 3, 4, 5, 7, 15, 43
assessment, 38, 308, 319, 321, 327
assets, 333, 335
ataxia, 271
atherosclerosis, 205
attribution, 43
audits, 17
Australasia, 374
Austria, 317
automobiles, 271, 334
autopsy, 316
av block, 204
azotemia, 9

B

back pain, 3, 4, 36, 43, 325
baggage, 67
barbiturates, 33, 39, 262, 316, 338
barriers, 43, 324, 341, 374
basal metabolic rate, 307
batteries, 320
behaviors, 267, 283, 288, 295, 298, 349
belladonna alkaloids, 33

benzodiazepine, 3, 266, 270, 315, 317, 321, 323, 324, 325, 336, 337, 347
benzodiazepines, 1, 5, 9, 10, 270, 315, 316, 317, 323, 325, 326, 327, 336, 337, 338
beta blocker, 266, 281, 283, 346, 349
bias, 11, 13, 33, 341
blind spot, 354, 355, 356
blood flow, 307
blood plasma, 324
blood pressure, 7, 9, 15, 271, 273, 283, 307, 308, 328, 329, 348, 353
blood vessels, 307, 345
body fat, 307
bradycardia, 204
breakdown, 15
breathing, 37
bronchitis, 206
bronchospasm, 34
bulimia, 317

C

calcium, 266, 281, 283, 327, 349
calcium channel blocker, 266, 281, 283, 327, 349
cancer, 269, 320, 321, 346
cancer care, 346
candidates, 266, 330, 331, 347
cannabinoids, 315
cannabis, 317
carbon, 72, 75
carbon monoxide, 72, 75
cardiac arrhythmia, 36
cardiac output, 307
cardiomyopathy, 205
cardiovascular adverse effects, 266, 347
cardiovascular disease, 5, 7, 337
cardiovascular system, 337
carotid sinus, 328, 329
Case Control Analysis, 3, 33
case study, 267, 300, 302, 313, 349
cataract, 7
category b, 338
Census, 268
central nervous system, 7, 8, 9, 15, 270, 271, 273, 326, 337
cholesterol, 281, 284, 307, 350, 351, 353
cholesterol-lowering drugs, 307
cholinesterase, 338
cholinesterase inhibitors, 338
chronic diseases, 4, 43, 260
citalopram, 322
class, 14, 26, 28, 31, 273, 283, 286, 295, 307, 322, 331, 334, 341, 348, 367, 368, 369, 373

cleaning, 12, 17, 339, 348, 368
closure, 287, 299, 305, 306
CNS, 24, 30, 34, 36, 41, 42, 46, 47, 86, 91, 98, 99, 100, 101, 141, 143, 145, 146, 148, 149, 151, 153, 155, 156, 159, 160, 162, 164, 165, 167, 169, 170, 172, 173, 175, 177, 178, 195, 196, 198, 203, 264, 270, 296, 324, 325, 326, 337
cocaine, 315, 316, 317
coding, 14, 43, 262, 263, 290, 295, 300, 301, 311, 333, 334, 336, 339, 340, 341, 343, 372, 373
cognitive ability, 287, 299, 306
cognitive deficit, 307, 308
cognitive deficits, 307, 308
cognitive function, 6, 283, 306, 366
cognitive impairment, 9, 30, 42
collateral, 43
collisions, 260, 272, 324
coma, 7, 15, 39
combined effect, 322
community, 9, 260, 266, 270, 284, 286, 288, 291, 293, 302, 304, 319, 325, 327, 342, 347, 375
comorbidity, 261
compensation, 286, 294, 301
complement, 292, 340
compliance, 273, 334
complications, 8, 327, 336
composition, 302
compounds, 270
conference, 315
confidentiality, 286
conflict, 3, 10, 38, 39, 41, 291, 293
confounders, 326
congruence, 313
consciousness, 35, 38, 351
consumption, 12, 13, 270
continuous data, 295
control group, 32, 320
coordination, 271, 318, 320
COPD, 36, 37, 42, 46, 99, 101, 142, 146, 151, 156, 162, 165, 171, 175, 197, 205
coronary artery disease, 3, 37
correlation, 301, 302, 304, 311, 312
correlations, 302
corticosteroids, 83, 84, 85, 86, 87, 88, 89, 90, 91
cost, 12, 43, 294, 334, 339, 340, 341, 343, 344, 348, 368, 369, 370, 373
counseling, 323, 368
covering, 340
crash involvement, vii, 1, 6, 36, 261, 266, 268, 271, 327, 330, 348
cues, 312, 356
curriculum, 377

D

daily living, 6
damages, iv
data analysis, 260, 339, 368
data collection, 2, 10, 14, 268, 283, 286, 287, 288, 290, 293, 294, 318
data mining, vii, 265, 266, 268, 278, 283, 330, 344, 346, 348, 350
data set, 13, 332, 335, 338, 343, 344
database, 2, 3, 11, 12, 13, 15, 16, 17, 18, 21, 260, 266, 268, 270, 271, 272, 273, 276, 279, 280, 281, 313, 314, 315, 316, 325, 329, 330, 331, 332, 333, 334, 335, 336, 337, 338, 339, 340, 341, 342, 343, 344, 346, 347, 348, 367, 370, 372, 373, 377
datasets, 12, 14, 336, 340, 342, 344
death rate, 261
deciliter, 319
deficiency, 351
deficit, 299, 300, 304, 305, 306, 308, 366
demographic characteristics, 2, 11
demographic data, 12, 327, 332
demographic factors, 336
dentist, 285
Department of Health and Human Services, 345
Department of Veterans Affairs, 338
depressants, 316
depression, 3, 4, 7, 8, 9, 30, 34, 36, 43, 203, 270, 351
Dermatologic, 269
detection, 262
detection system, 262
deviation, 318, 323, 324, 325
diabetes, 2, 3, 4, 5, 7, 10, 12, 13, 37, 42, 43, 269, 326, 327, 328, 350
diabetic patients, 328
diagnosis, 2, 7, 11, 13, 16, 31, 272, 333, 336, 337, 341, 347, 372
diagnostic procedures, 2, 11
diastolic blood pressure, 329
diphenhydramine, 315
discharges, 336, 340, 342, 368, 369, 372
discrimination, 272
disorder, 35, 43, 202, 317, 318, 351
dissociation, 324
District of Columbia, 332
disturbances, 4, 9, 43, 205
diuretic, 267, 297, 307, 308, 349
dizziness, 7, 8, 9, 15, 30, 33, 34, 38, 271, 308, 317, 324, 328
doctors, 260, 372
DOP, 206, 207, 208, 209, 211, 213, 221, 223, 224, 231
dosage, 318, 320, 321, 340

dose-response relationship, 319
dosing, 266, 315, 318, 323, 336, 338, 347
draft, 376
driving ability, 1, 3, 4, 6, 323
drug action, 308
drug interaction, vii, 2, 3, 4, 8, 10, 15, 21, 24, 28, 32, 33, 41, 44, 260, 345
drug metabolism, 308, 310
drug reactions, 12, 327, 328, 346
drug resistance, 345
drug safety, 338
drug side effects, 7
drug therapy, 4
drug treatment, 328
drug use, 1, 3, 8, 14, 21, 268, 274, 278, 315, 316, 337, 338, 345
drugs, vii, 1, 2, 3, 4, 5, 7, 8, 9, 10, 11, 12, 15, 16, 18, 19, 21, 23, 26, 28, 29, 30, 32, 39, 40, 42, 44, 261, 262, 265, 266, 267, 268, 269, 270, 273, 278, 279, 284, 295, 296, 297, 303, 304, 306, 308, 310, 315, 316, 317, 319, 323, 324, 325, 326, 327, 328, 329, 332, 334, 335, 337, 338, 341, 345, 346, 347, 348, 349, 350, 373, 377
dysphoria, 319, 377

E

eating disorders, 317
edema, 38, 204
educational materials, 350
educational programs, 4, 44
elderly population, 9
elders, 333
encoding, 343
enforcement, 316
engineering, 304, 315, 347
enrollment, 16, 17, 19, 20, 272, 332, 335, 343
enteritis, 205
environmental conditions, 6
enzymes, 8
epidemiologic studies, 11
epidemiology, 263
epilepsy, 2, 10, 351
equipment, 288, 289, 291, 294, 304, 357
ergonomics, 315, 347
esophagitis, 204
EST, 361
ethnicity, 5
etiology, 343, 369
exercise, vii, 265, 266, 273, 278, 302, 348
expenditures, 332, 335
experiences, 329
expertise, 286

exposure, 4, 6, 33, 267, 268, 271, 278, 288, 295, 301, 313, 325, 326, 348, 350, 373
extraction, 334, 367
eye movement, 317

F

fabrication, 289
fainting, 7, 15, 271, 308, 328, 377
family members, 372
family support, 335
fatality, 6, 268, 269, 375
FDA, 317, 346
FDA approval, 317
feedback, 284, 287, 352
fitness, 322, 323
flexibility, 299, 304
fluoxetine, 33
Ford, 286, 288, 290
fractures, 333
France, 323
freedom, 41
frequencies, 16, 18, 31, 272, 278, 330

G

gastritis, 204
Gastrointestinal tract, 269
general practitioner, 340
Georgia, 345
Germany, 320
glucose, 327
Google, 290
GPS, 264, 267, 283, 288, 290, 291, 294, 302, 313, 349
graph, 274
guidance, 312, 340
guidelines, 322

H

hair, 2, 10
half-life, 33, 266, 315, 323, 324, 347
Hawaii, 262, 346
hazards, 322, 354, 355, 356
HE, 145, 153, 159, 163, 174, 178, 194
head trauma, 35, 262
headache, 34, 203
health care system, 338
health insurance, 12, 262, 335
health services, 335

health status, 5, 7, 335
healthy older drivers, 266
heart attack, 281, 346
heart disease, 3, 4, 37, 42, 43, 269, 326, 327
heart failure, 37
heart rate, 328
Hébert, Bravo, Korner-Bitensky, and Boyer, 270
hemorrhage, 38, 204, 205
Henry Ford, 346
heroin, 316
high blood pressure, 2, 13, 295, 350, 353
highways, 286, 341
hip fractures, 270
HIV, 52, 59, 99, 101, 141, 147, 152, 160, 166, 171, 177, 201, 212, 221
Hong Kong, 327
Hormones, 269
hospitalization, 326
household income, 369
husband, 285
hyperactivity, 83, 84, 85, 86, 87, 88, 89, 90, 91
hypercholesterolemia, 2, 13
hyperkalemia, 9
hyperlipidemia, 7
hypernatremia, 9
hypersensitivity, 328
hypertension, 7, 34, 269, 307, 326
hypoglycemia, 4, 8, 9, 43, 271, 317, 327
Hypoglycemics, 269, 282
hypokalemia, 9, 205
hypomagnesemia, 205
hyponatremia, 9
hypotension, 8, 204, 205, 271, 308, 328
hypotensive, 26
hypotensive drugs, 26
hypothesis, 13

I

ideal, 266, 324, 330, 331, 347
Immunomodulators, 270
impacts, 335
impairing effects, vii, 2, 4, 5, 23, 24, 32, 38, 308, 325
impairments, 36, 260, 261, 323
inattention, 71
incidence, 10, 260, 266, 306, 325
Independence, 330, 331, 343
individual differences, 310
inferiority, 320
inflammation, 351
information processing, 287, 299, 306, 319
information processing speed, 287, 299, 306
informed consent, 286

infrastructure, 313, 330
inhibitor, 267, 307, 308, 322, 349, 353
initiation, 4, 33
Injury, 315, 374, 375, 376, 377
injury claims, 370
insomnia, 7, 36, 42, 323
insulin, 37, 39, 326, 327
interaction effect, 5
interaction effects, 5
interface, 301
International Classification of Diseases, 264
Internet, 290, 373
intervention, 10, 18, 294, 298, 299, 309, 354
intoxication, 316
irritability, 36

K

ketoacidosis, 4, 37, 43
kidney, 5

L

laboratory tests, 318, 319, 320
law enforcement, 315, 347
legislation, 43, 320
lethargy, 8
licensed drivers, vii, 1, 6, 265, 268
Limitations, 367
linear model, 295, 349
linear modeling, 295
lipotropics, 266, 281, 283, 284, 349
liquids, 287
lithium, 326
liver, 5, 8, 307, 318
liver damage, 318
living arrangements, 335
loss of appetite, 8
loss of consciousness, 317, 326, 328

M

machinery, 5, 67, 73, 317
macular degeneration, 285
majority, 5, 307, 318, 328
management, 2, 7, 11, 283, 318, 337, 349, 353
mania, 203
manipulation, 12
marijuana, 316
marital status, 336
markers, 341, 369

marketing, 12
MAST, 49, 52, 190, 193, 209, 212, 224
mast cell stabilizer, 262
median, 302, 318, 319, 323
Medicaid, 11, 260, 261, 264, 265, 330, 331, 332, 333, 334, 335, 342, 344, 345, 367, 373, 374
medical care, 11, 14, 335, 336
Medicare, 20, 43, 264, 269, 330, 331, 332, 333, 334, 335, 338, 339, 342, 344, 347, 367, 373
medicines, 3, 12, 13, 34, 39, 270, 271, 287, 339
membership, 343
memory, 299, 305, 306, 318
mental retardation, 322
metabolism, 5, 24, 29, 84, 89, 308
metformin, 326, 327
methamphetamine, 315
methodology, 35, 262, 267
migraine headache, 317
milligrams, 336
miniature, 267, 350
mining, vii, 265, 334, 341, 342, 347
modeling, 267, 350
monitoring, 267, 323, 346
mood change, 318, 319
morbidity, 340
morphine, 316, 317, 320
motor vehicle crashes, vii, 1, 2, 3, 5, 6, 10, 11, 13, 15, 16, 19, 24, 33, 35, 36, 37, 41, 42, 43, 260, 261, 268, 270, 272, 315, 316, 317, 325, 326, 327, 330, 333, 334, 335, 336, 340, 342, 343
motor vehicle crashes (MVC), 1
multiple medication use, vii, 2, 4, 5, 329
multiple PDI medications, vii, 4, 265, 266, 273, 278, 348
multiplier, 278
muscle relaxant, 21, 23, 316, 323, 326, 337
Muscle relaxants, 269
musculoskeletal system, 337

N

narcotic, 1, 5, 10, 23, 26, 28, 31, 33, 39, 83, 84, 85, 86, 87, 88, 89, 90, 91, 270, 271
narcotic analgesics, 2, 5, 10, 23, 26, 33, 39, 270, 271
narcotic antitussive, 33
narcotics, 29, 270, 316, 338
National Ambulatory Medical Care Survey [NAMCS], 2
National Health Service, 264, 340
National Highway Traffic Safety Administration (NHTSA), 1, 5
National Survey, 315
nausea, 205

negotiating, 301
nervous system, 15
nervousness, 36, 203
neuroleptics, 329, 338
neuropathic pain, 317
neuropathy, 327
nicotinic acid, 329
nitrate, 328
nitrates, 327, 329
non-institutionalized, 269
Nonopioid analgesics, 269
non-steroidal anti-inflammatory drugs, 9
norepinephrine, 39, 322
normal distribution, 310
Norway, 325
NSAIDs, 9, 29, 35, 265, 270, 271, 284
null hypothesis, 19
nursing, 315, 347
Nutrients/supplements, 269

O

obesity, 284, 317
obstacles, 355, 357
occupational therapist, vii, 265, 267, 283, 286, 349
olanzapine, 317
old age, 269
older adults, vii, 1, 2, 3, 4, 5, 6, 7, 8, 9, 24, 30, 33, 36, 42, 43, 260, 268, 329, 346
Ophthalmics, 269
opiates, 317, 319
opioids, 266, 315, 320, 337, 347
opportunities, 354
oral hypoglycemic agents, 37
organ, 342
orthostatic hypotension, 30, 328
osteoarthritis, 2, 13
Osteoporosis, 269, 297
outpatients, 260, 329
overlap, 273, 307

P

Pacific, 344, 370
pain, 4, 7, 15, 21, 36, 43, 204, 205, 284, 318, 319, 320, 327, 337, 338, 351
PAN, 47, 144, 150, 153, 159, 163, 169, 173, 178, 201
panic disorder, 324
parallel, 319, 345
paranoia, 203
parkinsonism, 30, 42

paroxetine, 322
pass/fail, 349
patents, 340
pathology, 11, 343, 369
patient care, 11
patient-level database, 17, 268
pedal, 16, 68, 70, 75, 76, 77
peptidase, 296
percentile, 320
performance, 5, 267, 270, 271, 273, 283, 292, 295, 297, 298, 299, 303, 304, 306, 307, 310, 317, 318, 319, 320, 321, 322, 323, 324, 325, 326, 348, 349
peripheral neuropathy, 327
permit, 294, 342
pharmaceuticals, 43
pharmacokinetics, 8
pharmacology, 9
PharMetrics Patient-Level Database, 2, 16, 271, 348
phenytoin, 316
physical therapy, 18
physiology, 315, 347
pilot study, vii, 265, 266, 267, 268, 271, 283, 346, 348
placebo, 318, 319, 321, 322, 323, 324
platelet aggregation, 33
police, 2, 10
population group, 344
postural hypotension, 9, 36
potentially driver-impairing (PDI) medications, vii, 265, 346
predictor variables, 295
prescription medications, vii, 12, 265, 271, 287, 304, 324, 346, 348, 350
prevention, 34, 266, 315, 317
probability, 14, 293, 310, 333
programming, 334, 367
project, 5, 10, 11, 14, 263, 265, 266, 268, 271, 272, 283, 286, 287, 299, 315, 329, 332, 333, 338, 345, 346, 347, 348, 349, 350, 370
proliferation, 346
proprietary insurance claims database (PharMetrics), 2
psychiatric disorders, 317, 318
psychoactive drug, 319
psychology, 315, 347
psychotropic drugs, 8, 328
public domain, 345
public health, 315, 347
public policy, 43
public safety, 5, 315, 347
pulmonary edema, 37
P-value, 262

Index

Q

quality control, 12, 13, 14, 17
quartile, 304, 307, 308
query, 18, 304, 340

R

Radiation, 41
radio, 300, 311
rate of fatality, vii, 1
rating scale, 321
reaction time, 294, 295, 298, 321
reactions, 23, 308
reactivity, 322
recall, 6, 11, 12, 285, 352
reception, 313
recognition, 262
recommendations, 268, 293, 330, 347
recruiting, 284, 285, 349
reflexes, 355
reflux esophagitis, 204
Registry, 265, 325
regression, 2, 3, 11, 18, 19, 20, 41, 267, 297, 299, 308, 309, 310, 326, 333, 349
regression analysis, 2, 3, 18, 19
regression model, 20, 41, 297, 299, 309
rehabilitation, 267, 283, 286, 310, 349
relaxant, 28, 31, 266, 315, 316, 323, 337, 347
reliability, 291, 310, 311
replacement, 266, 347
resolution, 290, 313
resources, 340, 345
respiratory disorders, 30, 37, 261
Respiratory tract, 269
response time, 267, 283, 291, 292, 293, 299, 304, 307, 308, 309, 349
retinopathy, 327
risk assessment, 337
risk factors, 6, 267
rubber, 319

S

saliva, 2, 10
sample survey, 14
satellites, 290
schizophrenia, 203, 317
sciatica, 204
screening, 287, 304, 305, 307, 308
seasonal factors, 19
secretion, 8, 29, 266, 283, 284, 297, 307, 349
sedative, 8, 39, 266, 315, 323, 347
sedatives, 266, 316, 326, 328, 329, 347
Sedatives/hypnotics, 269
seizure, 30, 42, 266, 315, 317, 347, 351
selective attention, 322
selective serotonin reuptake inhibitor, 322
self-monitoring, 311
self-reports, 303
sensitivity, 8, 12, 19
serum albumin, 8
settlements, 333
sex, 2, 12, 13, 14, 16, 17, 18, 19, 25, 41, 326, 337, 340
ships, 77
shock, 41, 205
sickle cell, 206
side effects, 4, 8, 9, 15, 24, 30, 32, 33, 36, 42, 44, 273, 308, 317, 318, 324, 325, 328, 329
signals, 354, 355, 356, 357, 362
signs, 8, 355, 356, 362
simulation, 323, 324
single test, 320
sinusitis, 206, 269
skeletal muscle, 26, 28, 29, 31, 33, 266, 270, 271, 315, 347
sleep apnea, 3
sleep disturbance, 7
snippets, 290
Social Security, 265, 334
software, 301, 304, 311, 337, 340, 373, 375
source code, 367
speech, 318
spinal cord, 336
spinal cord injury, 336
standard deviation, 318, 323, 325
statistics, 2, 11, 262, 302, 309, 332, 351, 374
steroids, 83, 86, 87, 88, 90, 91
Steroids, 29, 269
stimulant, 39, 316
stimulus, 293, 298
stroke, 3, 37, 327, 353
subgroups, 268, 271, 320, 329
subsidy, 43
substance abuse, 322
sulfonylurea, 326, 327
surface area, 8
surrogates, 267, 283, 308, 349
surveillance, 12
survey, 2, 3, 11, 14, 15, 21, 23, 270, 284, 335
survey design, 11
sweat, 2, 10
Sweden, 338

symptoms, 8, 11, 26, 42, 269, 328
synergistic effect, 308
systolic blood pressure, 329

T

teenagers, vii, 1, 6, 268
test procedure, 316, 377
test statistic, 278
testing, 278, 286, 287, 288, 304, 315, 316, 317, 318, 323, 324, 328, 329
therapeutic intervention, 295
therapeutics, 346
therapy, 7, 33, 317, 323, 326, 327, 341, 346
thiazide, 267, 308, 349
thiazide diuretics, 308
threats, 322
thrombocytopenia, 206
thrombosis, 205
thyroid, 351
Thyroid, 23, 24, 36, 269, 281, 282, 296
time frame, 355
time series, 332
tissue perfusion, 307
toxicology, 318
tracks, 362
traffic control, 293, 356
traffic stops, 316
training, 287, 324, 340
tranquilizers, 326
TransAnalytics, LLC, vii, 265
transformation, 320
transient ischemic attack, 37
transplantation, 334, 342
transport, 66, 67, 70, 77
transportation, 262, 268, 337, 341
Transportation in an Aging Society, 268, 377
trauma, 10, 35, 38, 41, 262, 317, 372
tricyclic antidepressant, 39, 322, 338
tricyclic antidepressants, 39, 322, 338
trucks, 334

U

UK, 340
ulcer, 205
ulcerative colitis, 205

uninsured, 342
United Kingdom, 330, 331, 338, 340, 341, 369
United States, vii, 5, 11, 14, 265, 268, 270, 287, 290, 323, 338, 341, 342
updating, 340
urinary retention, 9
urinary tract, 86, 90
urine, 2, 10
urticaria, 203

V

validation, 12, 43, 332
vasovagal syncope, 328
vehicles, 5, 15, 66, 67, 68, 70, 73, 273, 286, 290, 291, 294, 295, 301, 311, 319, 324, 326, 346, 355, 356, 357, 362, 371
venlafaxine, 322
vertigo, 34
victims, 316
video, 263, 267, 283, 286, 288, 289, 290, 294, 295, 300, 301, 302, 310, 311, 312, 323, 349
vision, 7, 8, 9, 15, 30, 34, 38, 271, 273, 287, 327
visual acuity, 6, 299, 317
visual field, 323
vitamins, 284, 287
Volunteers, 376
vomiting, 34, 205

W

walking, 328, 329
weakness, 30, 34, 36, 308
Web page, 377
weight gain, 317
weight reduction, 12
West Virginia, 316, 375
wheezing, 203, 205
withdrawal, 266, 328, 329, 347
working memory, 287, 299, 306

Y

yes/no, 319